Dahlem Workshop Reports
Life Sciences Research Report 30
Leukemia

The goal of this Dahlem Workshop is:
to elucidate the factors leading
to the leukemic state

Life Sciences Research Reports
Editor: Silke Bernhard

Held and published on behalf of the
Stifterverband für die Deutsche Wissenschaft

Sponsored by:
Hermann und Lilly Schilling-Stiftung für Medizinische Forschung
im Stifterverband für die Deutsche Wissenschaft

Leukemia

I. L. Weissman, Editor

Report of the Dahlem Workshop on
Leukemia
Berlin 1983, November 13 – 18

Rapporteurs:
D. Boettiger · C. G. Fathman · P. K. Vogt
O. N. Witte

Program Advisory Committee:
I. L. Weissman, Chairperson · D. Baltimore
J. M. Bishop · M. D. Cooper · M. Essex · T. Graf
R. Jaenisch · F. Melchers · M. A. S. Moore

Springer-Verlag
Berlin Heidelberg New York Tokyo

Copy Editors: K. Geue, J. Lupp
Text Preparation: M. Böttcher, J. Lambertz, M. Lax, D. Lewis
Photographs: E. P. Thonke

With 4 photographs, 15 figures and 19 tables

ISBN-13:987-3-642-69724-1 e-ISBN-13:987-3-642-69722-7
DOI: 10.1007/987-3-642-69722-7

CIP-Kurztitelaufnahme der Deutschen Bibliothek

Leukemia
report of the Dahlem Workshop on Leukemia
Berlin 1983, November 13-18
I.L. Weissman, ed. Rapporteurs: D. Boettiger...
(Held and publ. on behalf of the Stifterverb. für d. Dt. Wiss.
Sponsored by: Hermann-and-Lilly-Schilling-Stiftung
für Med. Forschung im Stifterverb. für d. Dt. Wiss.).
Berlin; Heidelberg; NewYork; Tokyo: Springer 1985
(Life sciences research report;30)

NE: Weissman, Irving L. (Hrsg.); Boettiger, D. (Mitverf.)
Workshop on Leukemia (1983, Dahlem, Berlin); GT

2131/3020-5 4 3 2 1 0

Table of Contents

The Dahlem Konferenzen
S. Bernhard ix

Introduction
I.L. Weissman 1

Specificity of Hemopoietic Growth Factors
N.N. Iscove 5

T Cell Proliferation and Differentiation
W. Haas and H. von Boehmer 21

Regulatory Defects in Leukemia: In Vitro Analysis
M.A.S. Moore 31

Induction of B Cell Proliferation and Differentiation
W.E. Paul 69

Lymphoid Tumor Stem Cells and Their Regulation
R.G. Lynch 83

Phenotypic Heterogeneity and the Origins of Lymphoid Malignancy in Man: Biological and Clinical Implications
M.F. Greaves 95

Differentiation of T Lymphocytes
J.J.T. Owen 111

Effects of Acute Leukemia Viruses on the Differentiation of Hematopoietic Cells
T. Graf 131

Multiple Mechanisms of Oncogene Activation in Viral and Nonviral Neoplasia
W.S. Hayward 147

Oncogenes of Avian Leukemia Viruses
M.J. Hayman 163

Significance of Chromosome Rearrangements in Leukemia and Lymphoma
J.D. Rowley 179

Tracing Development and Cell Lineages in Human Hemopoietic Neoplasia
P.J. Fialkow and J.W. Singer 203

The Preleukemic State in Virus-induced Leukemia
M. Essex 223

The Receptor-mediated Leukemogenesis Hypothesis: A Model of Retroviral Oncogenesis by Viral Stimulation of Cell-surface Receptors
I.L. Weissman, M.S. McGrath, and G. Tamura 235

Regulation of Hematopoietic Differentiation and Its Disruption
Group Report
C.G. Fathman, Rapporteur
A. Ganser, N.N. Iscove, M. Karpowicz, T. Kishimoto, E. Klein, P.H. Krammer, F. Lilly, F. Melchers, D. Metcalf, P.A. Meyer, M.A.S. Moore, W.E. Paul 251

Problems in Differentiation Pathways and Cellular Targets for Leukemogens
Group Report
D. Boettiger, Rapporteur
M.D. Cooper, T. Graf, M.F. Greaves, A.U. Harlozinska-Szmyrka, R. Jaenisch, R.G. Lynch, J.J.T. Owen, M. Potter 263

Genes and Viruses Able to Transform Hematopoietic Cells
Group Report
P.K. Vogt, Rapporteur
K. Bister, A.L. Burny, C.M. Croce, W.A. Haseltine, M.J. Hayman, W.S. Hayward, G. Klein, K. Moelling, R.D. Neth, I.B. Pragnell, J.D. Rowley 275

Evolution of the Leukemic State
Group Report
O.N. Witte, Rapporteur
J. Allison, M. Essex, P.J. Fialkow, N. Haran-Ghera, J. Howard, W. Ostertag, V. Schirrmacher, H.J. Seidel, I.L. Weissman 295

List of Participants with Fields of Research 301

Subject Index 307

Author Index 316

The Dahlem Konferenzen

Founders
Recognizing the need for more effective communication between scientists, especially in the natural sciences, the Stifterverband für die Deutsche Wissenschaft*, in cooperation with the Deutsche Forschungsgemeinschaft**, founded Dahlem Konferenzen in 1974. The project is financed by the founders and the Senate of the City of Berlin.

Name
Dahlem Konferenzen was named after the district of Berlin called "Dahlem", which has a long-standing tradition and reputation in the arts and sciences.

Aim
The task of Dahlem Konferenzen is to promote international, interdisciplinary exchange of scientific information and ideas, to stimulate international cooperation in research, and to develop and test new models conducive to more effective communication between scientists.

Dahlem Workshop Model
Dahlem Konferenzen organizes four workshops per year, each with a limited number of participants. Since no type of scientific meeting proved effective enough, Dahlem Konferenzen had to create its own concept. This concept has been tested and varied over the years, and has evolved into its present form which is known as the *Dahlem Workshop Model*. This model provides the framework for the utmost possible interdisciplinary communication and cooperation between scientists in a given time period.

**The Donors Association for the Promotion of Sciences and Humanities*
***German Science Foundation*

The main work of the Dahlem Workshops is done in four interdisciplinary discussion groups. Lectures are not given. Instead, selected participants write background papers providing a review of the field rather than a report on individual work. These are circulated to all participants before the meeting to provide a basis for discussion. During the workshop, the members of the four groups prepare reports reflecting their discussions and providing suggestions for future research needs.

Topics
The topics are chosen from the fields of the Life Sciences and the Physical, Chemical, and Earth Sciences. They are of contemporary international interest, interdisciplinary in nature, and problem-oriented. Once a year, topic suggestions are submitted to a scientific board for approval.

Participants
For each workshop participants are selected exclusively by special Program Advisory Committees. Selection is based on international scientific reputation alone, although a balance between European and American scientists is attempted. Exception is made for younger German scientists.

Publication
The results of the workshops are the Dahlem Workshop Reports, reviewed by selected participants and carefully edited by the editor of each volume. The reports are multidisciplinary surveys by the most internationally distinguished scientists and are based on discussions of new data, experiments, advanced new concepts, techniques, and models. Each report also reviews areas of priority interest and indicates directions for future research on a given topic.

The Dahlem Workshop Reports are published in two series:
1) Life Sciences Research Reports (LS), and
2) Physical, Chemical, and Earth Sciences Research Reports (PC).

Director
Silke Bernhard, M.D.

Address
Dahlem Konferenzen
Wallotstrasse 19
1000 Berlin (West) 33

Leukemia, ed. I.L. Weissman, pp. 1-3. Dahlem Konferenzen 1985. Berlin, Heidelberg, New York, Tokyo: Springer-Verlag.

Introduction

I.L. Weissman
Dept. of Pathology
Stanford University School of Medicine
Stanford, CA 94305, USA

It is not possible to consider the scientific issues presented by leukemia without first remembering the great human tragedies that result from its presence as a set of human diseases. The leukemias are diseases primarily found in younger people, and therefore, unlike cardiovascular diseases, do not serve as a somewhat accelerated, albeit unexpected, end to a life nearly fully lived. The myeloid leukemias strike young adults, as do the lymphomas, while the acute lymphocytic leukemias, up until recently, are tragedies of childhood. Leukemias and lymphomas are not rare diseases, and it is likely that every reader of this volume has a friend, relative, or close acquaintance who has fallen victim. With development of our modern industrial and militaristic society we have found ways to increase the incidence of leukemia on a worldwide basis, and I expect that epidemiological studies shall continue to find those agents made by man which are implicated in the development of this set of diseases.

Frightening, however, is the recent emergence of an epidemic of adult-onset, rapidly fatal, acute T cell leukemias and lymphomas. This epidemic is spreading rapidly throughout the world, almost certainly by means of transfer of a virus related to the slowly transforming lymphotropic retroviruses - the type present in many of our animal models and in animal communities. It is striking that the lethal event in most of these adult-onset HTLV-related leukemias is overwhelming infection, as these patients have an underlying profound immunodeficiency of the T cell system itself. Even more frightening are the series of studies which provide epidemiological and virological evidence that the concurrent epidemic of Acquired Immunodeficiency Syndrome (AIDS) coincides in type, place, and time with the lymphoma/leukemia epidemic.

Thus we are faced with two major new pathogenic problems of the T lymphocyte system: profound loss of selected functional T cell sets, with or without an associated neoplastic proliferation, both apparently caused by a related series of viruses, and both causing uniformly lethal diseases. It is with this dreadful knowledge that we gathered in Berlin to consider the leukemias and lymphomas within the context of the normal control of proliferation and differentiation of cells of the hematolymphoid system. We ended our discussions with a clearer view of the factors which lead to the normal proliferation and differentiation of these cells and therefore to the factors which might lead to the emergence of the leukemic state.

We concentrated our discussions on the normal cell lineages which lead to stem cells and progenitor cells of more and more limited differentiation potential, and of greater and greater control of proliferation potential, studying in detail the cell-to-cell interactions and the cell-produced polypeptide factors which apparently control proliferation and differentiation among these lineages. From this we hope has emerged a clearer story of what areas might be important to study in terms of failed differentiation or unceasing proliferation.

Within the context of hematolymphoid differentiation, we also discussed and studied the various leukemogens and how they might disrupt the pathways of normal proliferation and differentiation of cells in each of these series. We looked to evidence from human leukemias and lymphomas as to their predominant qualities and their implied targets for leukemogenesis. Central to the analysis of both animal and human models of leukemogenesis and normal cell proliferation was an analysis of those receptor systems used both by normal and leukemic hematolymphoid cells for cell-to-cell interactions, for mitogenesis, for cell differentiation, for homing and metastasis, as targets of immunity, and those which are products of known oncogenic elements. The oncogenic elements of interest were first discovered as viral genes which encode the neoplastic state, contained within those rapidly transforming viruses which have been the focus of study for the past eighty years. We considered at this workshop the full story of how these viral genes promote leukemogenesis, and how the known vertebrate homologues of these genes are expressed normally in differentiation and proliferation pathways as well as abnormally in well-defined lymphomagenic and other oncogenic pathways. What emerged from this meeting are a better understanding of the evolution of these gene systems themselves and an elucidation of simpler systems open to more rapid genetic and molecular genetic analysis to reveal the normal functions of these genes and their gene products.

Thus we sought new answers to several old questions concerning differentiation, proliferation, and neoplastic transformation. We gathered together in an unusual format - that of the unique Dahlem Workshops - not just to reiterate data which has recently emerged but to think about how these findings might lead to new approaches for the understanding and therapy of the leukemias and lymphomas. We deliberately chose experts from several different disciplines, ranging from the clinicians who diagnose, describe, and treat these maladies, to the molecular geneticists trying to reduce the analysis of the problem to its simplest variables in the simplest systems possible.

This volume contains the background papers written especially for this workshop, giving an overview of special areas of primary concern to us, which were distributed to all participants before the meeting and serve as the basis for the four group reports, which reflect the productive discussions that emerged during our week in Berlin and indicate the direction we need to go in future research in order to understand and control the factors leading to the leukemic state.

Leukemia, ed. I.L. Weissman, pp. 5-20. Dahlem Konferenzen 1985. Berlin, Heidelberg, New York, Tokyo: Springer-Verlag.

Specificity of Hemopoietic Growth Factors

N.N. Iscove
Basel Institute for Immunology
4005 Basel, Switzerland

Abstract. The growth of hemopoietic cells in culture is dependent on growth factors having lineage and maturational stage specificity. In the mouse model, seven factors of differing specificity patterns on normal cells have been described and sufficiently characterized chemically to be considered as separate entities. The interpretation of apparent specificities can be complicated by the presence in the cultures of serum and of factor-producing cells from hemopoietic tissue. Factor-dependent established cell lines have been described but may not be reliable as indicators of factor specificity for normal cells. Factors with lineage specificity might influence precursor development by either instructive or selective mechanisms; experiments which can distinguish between these are difficult but feasible. Finally, strong requirements in culture, even of lineage-specific nature, do not necessarily imply regulatory roles for the factors concerned in the whole animal. Such roles remain to be demonstrated for most of the factors considered.

INTRODUCTION

The survival, growth, and maturation of mammalian hemopoietic cells in culture depend on specific "growth factors," most or all of which are glycoprotein in nature. This article is intended to summarize current knowledge about the identity and number of these factors, and to provide a framework for consideration of their specificity and role in regulation of blood cell production. Because information is most complete in the mouse model, and because important insights are to be gained from comparisons of specificities among factors, only data derived from that system will be addressed here.

Table 1 lists seven factors which are required for formation of colonies of various differentiated cell types by mouse hemopoietic precursors in semisolid culture. The table incorporates a proposal for a rationalized "growth factor" nomenclature which has the advantage of comprehensibility to biologists outside the field of hemotalogy and which avoids the technique-specific "colony-stimulating" terminology. Other names in common use are also indicated. Inspection of the properties of the factors, presented in Table 2, shows most of them to be unique and mutually separable. They also differ one from another in the range of cell types which are responsive to them.

In the section to follow, target specificity of each factor is inferred from the kinds of cells contained in the colonies they stimulate in semisolid cultures. Action on early versus late stages in a particular lineage is

TABLE 1 - Nomenclature for hemopoietic growth factors.

Suggested name	acronym	lineage specificity	synonyms
erythropoietin	EP	erythroid	
megakaryocyte differentiation factor	MkDF	megakaryocyte	Mk-potentiator
macrophage growth factor	MGF	macrophage	CSF-1, M-CSF
neutrophil growth factor	NeuGF	neutrophil	G-CSF, MGI-2
neutrophil/macrophage growth factor	NMGF	neutrophil macrophage	GM-CSF, MGI-1
multilineage hemopoietic growth factor	MultiHGF	all hemopoietic lineages	BPA, BFA, BEF EPA, IL-3, Mk-CSA, MCGF, PSF, E-CSF, HCGF, Hemopoietin-2, Multi-CSF
synergistic activity	SA	macrophage ?others	

TABLE 2 - Distinguishing characteristics of mouse hemopoietic growth factors.

factor	source characterized	estimated size GPC	SDS-PAGE	charge	subunits	references
EP	human urine	60,000	39,000	pI 4.5-5.5	1	(21)
MkDF[1]	WEHI-3B(D^-)	100,000				(28)
MGF	L-929	100,000	70,000	pI 3.7-4.9	2	(25)
NeuGF[1,2]	lung CM	20,000	25,000		1	(22)
NMGF	lung CM	29,000	23,000	pI 5.0 retarded on DEAE pH 7.4	1	(3,4)
MultiHGF	WEHI-3B(D^-)	33,000	26,000	pI 4.7-8.0 unretarded on DEAE pH 7.4-9.0	1	(1,5,12, 13,15)
SA[1]	WEHI-3B(D^-)	17,000		pI 4.0-6.5		(17)

1 insufficiently characterized to exclude possible identity with one another

2 more hydrophobic than NMGF and MultiHGF

deduced from the ultimate size of the colonies, the time from inception of a culture to the appearance within colonies of markers of terminal maturation, and delayed factor addition experiments which directly determine the stage of colony development during which the factor is required.

LINEAGE SPECIFICITY OF THE HEMOPOIETIC GROWTH FACTORS

Erythropoietin

The restriction of activity of this factor to later stages in the erythroid lineage and the lack of responsiveness of the preceding stages have been documented before (reviewed in (15)). A highly purified preparation of human urinary erythropoietin has shown activity on terminal stages in the platelet pathway (29), but not all erythropoietin preparations have this activity (N. Williams, personal communication), and the observation may be explainable by endotoxin contamination of the active erythropoietin sample.

Megakaryocyte Differentiation Factor (MkDF)

This macrophage product appears to be required for the endomitotic stages of megakaryocyte differentiation but does not support earlier proliferative stages (28). Its production by the $P388D_1$ macrophage cell line is enhanced by bacterial lipopolysaccharide (30). The factor has yet to be extensively purified and characterized, and it is not yet known whether its action is restricted to the megakaryocyte lineage.

Macrophage Growth Factor (MGF)
This factor supports growth of pure macrophage colonies in semisolid cultures of mouse bone marrow. Experiments with single micromanipulated precursor cells (18) and partially purified MGF suggest that growth of a small proportion of cells with neutrophil potential may also be supported.

That mature macrophages are also among the targets of MGF is indicated by MGF-induced proliferation of a subset of peritoneal cells (referenced in (27)), induction of plasminogen activator (9), and requirement of MGF for macrophage survival in certain circumstances (27). Binding of radio-labeled MGF by mouse bone marrow cells is confined to macrophages/monocytes, a small number of more primitive cells, and a small proportion of the marrow population having ring-shaped nuclei (8). The observations taken together indicate that MGF acts mainly on cells of the macrophage lineage down to and including the mature macrophage, and possibly also on some precursors with dual neutrophil and macrophage potential.

Neutrophil Growth Factor (NeuGF)
This factor in highly purified form supports growth of small neutrophilic colonies from marrow and fetal liver (20). It also appears to support initial proliferation of cells with dual macrophage and neutrophil potential but does not support the subsequent growth of cells within the clones which have progressed into the macrophage pathway (20). Its proliferative effect therefore appears confined to neutrophilic cells and their immediate bipotent precursors.

Neutrophil/Macrophage Growth Factor (NMGF)
This factor supports the growth of neutrophil, macrophage, and mixed neutrophil/macrophage colonies. Mature macrophages respond to highly purified material by increased production of plasminogen activator (9). In addition, purified NMGF appears to support initial cell divisions of a proportion of single micromanipulated pluripotential or committed erythroid progenitors (19). However, subsequent proliferation and differentiation of cells further into the erythroid lineage is not supported, so that pure or mixed erythroid bursts do not develop even in the presence of erythropoietin (15). A low level of responsiveness to NMGF therefore

appears to be a feature of pluripotential and very early erythroid-committed precursors. Responsiveness is greatest among partially committed granulocyte/macrophage precursors and all their progeny in those lineages including the end cells, but is lost quickly as cells develop along the erythroid and megakaryocyte pathways. Eosinophil precursors from adult marrow (but not fetal liver (20)) and mast cells are unresponsive to NMGF (5).

Multilineage Hemopoietic Growth Factor (MultiHGF)
Conditioned media from cultures of stimulated lymphocytes, from some T cell hybridomas, and from the WEHI-3B(D$^-$) macrophage cell line contain growth factor activity effective on all hemopoietic lineages, including pluripotential cells as well as committed cells in the erythroid, megakaryocyte, macrophage, neutrophil, eosinophil, mast cell, and basophil lineages. It was widely assumed initially that this broad spectrum of activities reflected the presence of several distinct growth factors. Indeed, there is evidence that more than one factor is present in these conditioned media. MGF is detectable serologically in both spleen- and WEHI-3B(D$^-$)-conditioned medium (24), and molecules with biochemical and biological properties very similar to NMGF can be identified in conditioned medium from some T cell hybridomas (3) and from lectin-stimulated spleen cells (13).

However, despite the fact that these conditioned media contain several chemically distinct hemopoietic factors, one of the factors, distinct from NMGF, does appear to have multilineage activity by itself. This conclusion is based on the copurification of activity on various hemopoietic lineages through separation procedures based on size, charge, hydrophobicity, and hydroxyapatite affinity applied sequentially to WEHI-3B(D$^-$)-conditioned medium (1, 13, 15). The activity of the factor in several different hemopoietic cell growth assays has led to a plethora of operational names for it (BPA, Mast Cell Growth Factor, Hemopoietic Cell Growth Factor, etc., see Table 1). Several groups agree on its distinguishing chromatographic properties (Table 2).

In semisolid cultures MultiHGF supports early but not late stages of erythroid and megakaryocyte colony development, and growth of mixed myeloid/erythroid, macrophage, neutrophil, eosinophil, and basophil colonies. In liquid cultures of bone marrow or spleen it supports long-term growth of mast cells. It can be inferred that the range of cells responsive to MultiHGF includes pluripotential hemopoietic precursors, all their more committed progeny, and cells all the way along the granulocytic (including mast cell) and mononuclear phagocytic pathways. The only hemopoietic cells which appear unresponsive to MultiHGF are late-stage erythropoietin-responsive erythroid cells (15) and later megakaryocyte precursors at the stage of endomitotic maturation (15, 28).

Ihle and co-workers (13) have raised the question of possible action of this factor on T lymphoid cells or their precursors. They have called the factor "IL-3." The evidence for action on T lymphocyte precursors includes the induction of increased activity of 20-α-steroid dehydrogenase in nu/nu spleen cell cultures, and the capacity of the factor to support survival and proliferation of spleen-derived cell lines which bear T lymphocyte-associated antigens, notably Thy-1. The evidence is open to alternative interpretations. 20-α-steroid dehydrogenase, while apparently present in T thymocytes, is also abundant in granulocytic cell lines (7, 12) and possibly in mast cells which are known to be targets of MultiHGF. Furthermore, Thy-1 can coexist in established cell lines with other markers typical of granulocyte or macrophage lineages (e.g., FDC-P lines 1-5 (6) or WEHI-3B(D^-) (Forni and Iscove, unpublished), respectively).

Additional evidence for action of MultiHGF of T lymphocyte precursors was claimed in experiments in which lines of Thy-1^+, Lyt-1^+ cells emerged from nylon wool nonadherent spleen cells passaged for 6-8 weeks in medium containing partially purified factor from spleen-conditioned medium (10). However, when Thy-1 and Lyt-1 became identifiable, the lines were no longer factor-dependent. The dependence of the precursors of these lines on factor was assumed but not demonstrated in these experiments. In the absence of evidence showing normal unselected T lymphocytes or their precursors to be MultiHGF-responsive, the case for action on the T lymphocyte lineage is not compelling.

The known target specificity of each of the above factors is summarized in Fig. 1.

Synergistic Activity

When normal mouse bone marrow is cultured with a source of MGF (e.g., pregnant mouse uterus extract), macrophage colonies grow up to a maximum size of 5,000 cells per colony ("small colonies"). If the MGF is supplemented with unstimulated human spleen- or placenta-conditioned medium, the colony number increases about 10%, and 10% of the colonies contain between 5,000 and 50,000 cells ("large colonies") (2). If mice are treated with 5-fluorouracil and their marrow is plated 48-72 h later with MGF alone, the number of macrophage colony-forming cells per

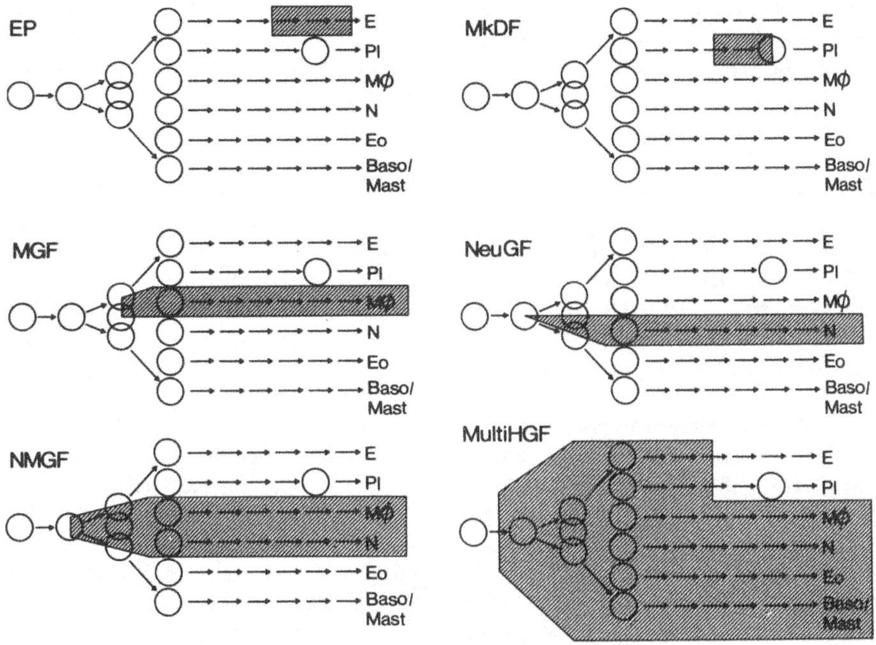

FIG. 1 - Specificity of hemopoietic growth factors. The cells within the shaded areas on each of the six lineage diagrams are responsive to the factor indicated. Each lineage diagram begins on the left with an early and then later pluripotential cell, followed by partially determined cells of more than one potential, which in turn are followed by unipotential cells which differentiate down their respective lineages (E, erythroid; Pl, platelet immediately preceded by a megakaryocyte; MØ, macrophage; N, neutrophil; Eo, eosinophil; Baso/Mast, basophil and mast cell).

femur falls below 1% of the original frequency. However, if the cultures contain both MGF and spleen- or placenta-conditioned medium, the frequency of large (but not small) macrophage colonies is close to that of untreated mice. The differential sensitivity of precursors of small and large colonies to 5-fluorouracil, their differing kinetics of regeneration in such treated animals, and their differing kinetics in liquid culture support the notion that the precursors of the large and small colonies are distinct cells and that the former are precursors of the latter (2).

Marrow from 5-fluorouracil-treated mice thus provides a convenient assay for an activity distinct from MGF. Semisolid cultures are set up with MGF. If nothing else is added, very few background colonies form. If certain conditioned media are added, large macrophage colonies develop. The additional activity which permits them to develop is operationally designated as "synergistic activity."

Synergistic activity has been detected in the conditioned medium from WEHI-3B(D^-) cells (17) as well as in human placental and unstimulated human and mouse spleen (16). Some characteristics of the WEHI-3B(D^-) product are given in Table 2 and distinguish it clearly from MultiHGF derived from the same source. Partially purified preparations of synergistic activity from this source lack direct colony-stimulating activity when tested alone in marrow cultures.

These observations suggest that early but not later cells in the macrophage lineage require synergistic activity for survival or growth in culture. In addition, if marrow cells from 5-fluorouracil-treated mice are incubated in liquid culture before plating in agar, persistence of precursors of large macrophage colonies for four days in the liquid cultures requires the combined presence of MGF and synergistic activity (2). This observation suggests that at least some of the early cells may already have MGF receptors in addition to their requirement for synergistic activity. Whether or not the targets of synergistic activity which form large macrophage colonies in the presence of MGF are all macrophage-committed, or whether they include earlier pluripotential precursors remains to be seen. The published experiments do not provide an answer since they were not performed with culture conditions which would have permitted expression of erythroid or granulocytic potential (i.e., the cultures did not contain added erythropoietin, NMGF, or NeuGF). For the same reason, we do not yet know whether a similar requirement for synergistic activity exists in any of the other hemopoietic lineages, or indeed for other non-hemopoietic cells.

SOURCES OF UNCERTAINTY IN ASSIGNMENT OF SPECIFICITY

In the preceding sections, the target cells of each factor were inferred from the character of the clones whose growth the factors appear to support. Where a factor appears to lack effectiveness on a particular lineage or stage, interpretation is reasonably straightforward. However, the interpretation of positive findings can be complicated if the intentionally added factor is not the only one present in the cultures. For example, when purified MGF is added to a bone marrow culture, a minority population of neutrophil or mixed neutrophil/macrophage colonies is sometimes observed in addition to the majority of pure macrophage colonies. The interpretation of the observation depends critically on whether or not MGF is the only factor available to the cells.

There are two major, interrelated sources of unwanted and quantitatively uncontrolled factors in hemopoietic cell cultures: the serum component of the medium, and factor-producing cells. The two are interrelated in the sense that serum components may provoke factor release by the producing cells. The data on which the preceding sections were based were for the most part obtained in culture medium containing serum.

Each of the hemopoietic factors can be presumed to be present in serum in some finite concentration. Whether or not their presence leads to significant noise in an experiment will depend on the final concentration of the contaminant in the culture and on the effectiveness of the factor across the species boundary in question (e.g., bovine factor on mouse hemopoietic cells).

Similarly, marrow can be presumed to be a potential source of factor release, at least by virtue of its content of T cells, of appropriate accessory cells, and of precursors of these two kinds of cell. Besides providing some background level of hemopoietic factor to the cultures, these cells could be provoked to additional factor release by substances in serum. Worse still, a growth factor presumed to act directly on hemopoietic precursors might in fact exert its action indirectly by induction of release of directly acting growth factor. The production of megakaryocyte differentiation factor by macrophages provides a possible illustration. In this case, it could be imagined that the 100,000 dalton product of WEHI-3B(D^-) cells (Table 2) might in fact be macrophage growth factor, providing the cultures with sufficient macrophages to supply an essential macrophage product to the developing megakaryocytes.

It is now possible to perform experiments in which the serum component of the cultures is greatly reduced if not eliminated entirely. The conditions originally optimized for the later stages of erythropoiesis (detailed in (14)) have since proven to support efficiently the growth of granulocyte, macrophage, megakaryocyte, and mixed lineage colonies as well (N. Iscove, unpublished observations).

The problem of excluding factor-producing marrow cells from the cultures has been approached in three main ways: purification of precursor cells, culture of single precursor cells isolated by micromanipulation, and development of permanently established factor-dependent cell clones. The last of these is discussed in the section that follows. Of the first two, only the culture of single isolated cells can provide definitive demonstration of direct factor action, since no separated population can be 100% pure. Direct action on single isolated precursor cells has been demonstrated for erythropoietin (Iscove, unpublished observations), macrophage growth factor (18), neutrophil growth factor (20), neutrophil/macrophage growth factor (18), and multilineage hemopoietic growth factor (Iscove, experiments in progress).

FACTOR-DEPENDENT CELL LINES AND FACTOR SPECIFICITY

Practically all nonadherent cells in mouse hemopoietic or lymphoid tissue will normally die out in a matter of weeks of passage in culture medium that is not supplemented with specific growth factors. If T cell growth factor is included and T cells are appropriately activated at the initiation of culture, the passaged cultures soon come to consist exclusively of growing T cells. Similarly, if spleen or bone marrow is passaged in the presence of MultiHGF from spleen or WEHI-3B(D^-) cells, the cultures soon consist entirely of growing mast cells (5, 11, 26). In both instances, the most common fate of the growing lines is ultimate "senescence" and extinction. However, some lines may progress to permanent established lines which retain their factor dependence. Such lines are frequently of abnormal chromosomal composition. In cultures passaged in MultiHGF, permanent lines of other than the usual mast cell character may finally emerge. Some such lines may bear markers of T lymphoid differentiation despite their non-lymphoid character (6, 12). Emergence of MultiHGF-dependent cells bearing several markers of the B lymphocyte lineage has also recently been observed (Palacios, personal communication).

The emergence of lymphoid cell lines dependent on MultiHGF, a factor not yet shown to affect directly normal T or B lymphocytes or their immediate precursors, raises questions as to the significance of the cell line findings. Since normal cells die when passaged in medium lacking their appropriate growth factors, the passage of cells in medium containing a growth factor constitutes a powerful positive selection for cells able to respond to the factor used.

We know little about the "fidelity" or accuracy of gene activation in developmental programs. It is possible that there is a low but finite "error" rate, for example, among cells in the lymphocytes lineage that results in "inappropriate" expression of receptors for MultiHGF in, say, $1/10^6$ lymphocytes. Such errors might be of no particular consequence in the intact animal and would normally escape detection in short-term tests for responsiveness in vitro. However, in view of the large numbers of cells used in initiating cultures for passage with factor, there would be finite numbers of such "aberrant" cells available for selection and expansion. It will not be easy to demonstrate the validity of this suggestion. However, it does not seem farfetched and provides reason for giving greater weight to data obtained with cells fresh from the animal than to evidence obtained from passaged cell lines. Clonal assays for normal cells at early stages of lymphocyte differentiation will provide decisive information on this issue, and there is an urgent need for their development.

THE PHYSICAL BASIS FOR FACTOR SPECIFICITY, INSTRUCTION, AND SELECTION

In view of the precedents with other, more intensively studied polypeptide effectors such as epidermal growth factor and insulin, and more recent evidence with the MGF-macrophage system, it seems safe to assume that some or all of the factors discussed here will turn out to exert their effects via interaction with receptors on the surface of their target cells. If so, then the patterns of responsiveness illustrated in Fig. 1 should correspond to the distribution of factor-specific receptors in the hemopoietic family tree.

It will be of particular interest to work out the mechanisms of response in those cells that bear receptors for more than one factor, for it is in those cells where the question of instructive versus selective factor-mediated regulation arises. Two scenarios can be envisaged:

1 - On a given cell, occupancy of any receptor, regardless of its factor specificity, would have identical intracellular consequences. For example, occupied receptors might have protein kinase activity. In this scenario the substrate specificity of the various kinds of receptor would be identical.

2 - On a given cell, occupancy of receptors of different factor specificities would have different intracellular consequences. If occupied receptors had, for example, kinase activity, then this scenario would require that different receptor types would have different substrate specificities.

Where scenario 1 holds, factors can have specificity only on a selective basis, i.e., specificity of response will be determined solely by which kinds of cells in the population have appropriate receptors. In the presence of a given factor, those with receptors for it will survive and grow, those without will die. The character of the clone derived from a cell bearing more than one kind of receptor and exposed to a given factor will be determined in part by the presence or absence of receptors for that factor among the various kinds of progeny of the original cell.

Where scenario 2 applies, factors might also act by instructive mechanisms. A cell with more than one kind of receptor might be biased in one direction of development by one kind of factor, in another direction by another factor. Both biochemical and biological experiments will be required to identify where and how instructive and selective mechanisms operate.

BIOLOGICAL EXPERIMENTS CAPABLE OF DISTINGUISHING INSTRUCTIVE FROM SELECTIVE PHENOMENA

This discussion will examine the hypothetical case where the target of factor-mediated instruction involves cells capable of response to more than one kind of factor. The essence of instruction (or "induction") is that the state (e.g., future developmental potential) of the target cell after interaction with one kind of factor is different from the state it would have if it interacted with a different factor. Formal demonstration of instruction will require examination of the fates of initially identical cells after exposure to different factors. The experimental requirements for the exclusion of selective mechanisms differ according to how quickly induction can take place.

If induction can occur before the target cell divides, the experiment is straightforward. Some cells are exposed to factor A, and counterparts (known from control experiments to have a high chance of being identical) are exposed to factor B. Then, before the cells have divided, they are washed and plated in identical growth conditions. If the ultimate differentiative potential is influenced by the initial exposure to A or B, induction is formally demonstrated.

If, on the other hand, induction takes longer than the time it takes the cell to divide, the experiment becomes complicated by the necessity to exclude selective mechanisms (death of non-responsive cells, growth of responsive cells) operating at the level of the daughter cells.

To do this, it is now necessary to grow the cells in the initial conditions (factor A or B) as discrete clones and to follow the fates of all individual cells in the derivative lineages. This is probably feasible by combining the use of time-lapse photography with a semisolid culture technique which confines the growing cells to a layer only one cell diameter in thickness.

There are published experiments on precursors with dual granulocyte/macrophage potential which show the feasibility of working with single identical paired precursors (17). However, experiments which are decisive on the issue of induction versus selection in hemopoietic precursors have yet to be reported.

REGULATORS AND TISSUE CULTURE REQUIREMENTS

When polypeptide growth requirements are identified for lymphocytes or hemopoietic cells, terms such as "regulator," "inducer," "modulator," and the like rapidly enter common usage. If a "regulator" is defined as a factor whose locally available concentration in the whole animal is subject to change and is limiting for the cells in question in normal steady-state conditions, then only erythropoietin has an established regulatory role among the lymphopoietic and hemopoietic factors.

Furthermore, only in the case of MGF (8) and T cell growth factor (23) have there been satisfactory demonstrations of lineage-specific cell surface receptors for the respective factor. Similar demonstrations for other factors are likely to come as factors become suitably purified and labeled.

However, in the meantime it seems prudent to be alert to the possibility that a particular in vitro requirement may be neither regulatory in the animal nor necessarily receptor-mediated in its action. The tissue culture environment has many potential hazards for cells, and it is easy to imagine possible roles for enzymes which eliminate inhibitors (e.g., catalase, adenosine deaminase) or provide nutrients (e.g., asparagine synthetase in an asparagine-free medium), or for nutrient carriers (e.g., transcobalamin II). Lineage or stage specificity do not by themselves argue against this sort of possibility. Finally, even where a requirement for a lineage-specific, receptor-mediated factor exists in vitro, the factor in question may be present in vivo at an invariant, high concentration disqualifying it as a physiologically important regulator. These issues require clarification for most of the known hemopoietic growth factors.

Acknowledgements. I thank B. Fagg, G. Keller, J. McCarty, and C. Paige for critical readings of the manuscript. The Basel Institute for Immunology was founded and is supported by F. Hoffmann-La Roche, Limited Company,

Basel, Switzerland.

REFERENCES

(1) Bazill, G.W.; Haynes, M.; Garland, J.; and Dexter, T.M. 1983. Characterization and partial purification of a haemopoietic cell growth factor in WEHI-3 cell conditioned medium. Biochem. J. 210: 747-759.

(2) Bradley, T.R.; Hodgson, G.S.; and Bertoncello, I. 1980. Characteristics of primitive macrophage progenitor cells with high proliferative potential: Relationship to cells with marrow repopulating ability in 5-fluorouracil treated mouse bone marrow. In Experimental Hematology Today 1980, eds. S.J. Baum, G.D. Ledney, and D.W. van Bekkum, pp. 285-297. Basel: Karger.

(3) Burgess, A.W.; Bartlett, P.F.; Metcalf, D.; Nicola, N.A.; Clark-Lewis, I.; and Schrader, J.W. 1981. Granulocyte-macrophage colony-stimulating factor produced by an inducible murine T-cell hybridoma: Molecular properties and cellular specificity. Exp. Hemat. 9: 893-903.

(4) Burgess, A.W.; Camakaris, J.; and Metcalf, D. 1977. Purification and properties of colony-stimulating factor from mouse lung-conditioned medium. J. Biol. Chem. 252: 1998-2003.

(5) Clark-Lewis, I., and Schrader, J.W. 1981. P cell-stimulating factor: Biochemical characterization of a new T cell-derived factor. J. Immunol. 127: 1941-1947.

(6) Dexter, T.M.; Garland, J.; Scott, D.; Scolnick, E.; and Metcalf, D. 1980. Growth of factor-dependent hemopoietic precursor cell lines. J. Exp. Med. 152: 1036-1047.

(7) Garland, J.M.; Lanotte, M.; and Dexter, T.M. 1982. Expression of 20 -hydroxysteroid dehydrogenase in non-lymphoid hemopoietic cell lines. Eur. J. Immunol. 12: 332-336.

(8) Guilbert, L.J., and Stanley, E.R. 1980. Specific interaction of murine colony-stimulating factor with mononuclear phagocytic cells. J. Cell. Biol. 85: 153-159.

(9) Hamilton, J.A.; Stanley, E.R.; Burgess, A.W.; and Shadduck, R.K. 1980. Stimulation of macrophage plasminogen activator activity by colony-stimulating factors. J. Cell. Physiol. 103: 435-445.

(10) Hapel, A.J.; Lee, J.C.; Farrar, W.L.; and Ihle, J.N. 1981.

Establishment of continuous cultures of Thy 1.2^+, Lyt $1^+,2^-$ T cells with purified Interleukin 3. Cell 25: 179-186.

(11) Hasthorpe, S. 1980. A hemopoietic cell line dependent upon a factor in pokeweed mitogen-stimulated spleen cell conditioning medium. J. Cell. Physiol. 105: 379-384.

(12) Ihle, J.N.; Keller, J.; Greenberger, J.S.; Henderson, L.; Yetter, R.A.; and Morse, H.C. 1982. Phenotypic characteristics of cell lines requiring Interleukin 3 for growth. J. Immunol. 129: 1377-1383.

(13) Ihle, J.N.; Keller, J.; Oroszlan, S.; Henderson, L.E.; Copeland, T.D.; Fitch, F.; Prystowsky, M.B.; Goldwasser, E.; Schrader, J.W.; Palaszynski, E.; Dy, M.; and Lebel, B. 1983. Biologic properties of homogeneous Interleukin 3. J. Immunol. 131: 282-286.

(14) Iscove, N.N. 1983. Culture of lymphocytes and hemopoietic cells in serum-free medium. In Methods for Serum-free Culture of Neuronal and Lymphoid Cells, eds. D. Barnes, D. Sirbasku, and G. Sato, pp. 169-185. New York: Liss.

(15) Iscove, N.N.; Roitsch, C.A.; Williams, N.; and Guilbert, L.J. 1982. Molecules stimulating early red cell, granulocyte, macrophage, and megakaryocyte precursors in culture: Similarity in size, hydrophobicity, and charge. J. Cell. Physiol. Suppl. 1: 65-78.

(16) Kriegler, A.B.; Bradley, T.R.; Januszewicz, E.; Hodgson, G.S.; and Elms, E.F. 1982. Partial purification and characterization of a growth factor for macrophage progenitor cells with high proliferative potential in mouse bone marrow. Blood 60: 503-507.

(17) McNiece, I.K.; Bradley, T.R.; Kriegler, A.B.; and Hodgson, G.S. 1982. A growth factor produced by WEHI-3 cells for murine high proliferative potential GM-progenitor colony forming cells. Cell Biol. Int. Rep. 6: 243-251.

(18) Metcalf, D., and Burgess, A.W. 1982. Clonal analysis of progenitor cell commitment to granulocyte or macrophage production. J. Cell. Physiol. 111: 275-283.

(19) Metcalf, D.; Johnson, G.R.; and Burgess, A.W. 1980. Direct stimulation by purified GM-CSF of the proliferation of multipotential and erythroid precursor cells. Blood 55: 138-147.

(20) Metcalf, D., and Nicola, N.A. 1983. Proliferative effects of purified granulocyte colony-stimulating factor (G-CSF) on normal mouse hemopoietic cells. J. Cell. Physiol. 116: 198-206.

(21) Miyake, T.; Kung, C.K.-H.; and Goldwasser, E. 1977. Purification of human erythropoietin. J. Biol. Chem. 252: 5558-5564.

(22) Nicola, N.A.; Metcalf, D.; Matsumoto, M.; and Johnson, G.R. 1983. Purification of a factor inducing differentiation in murine myelomonocytic leukemia cells. J. Biol. Chem. 258: 9017-9023.

(23) Robb, R.J.; Munck, A.; and Smith, K.A. 1981. T cell growth factor receptors. J. Exp. Med. 154: 1455-1474.

(24) Stanley, E.R. 1979. Colony-stimulating factor (CSF) radioimmunoassay: Detection of a CSF subclass stimulating macrophage production. Proc. Natl. Acad. Sci. USA 76: 2969-2973.

(25) Stanley, E.R., and Heard, P.A. 1977. Factors regulating macrophage production and growth. J. Biol. Chem. 252: 4305-4312.

(26) Tertian, G.; Yung, Y.-P.; Guy-Grand, D.; and Moore, M.A.S. 1981. Long-term in vitro culture of murine mast cells. J. Immunol. 127: 788-798.

(27) Tushinski, R.J.; Oliver, I.T.; Guilbert, L.J.; Tynan, P.W.; Warner, J.R.; and Stanley, E.R. 1982. Survival of mononuclear phagocytes depends on a lineage-specific growth factor that the differentiated cells selectively destroy. Cell 28: 71-81.

(28) Williams, N.; Eger, R.R.; Jackson, H.M.; and Nelson, D.J. 1982. Two-factor requirement for murine megakaryocyte colony formation. J. Cell. Physiol. 110: 101-104.

(29) Williams, N., and Jackson, H. 1983. The role of erythropoietin, thrombopoietic stimulating factor and myeloid colony stimulating factors on murine megakaryocyte colony formation. Exp. Hemat. 11 (Suppl. 14): 11.

(30) Williams, N.; Jackson, H.; Ralph, P.; and Nakoinz, I. 1981. Cell interactions influencing murine marrow megakaryocytes: Nature of the potentiator cell in bone marrow. Blood 57: 157-163.

Leukemia, ed. I.L. Weissman, pp. 21-30. Dahlem Konferenzen 1985. Berlin, Heidelberg, New York, Tokyo: Springer-Verlag.

T Cell Proliferation and Differentiation

W. Haas and H. von Boehmer
Basel Institute for Immunology
4005 Basel, Switzerland

Abstract. Antigens or lectins induce the production of a growth factor for T cells (IL-2) and T cell responsiveness to this growth factor. At least one of these steps is dependent on special stimulatory cells (S^+ cells). T cell proliferation can be maintained in long-term cultures. T cell effector functions such as cytolitic activity, help for B cells, or the production of various lymphokines and the requirements for their induction are poorly understood.

INTRODUCTION

The thymus is essential for the differentiation of T cells which originate from hemopoietic stem cells. Various types of cells in the bone marrow and within the thymus are suspected to be immature T cell progenitors (30). In the following we summarize information available about proliferation and differentiation of mature T cells. We use the terms "class I T cells" and "class II T cells" for the two major subpopulations of T cells which can be distinguished according to major histocompatibility complex (MHC) restriction, differentiation antigens, and functions (Table 1).

T CELL PROLIFERATION

Induction of DNA Synthesis in T Cells

There is a general agreement on three requirements for the induction of DNA synthesis in T cells: it requires antigen recognition, non-lymphoid stimulatory cells, and a growth factor.

TABLE 1 - The two major classes of T cells.

	Class I T cells	Class II T cells
MHC restriction	Class I MHC antigens	Class II MHC antigens
Surface markers		
mice	Lyt 2^+	Lyt 2^-
man	$T8^+$, $T4^-$	$T8^-$, $T4^+$
Functions	Cytolytic activity	Helper activity
	Delayed hypersensitivity	Delayed hypersensitivity

The induction of DNA synthesis of resting T cells is strictly controlled by the T cell's receptors for antigen. T cells recognize (i.e., respond) only to antigens in membranes which carry MHC antigens (MHC-restriction). Experiments suggesting that non-MHC antigens alone could activate T cells (5) have not been reproducible in other laboratories (18, 24). T cell activation by lectins may or may not involve antigen receptors and MHC antigens (for discussion see (16, 18)).

Induction of DNA synthesis of resting T cells requires viable non-lymphoid stimulatory cells (S^+ cells). In vitro induction of DNA synthesis in resting T cells has never been possible in the absence of non-lymphoid cells or factors from such cells. The non-lymphoid cells required must be special stimulatory cells (S^+ cells). Most non-lymphoid cells are S^- cells. Allografts consisting of only S^- cells are not rejected (4), indicating that the requirement for S^+ cells is not a tissue culture artefact. Various types of S^+ cells - macrophages, dendritic cells, Langerhans cells, and others - are distinguished according to differences in morphology, surface markers, enzymes, tissue localization, or migration. All these cells have a limited life span and are continuously produced from a dividing pool of precursor cells in the bone marrow. S^+ cells can "present" on their surface extrinsic antigens (including surface antigens of other cells (17)), express class I and class II MHC antigens (allowing specific interactions with both classes of T cells), and can be stimulated to produce a lymphocyte-activating factor (interleukin 1, or IL-1) (for references see (26)). A prominent feature of S^+ cells is their expression of class II MHC antigen - which is often used to eliminate them by antibody-mediated lysis - but there is no evidence for the view of some authors that class II MHC antigens have functions other than being recognized as restricting elements by T cells.

The induction of DNA synthesis of resting T cells requires a growth factor. Antigens or lectins do not induce T cell proliferation directly: they activate T cells to produce a growth factor and to become responsive to this growth factor. Proliferative responses of class I T cells (9) or class II T cells (25) could be inhibited completely by X-irradiated T cells able to absorb growth factor and the inhibition could be overcome by addition of exogenous growth factor. This observation suggests that any proliferative T cell response is growth factor-dependent. The in vivo relevance of growth factors is not known.

The following is a summary of information available about T cell growth factors:

1 - There is one known T cell-specific growth factor: interleukin 2 (IL-2). IL-2 is a polypeptide of 30Kd in mice and 15Kd in man. MRNA encoding human IL-2 has been identified and the corresponding cDNA cloned and sequenced (31).

2 - Non T cells have never been found to produce IL-2, and many T cell lines produce IL-2 in the absence of any other cells, indicating that IL-2 is produced by T cells. Both class I and class II T cells produce IL-2 (8, 15, 20). Class I T cells either produce less IL-2 or absorb more efficiently IL-2 than class II T cells, particularly in response to antigen and S^+ cells.

3 - S^+ cells are required to induce IL-2 production by lectin or antigen. S^+ cells produce interleukin 1 (IL-1) which facilitates or augments IL-2 production of antigen- or lectin-stimulated T cells (6, 19, 24). Some T cells, T lymphomas, or hybridomas maintained in long-term cultures produce IL-2 in the absence of exogenous IL-1.

4 - Small resting T cells do not bind and do not respond to IL-2. IL-2 responsiveness is induced by lectin or antigen in the presence of S^+ cells (13). However, lectin-mediated T cell contact with neuraminidase-treated S^- cells is sufficient to induce IL-2 responsiveness; in this case S^+ cell-derived factors are not required (12). In response to antigen, most S^- cells are less efficient inducers than S^+ cells. One could speculate that S^+ cells have surface properties facilitating interactions with T cells, but that S^- cells may be sufficient to activate some T cells, for example, memory cells with high affinity

receptors for antigen. Induction of IL-2 responsiveness by antigen in the absence of S^+ cells has been observed only with T cells from immunized mice (11, 22).

5 - Class I and class II T cells can become IL-2 responsive. IL-2 receptors are not induced by lectin in a minor population of human T cells from the blood. These cells produce and perhaps respond to interleukin 3 (IL-3) (Palacios, personal communication). IL-3 is not a T cell-specific growth factor; its biological significance is not clear (see below).

6 - IL-2 responsive T cells express receptors which bind IL-2 with high affinity (Kd = 10^{-12} mol l^{-1}) (28). Monoclonal anti-Tac antibodies bind to IL-2 receptors of human T cells: they inhibit IL-2-binding and IL-2-dependent growth (32). IL-2-binding to activated T cells does induce DNA synthesis. Apparently the binding leads to the expression of transferrin receptors known to control the growth of many cell types (21).

7 - T cell class-specific growth factors were postulated (18) but not demonstrated.

Maintenance of T Cell Proliferation

Continuous T cell lines were established in many laboratories. Growth of most of these cell lines depends on IL-2 which is produced by the lines or added to the medium. Most, though not all, T cell lines maintained in long-term cultures have abnormal chromosomes (14). Whether chromosomal rearrangements or morphologically undetectable gene translocations are required for continuous T cell growth remains to be seen. We distinguish different types of clones according to their growth requirements (Table 2).

TABLE 2 - Growth requirements of different types of clones.

Clones	Growth requirement
Type 1	Antigen and S^+ cells
Type 2	Antigen, S^+ cells, and exogenous IL-2
Type 3	Exogenous IL-2 only

IL-2-dependent growth of clones of class I T cells (for references see (3, 10))

Type 1 clones

The proliferation of about 30% of cytolytic class I T cell clones derived from short-term cultures could be maintained by regular restimulation with antigen and S^+ cells in the absence of exogenous IL-2, but only for one to several weeks ((3) and von Boehmer, unpublished data). Possibly the maintenance of the growth of these clones depends on non-cytolytic antigen-reactive cells which are eventually overgrown by cytolytic cells. Cytolytic cells could interfere with the growth of these clones because they do not produce IL-2 and/or because they eliminate viable S^+ cells required to induce IL-2 production.

Type 2 clones

The growth of all class I T cell clones derived from short-term cultures and of all type 1 clones (which ceased to grow) could be maintained by regular restimulation with antigen and S^+ cells in the IL-2 conditioned media. Cells of these clones express IL-2 responsiveness only if exposed to antigen or lectin in the presence of S^+ cells but do not produce IL-2 and do not mediate antigen-specific delayed hypersensitivity, a function retained by type 1 clones. Type 2 clones could be maintained in culture for more than one year.

Type 3 clones

Type 3 clones grow in IL-2 conditioned media in the absence of antigen and any other cells. Such clones are derived from rare T cell variants which do not need to recognize antigen to express IL-2 responsiveness but still express antigen specific cytolytic activity. We consider these variants and their progeny as tissue culture artefacts. Apparently, one type 3 clone could be adapted to grow in the absence of exogenous IL-2 (2).

IL-2-dependent growth of clones of class II T cells (for references see (7, 29))

Type 1 and type 2 clones

In contrast to clones of class I T cells, all class II T cell clones derived from short-term cultures could be maintained for several months by regular restimulation with antigen and S^+ cells in the absence of exogenous IL-2. Antigen and S^+ cells are required to induce both IL-2 production and IL-2 responsiveness of these clones. Although these clones could be maintained for more than one year in the absence of exogenous IL-2, their growth often became very slow but could then be enhanced considerably by feeding the cultures with exogenous IL-2. Many investigators maintain class II T cell clones by regular feeding with exogenous IL-2 at each or at every second restimulation with antigen and S^+ cells. The functional phenotypes of these clones appear to be stable whether grown with or without exogenous IL-2: they produced IL-2 and other lymphokines after exposure to antigen and S^+ cells, they transferred delayed hypersensitivity, and they could activate B cells under appropriate conditions.

Type 3 clones

Class II T cell clones which grow continuously in IL-2 conditioned media in the absence of any other cells were established in several laboratories. These lines are probably derived from rare T cell variants analogous to those of class I T cells described above.

Interleukin 3 (IL-3)-dependent cell lines

A recently purified 26 to 28Kd polypeptide factor (called interleukin 3 or IL-3) which is produced by lectin- or antigen-stimulated T lymphocytes or constitutively by the mouse tumor cell line WEHI-3 allowed the long-term growth of members of the T cell lineage and the B cell lineage ((23), and Palacios, personal communication). IL-3 is probably identical with previously described factors which stimulated the growth and differentiation of various immature hemopoietic cells and allowed the long-term growth of various non-lymphoid hemopoietic cell lines (1).

T CELL DIFFERENTIATION

Mature T cells are highly differentiated cells which lost the potential of their ancestors to become, for example, granulocytes or B lymphocytes. Class II T cells have the potential to become IL-2-responsive and to produce IL-2 as well as other lymphokines. Class I T cells have, in addition, the capacity to express cytolytic activity and to produce γ-interferon. Induction of all these functions does not require DNA synthesis. After stimulation of T cell populations with lectin or antigen in the presence of S^+ cells, usually all potential changes in T cell phenotypes are observed: class I T cells, for example, proliferate, secrete lymphokines, and express cytolytic activity. A culture of a T cell line that is clonally derived from a single ancestor can express all these properties. It is not clear, however, whether a single T cell can express all of these properties. It is not known, for example, whether or not a single class I T cell can express cytolytic activity and secrete γ-interferon, nor whether each of these functions can be selectively induced. There are examples for the expression of selected phenotypes: first, induction of IL-2 responsiveness of class I T cells is not necessarily associated with induction of IL-2 production (see above). Second, T cell populations could be induced by lectin to proliferate under certain conditions for a limited time period without expression of cytolytic activity. Eventually, after 3 to 4 days, cytolytic activity was always observed. Cytolytic activity could be induced before its "spontaneous" appearance by factor or factors distinct from IL-2 (27). An important future task will be the purification and characterization of differentiation-inducing factors and the development of assay systems allowing detection of T cell functions at the single cell level.

REFERENCES

(1) Bazil, G.W.; Haynes, M.; Garland, J.; and Dexter, T.M. 1983. Characterization and partial purification of a hemopoietic cell growth factor in WEHI-3 cell conditioned medium. Biochem. J. 210: 747-759.

(2) Benjamin, W.R.; Steeg, D.S.; and Farrar, J.J. 1982. Production of immune interferon by an IL-2 independent murine T cell line. Proc. Natl. Acad. Sci. USA 79: 5379-5383.

(3) von Boehmer, H., and Turton, K. 1983. Autonomously proliferating K/D-restricted cytolytic T cell clones. Eur. J. Immunol. 13: 176-179.

(4) Burdick, J.F., and Russell, P.S. 1982. Antigenic requirements for induced rejection of long-surviving murine heart transplants. J. Immunol. 128: 1551-1554.

(5) Durum, S.K., and Gershon, R.K. 1982. Interleukin 1 can replace the requirement for I-A positive cells in the proliferation of antigen-primed T cells. proc. Natl. Acad. Sci. USA 79: 4747-4750.

(6) Favata, M.; Smith, K.A.; Lachman, L.B.; and Oppenheim, J.J. 1980. The functional relationship of the interleukins. J. Exp. Med. 155: 1551-1556.

(7) Glasebrook, A.L.; Sarmiento, M.; Loken, M.R.; Dialynas, D.P.; Quintans, J.; Eisenberg, L.; Lutz, C.T.; Wilde, D.; and Fitch, F.W. 1981. Murine T lymphocyte clones with distinct immunological functions. Immunol. Rev. 54: 225-266.

(8) Guerme, P.A.; Piquet, R.F.; and Vasalli, P. 1983. Positively selected Lyt 2^+ and Lyt 2^- mouse T lymphocytes are comparable after ConA

stimulation in release of IL-2 and lymphokines acting on B cells, macrophages and mast cells but differ in interferon production. J. Immunol. 130: 2225-2230.

(9) Günther, J.; Haas, W.; and von Boehmer, H. 1982. Suppression of T cell responses through competition for T cell growth factor (interleukin 2). Eur. J. Immunol. 12: 247-249.

(10) Haas, W., and von Boehmer, H. 1982. Methods for the establishment of continuously growing cytolytic T cell clones. J. Immunol. Meth. 52: 137-148.

(11) Herrmann, S.H.; Weinberger, O.; Burakoff, S.J.; and Mescher, M.F. 1982. Analysis of the two-signal requirement for precursors of cytolytic T lymphocyte activation using $H\text{-}2K^{k}$ in liposomes. J. Immunol. 128: 1968-1974.

(12) Hünig, T. 1983. The role of accessory cells in polyclonal T cell activation II. Induction of interleukin 2 responsiveness requires cell-cell contact. Eur. J. Immunol. 13: 596-601.

(13) Hünig, T.; Loos, M.; and Schimpl, A. 1983. The role of accessory cells in polyclonal T cell activation I. Both induction of IL-2 production and of IL-2 responsiveness by ConA are accessory cell dependent. Eur. J. Immunol. 13: 1-6.

(14) Johnson, J.P.; Cianfriglia, M.; Glasebrook, A.L.; and Nabholz, M. 1982. Karyotype evolution of cytolytic T cell lines. In Isolation, Characterization and Utilization of T Lymphocyte Clones, eds. C.G. Fathman and F.W. Fitch, pp. 183-190. New York: Academic Press.

(15) Kelso, A., and McDonald, H.R. 1982. Precursor frequency analysis of lymphokine secreting alloreactive T lymphocytes. Dissociation of subsets producing IL-2, MAF and GM-CSF on the basis of Lyt 2 phenotype. J. Exp. Med. 156: 1366-1379.

(16) Kimura, A., and Ersson, B. 1981. Activation of T lymphocytes by lectins and carbohydrate-oxidizing reagents viewed as an immunological recognition of cell-surface modifications seen in the context of "self" major histocompatibility antigens. Eur. J. Immunol. 11: 475-483.

(17) Korngold, R., and Sprent, J. 1980. Selection of cytotoxic T cell precursors specific for minor histocompatibility determinants. I. Negative selection across H-2 barriers induced with disrupted cells but not with glutaraldehyde treated cells: evidence for antigen processing. J. Exp. Med. 151: 314-327.

(18) Larsson, E.L.; Coutinho, A.; and Martinez, C. 1980. A suggested mechanism for T lymphocyte activation: Implications on the acquisition of functional reactivities. Immunol. Rev. 51: 61-91.

(19) Larsson, E.L.; Iscove, N.N.; and Coutinho, A. 1980. Two distinct factors required for induction of T cell growth. Nature 283: 664-666.

(20) Meuer, S.C.; Hussey, R.E.; Penta, A.C.; Fitzgerald, K.A.; Stadler, B.M.; Schlossman, S.F.; and Reinherz, E.L. 1982. Cellular origin of IL-2 in man: Evidence for stimulus restricted IL-2 production by T4+ and T8+ lymphocytes. J. Immunol. 129: 1076-1079

(21) Neckers, L.M., and Cossman, J. 1983. Transferrin receptor induction in mitogen stimulated human T lymphocytes is required for DNA synthesis and cell division and is regulated by interleukin 2. Proc. Natl. Acad. Sci. USA 80: 3494-3498.

(22) Okada, M., and Henney, C.S. 1980. The differentiation of CTL in vitro. III. the role of helper cells and their products in the differentiation of CTL from memory cell populations. J. Immunol. 125: 850-857.

(23) Palacios, R. 1982. Cloned lines of IL-2 producer human T lymphocytes. J. Immunol. 129: 2586-2593.

(24) Palacios, R. 1982. Mechanisms of T cell activation: Role and functional relationship of HLA-DR antigens and interleukins. Immunol. Rev. 63: 73-110.

(25) Palacios, R., and Möller, G. 1981. T cell growth factor abrogates Concanavalin-A induced suppressor cell function. J. Exp. Med. 153: 1360-1365.

(26) Pugh, C.W.; MacPherson, G.G.; and Steer, H.W. 1983. Characterization of non lymphoid cells derived from rat peripheral lymph. J. Exp. Med. 157: 1758-1779.

(27) Raulet, D.H., and Bevan, M.J. 1982. A differentiation factor required for the expression of cytotoxic T cell function. Nature 296: 754-757.

(28) Robb, R.J.; Munck, A.; and Smith, K.A. 1981. T cell growth factor receptors. Quantitation, specificity and biological relevance. J. Exp. Med. 154: 1455-1474.

(29) Schreier, M.H.; Iscove, N.N.; Aarden, L.; and von Boehmer, H. 1980.

Clones of killer and helper T cells: growth requirements specificity and retention of function in long-term culture. Immunol. Rev. 51: 315-336.

(30) Scollay, R., and Shortman, K. 1983. Thymocyte subpopulations: An experimental review including flow cytometric cross-correlations between the major murine thymocyte markers. Thymus 5: 245-295.

(31) Taniguchi, T.; Matsui, H.; Fujita, T.; Takaoka, C.; Kashima, N.; Yoshimoto, R.; and Hamuro, I. 1983. Structure and expression of a cloned cDNA for human IL-2. Nature 302: 305-310.

(32) Warren, J.L.; Depper, J.M.; Uchiyama, T.; Smith, K.A.; Waldmann, T.A.; and Greene, W.L. 1982. A monoclonal antibody that appears to recognize the receptor for human T cell growth factor, partial characterization of the receptor. Nature 300: 267-269.

Leukemia, ed. I.L. Weissman, pp. 31-67. Dahlem Konferenzen 1985. Berlin, Heidelberg, New York, Tokyo: Springer-Verlag.

Regulatory Defects in Leukemia: In Vitro Analysis

M.A.S. Moore
Memorial Sloan-Kettering Cancer Center - Section 6136
New York, NY 10021, USA

INTRODUCTION

Studies of myeloid leukemic cell lines and primary cultures of leukemic bone marrow have yielded information on humoral regulation of growth and differentiation of myeloid cells and have revealed specific abnormalities in regulatory control that would appear to play important roles in the development and progression of hematopoietic neoplasia. Already considerable in vitro data have been accumulated to document the feasibility of the clinical application of such biological response modifiers as Retinoic acid, interferon, tumor necrosis factor, prostaglandin E, and differentiation-inducing proteins in a strategy designed to revert malignant hematopoietic cells to a pattern of normal proliferation and differentiation, or to mediate their selective ablation. Evidence that an effective cancer therapy can be based on induction of a phenotypic reversion of the tumor cell as well as by direct killing of tumor cells has been based on extensive studies on leukemic cell lines such as Friend mouse erythroleukemic cells (39), mouse myeloid (M1) and myelomonocytic (WEHI-3) cell lines (33, 71), and human HL-60 myeloid leukemic cells (40). These cell lines can be induced to differentiate and lose self-renewal and leukemogenic capacity following exposure to a variety of chemical agents, including some anticancer drugs (52, 109).

Fibach, Hayachi, and Sachs (33) reported that serum from mice injected with endotoxin induced granulocyte and macrophage differentiation of the mouse myeloid leukemic cell line M1. At that time it was unclear whether the differentiation-inducing factor was CSF (MGI). Metcalf (71) also reported that a pure preparation of GM-CSF has some capacity to induce differentiation of murine WEHI-3B(D+) myelomonocytic leukemic cells. More recently biochemical characterization of post-endotoxin serum has shown that the differentiation factor could be separated from GM-CSF (MGI-1) (66) (and was termed MGI-2) or could be separated from the bulk of serum CSF but co-eluted with a minor species of CSF that stimulated only granulocyte colony formation (12).

The cellular origin of proteinaceous differentiation factors (DF) for leukemic cells is diverse. Spleen lymphocytes and macrophages have been shown to produce the activity when treated with various mitogens including endotoxin (127). Conditioned medium from a variety of murine organs also contained DF, but much higher levels of activity were reported following endotoxin treatment (84). DF produced by the different organs in vitro and in vivo in endotoxin serum was distinguishable from the majority of granulocyte-macrophage (GM) and macrophage (M) CSF. DF was precipitated by 55% ammonium sulfate and did not bind to concanavalin A-Sepharose, whereas CSF required 85% saturation and bound to con A-Sepharose. DF also eluted later than CSF from Phenyl-Sepharose columns and could be distinguished from M-CSF by its apparent molecular weight (23,000) on native gels (84).

Induction of DF is radio-resistant and probably independent of T cells since nude mice respond normally (73). Repeated injections of endotoxin lead to depressed responsiveness as measured by serum DF and CSF levels, and sustained serum DF levels have not been obtained (73). This in part is due to the short serum half-life of GM-DF (1.5 - 2.3 hours) and the development of endotoxin "tolerance," which provide a possible major obstacle to the clinical value of endotoxin induction of endogenous mediators.

Endotoxin or other immunostimulants from microorganisms may also induce leukemic cell differentiation in vitro by inducing the leukemic cells to produce endogenous DF (2, 28, 121). The structure of microorganisms required for a direct effect on the differentiation of leukemic cells and for stimulation of DF production by normal spleen cells may differ, since BCG induced direct differentiation of M1 leukemic cells and spleen DF production; C. parvum had no direct effect on M1 cells but was a potent inducer of spleen cell DF production, and N-acetylmuramyl dipeptide, the minimal adjuvant-active subunit of the bacterial cell wall, had no direct effect on the differentiation of

Ml cells and only slightly stimulated the production of DF by spleen cells (127).

Expression of Ia-antigens relative to S-phase of the cell cycle is closely associated with the normal in vitro regulation of the proliferation of normal and leukemic stem and progenitor cells (CFU-GM, BFU-e, and CFU-GEMM) by prostaglandin E (PGE) and acidic isoferritins (AIF) (9, 89). In patients with leukemia, particularly those with chronic myeloid leukemia, abnormal expression of Ia-antigens and hyposensitivity to growth inhibition by prostaglandin E and acidic isoferritin are closely associated with leukemic transformation (9, 91-93).

A suspension preculture assay which represents an important improvement over agar or methylcellulose culture alone has enabled the investigation of cellular interactions which occur early in hemopoietic progenitor cell proliferation and which cannot be easily studied in a semisolid matrix (89). Using this culture system approach, there is a significant association between expression of HLA-DR antigen and control of hemopoietic cell proliferation. Furthermore, a new role for prostaglandin E in the control of hematopoietic progenitor cell cycle modulation of Ia-antigen expression was demonstrated. As a consequence, there is maintenance of the CFU-GM, BFU-e, and CFU-GEMM cell compartments in a state of responsiveness to subsequent growth regulation. Most significantly, in patients with chronic myeloid leukemia (CML), prostaglandin E mediates reversion of the overt leukemic phenotype displayed by Ph^{1+} cells to a normal one which is associated with normal Ia-antigen expression and normal response to regulation (94). These studies reaffirm a close association between Ia-expression and hematopoietic progenitor cell regulation.

The roles of prostaglandin E and also of accessory T lymphocytes in hematopoietic cell proliferation must also be considered in the context of marrow transplantation. Improved methods to ablate cell populations, particularly T cells, in an effort to reduce graft versus host disease may impair hemopoietic engraftment by removing accessory cells required for stem and progenitor cell proliferation.

Hematopoiesis occurs within a specialized physical and functional microenvironment consisting of a variety of cells, an architectural framework (the marrow matrix), and regulatory influences. This hematopoietic microenvironment ensures the lodgement, self-replication, and differentiation of hematopoietic stem cells. The functional integrity of the marrow microenvironment following transplantation or immune suppression is therefore critical for the occurrence and maintenance of sustained hematopoiesis.

The understanding of the nature and the function of marrow microenvironment has been greatly facilitated by the opportunity to examine and manipulate in vitro the marrow-derived heterogeneous adherent layer supporting the long-term culture of hematopoietic cells. Dexter and co-workers (20, 22) reported the first successful long-term bone marrow culture using mouse cells and provided perhaps the most compelling evidence supporting the existence of a hematopoietic microenvironment. Prolonged hematopoiesis could not be maintained in absence of the marrow-derived adherent layer. This adherent layer has been shown to be composed of fibroblasts, macrophages, endothelial cells, and lipid-containing cells (3, 14). Dexter and Moore (21) were able to reproduce in vitro the defect of the Steel mouse (Sl/Sl^d) in long-term marrow cultures and to cure it in vitro by inoculating marrow cells from W/W^v mouse.

It has been generally assumed that the expansion of donor hematopoietic elements and sustained hematopoietic recovery is supported by microenvironmental elements of the host marrow. This concept has been based on in vitro observations suggesting a relative insensitivity of the marrow microenvironment to high dose radiation and chemotherapy (106, 116) and on studies in murine models and humans documenting the host origin of marrow-derived fibroblastic cells in the post-transplant period (38, 44, 125). However, this concept has recently been challenged by studies demonstrating the relative radiosensitivity of marrow stromal cells and their donor origin in the post-transplant period. Castro-Malaspina et al. (13) have found that the in vitro radiosensitivity of human marrow fibroblast progenitors (CFU-F) is similar to that of granulocyte-macrophage progenitors (CFU-GM), which suggests that the resistance of critical elements of the stroma to in vivo radiation may be more limited than previously appreciated. Furthermore, Keating et al. (58) and others have shown the donor origin of heterogeneous adherent layers derived from marrow of sex-mismatched marrow transplant patients. Piersma et al. have demonstrated the transplantability of marrow fibroblast progenitors in CBA mice grafted with allogeneic marrow cells bearing the T6 chromosome marker. These as yet limited observations underscore the possibility that variations in the contribution of donor and host marrow microenvironmental elements to the development of donor hematopoietic progenitors may exist in different patients and at different times in the post-transplant course, which may serve to limit or foster hematologic recovery.

There are some observations in marrow transplant patients suggesting that the hematopoietic microenvironment may play a central role in the pathogenesis of certain cases of defective hematopoietic reconstitution. For instance, the fact that some patients with aplastic anemia exhibiting no evidence of abnormal suppressor cell activity fail to engraft following immunosuppression and syngeneic marrow transplantation suggests that the engraftment failure is due to the donor's unfavorable microenvironment. Furthermore, in our marrow transplant experience the recognition of a few patients among fifty transplanted for severe aplastic anemia who achieved complete engraftment of donor lymphoid elements yet remained aplastic suggested the possibility that these patients might have, as the basis for aplasia, a defect in the marrow microenvironment. Also, patients with isolated cytopenias, such as congenital agranulocytosis or Wiskott-Aldrich syndrome may, despite immunosuppression with cyclophosphamide, be engrafted only with lymphoid precursors unless myeloablation with agents such as busulfan or total body irradiation are also induced prior to transplantation (57). More overt examples of the limitations to hematopoietic recovery which may be imposed by the host environment are provided by analyses of the post-transplant course in patients grafted for chimeric forms of aplastic anemia and for the preleukemic disorder termed refractory anemia with excess blasts (RAEB). In our experience, such patients have consistently exhibited poor recovery of hematopoietic function in the post-transplant period, despite durable engraftment of donor lymphoid and hematopoietic elements, as confirmed by karyotypic analyses. The persistent and profound leukopenia and thrombocytopenia observed in the patients has not been attributable to viral infection or GvHD and has been refractory to secondary infusion of marrow from the original donor. The basis for this sustained dysfunction of the engrafted donor hematopoietic system in the post-transplant period is unexplained, but it may be due to persisting defects of the host marrow microenvironment.

Aplastic anemia was early recognized as a principle manifestation of graft vs. host disease in patients with severe combined immunodeficiency inadvertently transfused with unirradiated HLA-mismatched blood cells or transplanted with HLA-incompatible or even HLA-matched marrow grafts (43, 49, 87). Aplastic anemia has also developed as a complication of GvHD in heavily immunosuppressed patients treated for Hodgkin's disease or leukemia, who have been engrafted with allogeneic cells following transfusion of unirradiated blood (23, 120). Indeed, even patients transplanted with HLA-matched marrow for aplastic anemia or leukemia may develop persistent leukopenia and thrombocytopenia during GvHD, irrespective of whether the GvHD is treated with prednisone or not. The problem of GvH-associated leukopenia and thrombocytopenia has been a regular feature observed in our transplant experience of now over 300 allogeneic marrow grafts. It is not known, but clearly suspected, that macrophages, and possibly other cellular constituents of the marrow microenvironment of the host, display the minor allospecificities stimulating GvHD in the HLA-matched marrow transplant recipient. Furthermore, although it has been demonstrated that in vitro alloactivated T and non-T cell populations are capable of suppressing the growth of donor hematopoietic progenitors (19), they may also exert an equal and possibly more profound effect on the stromal cells which support their growth. Thus, studies are clearly needed to define the relative importance of marrow microenvironmental and hematopoietic cells, both in the stimulation of alloreactive T cells initiating GvHD and in the pathogenesis of the limited hematopoietic recovery which is its sequela.

It is obvious that for bone marrow transplantation appropriate stem and progenitor cells, accessory cells, and microenvironment cells must interact in specific ways in order to enable engraftment and to bring those cells which subsequently proliferate under appropriate regulatory control. Monitoring these parameters is important to insure that true normal hematopoietic reconstitution has occurred.

RESULTS

Induction of Serum GM-DF Activity and an Antineoplastic Cytotoxin (Tumor Necrosis Factor - TNF) in Mice and in Patients with Advanced Malignancy Receiving Purified Lipopolysaccharide

Sachs (66, 107) and Metcalf (73) have independently reported that serum from endotoxin-treated mice contains a factor which induces terminal granulocyte and macrophage differentiation of murine myeloid leukemia cell lines M1 and WEHI-3B(D+) (66, 72). In addition, serial reculture of WEHI-3B(D+) cells in the presence of this serum factor has been shown to lead to clonal extinction in 2-6 passages (72) and to suppress leukemogenicity when transplanted into syngeneic mice (73). We examined the ability of mouse serum obtained three hours after intravenous injection of 5 ug of endotoxin to induce differentiation of WEHI-3B(D+) cells cloned in semisolid agar. Dose response analysis indicated that 100% of leukemic colonies converted from tight undifferentiated pattern to diffuse, differentiated colonies composed of neutrophil and mature macrophages when exposed to 5-10% of post-endotoxin serum, and differentiation was still noted at 1:64 dilution of serum. Significantly, colony inhibition was not observed even at high serum concentrations. Tumor necrosis factor (TNF) serum (unfractionated serum from C. parvum + endotoxin-treated mice) inhibited 90% of leukemic colony growth when used at 10% concentration, but this presumed TNF-dependent inhibition rapidly titrated out. Significant levels of differentiation-inducing factor activity, comparable to levels in post-endotoxin serum, were also noted.

To determine further the independent actions of TNF and GM-DF on myeloid leukemic cell growth, TNF was subjected to batch elution on DEAE-A-50 gel. The serum fraction eluting with 0.2M NaCl was found to contain very little TNF activity but contained a major proportion of the differentiation-inducing factor activity; in contrast, the serum fraction eluted with 1.0M NaCl contained most of the TNF which was further purified on Sephadex G-100 columns. The TNF-rich peak was strongly inhibitory to WEHI-3B(D+) leukemic cloning but contained no significant differentiation-inducing activity.

The suggestion of Burgess and Metcalf (12) that differentiation-inducing protein for myeloid leukemic cells could be a subspecies of granulocyte CSF (G-CSF) is rendered unlikely by our studies on WEHI-3B(D+) leukemic cell differentiation in which the capacity of serum fractions or conditioned medium to stimulate WEHI-3 differentiation was compared to the capacity to stimulate normal mouse myeloid colony formation. The TNF serum fraction which induced WEHI-3 leukemic cell differentiation also stimulated normal GM-colony formation (CFU-GM).

In contrast, a more purified and active source of CSF from L cell-conditioned medium, induced differentiation in only a minority of leukemic colonies, and more significantly, conditioned medium from nondifferentiating WEHI-3 leukemic cells, which we have shown is a particularly rich source of G-CSF (123), stimulated extensive granulocyte colonies in normal marrow but had very little capacity to induce leukemic cell differentiation. These preliminary studies need to be extended by further biochemical characterization of differentiation protein, but at the present time the results suggest that the differentiation-inducing protein may be uniquely specific for leukemic target cells and may mediate an important surveillance role in suppressing emergent malignant clones.

In view of the evidence that potent macromolecules, such as GM-DF, can be induced following endotoxin administration in the mouse, serum from patients with advanced non-hematopoietic malignancies, treated with Novo-Pyrexal (a highly purified preparation of endotoxin extracted from S. Abortus equi) were analyzed in order to determine if such a differentiation-inducing protein could also be detected in man.

Serum was collected at time 0, 1/2 h, 2 h, 4 h, 6 h, 8 h, 12 h, and 24 h after a patient had received an intravenous injection of Novo-Pyrexal, beginning with a dose of 0.1 ug/m^2 and escalating at weekly or biweekly intervals. The serum was assayed at 10% and 1% in 1 ml agar cultures containing 300 WEHI-3B(D+) murine myelomonocytic leukemic cells. Time 0 serum had no significant effect on cloning efficiency or colony differentiation, as measured by tight versus diffuse colonies. A serum activity which induced up to 85% of leukemic colonies to differentiate to mature granulocytes and/or macrophages reached its peak at 2-4 h after Novo-Pyrexal administration and disappeared after 12-24 h. An acute decrease in white cell count was observed in every instance, as early as 30 min. after the completion of Novo-Pyrexal infusion, followed by a return to normal or a rebound leukocytosis by 24 h. In seven patients studied so far, induction of this differentiation factor has been seen with similar kinetics. Serum collected 30 min. after Novo-Pyrexal administration was inhibitory to leukemic colony formation but was not active in inducing differentiation. The relationship of this inhibitory activity to TNF is not known at this time.

The ability repeatedly to induce serum activities such as GM-DF following repeated endotoxin administration may be influenced by the development of tolerance. The mechanism of tolerance induction is not clear, and it is not simply due to the appearance of antibodies directed against the polysaccharide component of endotoxin. In an attempt to prevent endotoxin tolerance in patients receiving repeated dosages of highly purified endotoxin, clinical protocols were developed which involved escalating doses and biweekly or weekly schedules of drug administration. The results of one such study in a patient with advanced cancer is depicted in Fig. 1. In Fig. 1, serum obtained prior to and at various intervals following endotoxin administration was assayed for its ability to induce differentiation of WEHI-3B(D+) cells. Leukemia differentiation-inducing activity was elevated from essentially undetectable levels to a peak between 2-6 h following endotoxin, and the escalation of endotoxin at twice weekly intervals to a maximum of 30 ug/m^2 produced consistent re-induction of this response. Figure 1 illustrates that with repeated administration of a given dose of endotoxin, a degree of tolerance appears to occur with regard to the induction of GM-DF.

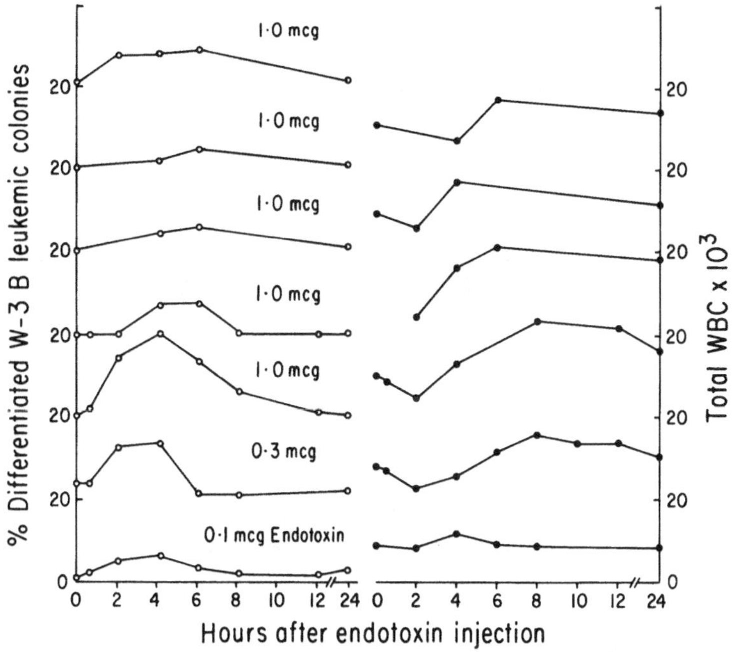

FIG. 1 - Induction of a differentiation-inducing factor (GM-DF) in the serum of a patient with advanced malignancy. Biweekly intravenous injections of increasing doses (expressed as dose per m^2) of highly purified endotoxin (Novo-Pyrexal) to the patient induced a regular biphasic leukocyte response with initial leukopenia followed by leukocytosis. Serum (10% v/v) was added to agar cultures containing WEHI-3D(D+) leukemic cells and the percent of colonies becoming diffuse (differentiated) by seven days was scored. Note the induction of GM-DF activity 2-4 h after endotoxin treatment.

The ability of endotoxin to induce human active CSF in the serum of these patients was confirmed by the assay of the patients' own serum on the patients' own bone marrow obtained prior to and 24 h following treatment with Novo-Pyrexal. Colony-stimulating activity (CSF) was observed in the serum at 4-8 h post-endotoxin. In addition, the pre-endotoxin marrow exhibited a greater responsiveness, i.e., contained a greater number of CFU-GM, than did the marrow obtained 24 h after treatment (Fig. 2). This might suggest, as one possibility, an in vivo depletion of marrow CFU-GM, which have moved further along the myeloid

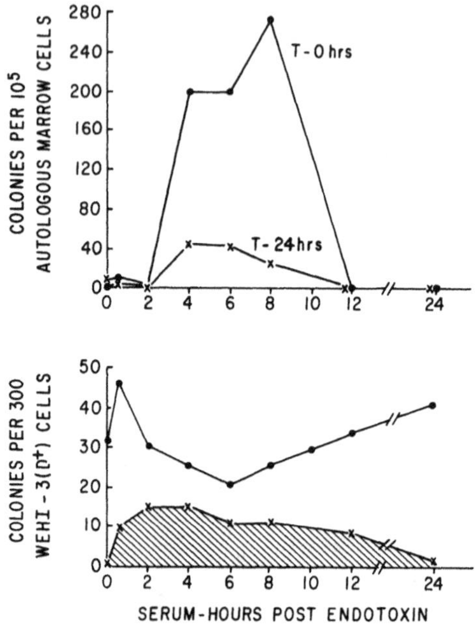

FIG. 2 - Leukemia-differentiating capacity and human CSF in human post-endotoxin sera. Sera collected after intravenous injection of 1 ug/m^2 and added 10% v/v to 1ml agar culture containing 300 WEHI-3B(D+) cells or to cultures of the patients' bone marrow obtained immediately prior to endotoxin treatment and 24 h post-endotoxin: human CFU-GM and differentiation agar culture assay were done in triplicate and scored on day 7.

differentiation pathway as a result of biological regulators of hematopoiesis released following endotoxin.

Endotoxin-induced Leukemia Differentiation Factor in the Serum of Patients with Preleukemia, Chronic Myelogenous Leukemia, or Acute Myelogenous Leukemia (ANLL)

Interest in host resistance factors in leukemia has continued for some decades, and for this reason incidences of spontaneous regressions or remissions have excited considerable attention. The majority of spontaneous regressions have occurred following streptococcal or prolonged staphylococcal infections. At Memorial hospital, patients with ANLL, who received pseudomonas vaccine to protect against pseudomonas infection were found to have improved survival as compared to patients who did not receive the vaccine (there was no difference in the incidence of pseudomonas morbidity). The therapeutic role of bacterial vaccine or endotoxins has been seen in the context of various mechanisms of anti-neoplastic defense with augmentation of host immune mechanisms. Our present work suggests that such therapy might be effective by virtue of the acute induction of factors promoting leukemic cell differentiation and/or an anti-proliferative factor with selectivity for transformed cells and suggests a possible therapeutic role in human myeloid leukemia. In view of the evidence that potent macromolecules such as GM-DF and TNF are found in post-endotoxin serum in man, and in light of the work by Lotem et al. (66), who have shown that injection of either endotoxin or murine-derived MGI-1 containing significant amounts of MGI-2 (GM-DF) can inhibit the development of myeloid leukemia in vivo and stimulate normal hematopoiesis, we have begun to treat patients with ANLL, all FAB classifications, in first or second relapse, CML patients in blast crisis or accelerated phase of their disease, and patients with preleukemia, with or without prior treatment, with Novo-Pyrexal.

At the present time we have treated three leukemic patients with Novo-Pyrexal. The diagnosis of these patients include myelodysplastic syndrome (patient #1), chronic myelogenous leukemia in lymphoblastic crisis (patient #2), and erythroleukemia (patient #3). Patients #2 and #3 had received several courses of chemotherapy prior to treatment with endotoxin; patient #1 had received no prior treatment. Patients were treated with either a weekly schedule of Novo-Pyrexal beginning at a dose of 0.2 ug/m^2 and escalating to a dose which produced significant clinical toxicity, i.e., fever and chills, or a daily schedule designed to induce physiological tolerance to fever and chills, commencing with the same dose and escalating once tolerance was induced at a given dose level. So far, patients #1 and #2 are evaluable for production of GM-DF: patient #3 is just being evaluated. The results demonstrate the presence of 70-100 units of GM-DF/0.1ml of undiluted serum (units being defined by Metcalf (73) as follows: 50 units equals the activity which renders 50% of WEHI-3B(D+) colonies differentiated in the clonal agar system). In patient #1, this activity could be repeatedly induced when treated on a weekly schedule with 0.6 ug/m^2; no factor production, however, could be detected in the patients' undiluted serum, when endotoxin was given daily, at a dose comparable to that employed on the weekly regimen, in the same patient. Although this is a phase I study of Novo-Pyrexal in this group of patients, and not designed to address the therapeutic benefit of such treatment, we have evaluated for evidence of therapeutic effect. Patient

#1's initial bone marrow revealed 29% Auer rod positive blasts plus promyelocytes: subsequently this dropped to 12% blasts plus promyelocytes, as documented on successive bone marrow aspirations. The number of Auer rod positive blasts also decreased and, in addition, the number of micromegakaryocytes was noted to have decreased. Patient #2 received two treatments with Novo-Pyrexal and soon thereafter was treated with high-dose Ara-C. He subsequently reverted to the chronic phase (in our series at Memorial hospital only one out of five patients with CML in blast crisis has reverted to the chronic phase with high-dose Ara-C alone). Whether or not treatment with endotoxin directly or indirectly affects the number of cells entering S-phase and possibly rendering them more susceptible to a cycle-specific agent such as Ara-C is of considerable interest, and we shall attempt to study this question in the future.

The Influence of Vitamins A, D, and Their Analogues on Normal and Leukemic Myelopoiesis

Vitamin A and its analogues (retinoids) affect proliferation and differentiation of normal and malignant hematopoietic cells. The extensively studied system has been the human promyelocytic leukemic cell line HL-60 which can be induced to differentiate to mature granulocytes (as measured morphologically by differentiation antigen expression and functionally by ability to reduce nitroblue tetrazolium) following exposure to Retinoic acid (8, 50, 86, 96). Maximum differentiation (approximately 90% of cells) occurs with 1 uM of Retinoic acid, a concentration 500-160,000-fold less than the concentration of butyrate and dimethyl-sulfoxide that promote a similar increase in differentiation. Continuous exposure to Retinoic acid is necessary for maximum differentiation which occurs after five days of incubation, and retinol (vitamin A), retinal acetate, and retinal are approximately 1000-fold less potent than Retinoic acid which can induce some differentiation at concentrations as low as 1 nanomole.

Retinoid induction of myeloid leukemic differentiation is not a universal phenomenon. While the murine myelomonocytic leukemic cell line WEHI-3 can be induced to mature neutrophil differentiation (80) and Retinoic acid induces the human malignant monoblast line U937 to monocyte-like cells with the capacity to reduce nitroblue tetrazolium (86), the human myeloid cell lines KG-1 and K562 cannot be induced to differentiate (24). The mouse myeloid leukemia, M1, can be induced to increase levels of lysomal enzyme production without induction of phagocytosis, locomotive activity, or morphological maturation (114). Indeed, Retinoic acid was a potent inhibitor of induction of these latter differentiation-associated properties. Fresh leukemic cells from patients with various myeloid leukemias have also been exposed to Retinoic acid in short-term primary suspension cultures, and morphological and function maturation was observed only in cases of acute promyelocytic leukemia (41). The differential sensitivity of various leukemias to Retinoic acid-induction of terminal differentiation may be attributed to whether or not the target cells contain cellular Retinoic acid-binding protein, but evidence on this point is conflicting (24, 114). Alternatively, the potential for terminal differentiation may be irreversibly lost in many cases of acute myeloid leukemia. This latter possibility does not negate the therapeutic value of Retinoic acid therapy in a wide range of leukemias since considerable evidence has accumulated to suggest that retinoids can selectively inhibit leukemic cell self-renewal independent of activation of a differentiation program in the leukemic stem cell. Retinoic acid is a potent inhibitor of the clonal growth in vitro of myeloid leukemic cells, and a 50% growth inhibitor of HL-60 was achieved by 25 nM Retinoic acid and the human myeloid leukemic line KG-1, which is not inducible to differentiate but was, nevertheless, extremely sensitive to Retinoic acid with 50% of the colonies inhibited by 2.4 nM concentrations of the drug (24). Retinoic acid also inhibited the clonal growth of leukemic cells from five of seven patients with acute myeloid leukemia.

The anti-proliferative action of retinoids upon leukemic cells is more general than the incidence of induction of terminal differentiation and is seen with retinoid concentrations readily attainable in vivo. The potential efficacy of Retinoic acid in the treatment of human leukemia is further suggested by the observation that Retinoic acid enhances colony-stimulating factor-induced clonal growth of normal human myeloid progenitor cells in vitro (25). Maximal stimulation occurred at a concentration of 3 x 10^{-7} Retinoic acid which increased the mean number of colonies by 213 8% over plates containing CSF alone. Retinoic acid has no direct CSF activity nor does it stimulate CSF production by the cultured bone marrow cells. This stimulation may be mediated by increased responsiveness of the granulocyte-macrophage progenitors and the action of CSF, possibly by increasing the number of CSF receptors per cell. Retinoids are reported to enhance the binding of epidermal growth factor (EGF) to fibroblasts with epidermal cells by increasing the number of EGF receptors per cell (55). Enhancement of normal myelopoiesis and inhibition of myeloid leukemic cell proliferation by Retinoic acid suggest that 13-cis Retinoic acid, significantly less toxic in vivo than Retinoic acid, could be effective in the therapy of patients with myelodysplastic syndrome because of the possibility of prevention of progression to overt leukemia of these preleukemic patients for whom no other effective treatment is currently available.

In a phase I clinical study of nineteen patients with various myelodysplastic syndromes (including refractory anemias with or without excess of blasts and chronic myelomonocytic syndrome) receiving dose-limiting hepatotoxicity only at the 125 mg/m^2 level, the most common toxic manifestation was hyperkeratosis which was mild and easily alleviated (Gold et al., submitted). Of sixteen evaluable patients, three were considered to have achieved a partial response and three others showed improvement in one or more hematologic parameters. The ability to sustain chronic levels of Retinoic acid in patients with only minor toxicity suggests that this may be a valuable adjunct either to conventional chemotherapy or to additional forms of biological response modification. In this context, leukemia differentiation-inducing factor (GM-DF) produced by mitogen-stimulated human leukocytes acts synergistically with Retinoic acid in inducing maturation of the human leukemic lines U*-937 and HL-60 (86), and compounds elevating intracellular levels of cAMP, such as dibutryl cAMP, prostaglandin E, and choleratoxin, acted synergistically with Retinoic acid to induce maturation of both cells' lines. In contrast to the requirement for continuous presence of Retinoic acid for up to five days in order to achieve terminal differentiation of HL-60 cells, differentiation proteins or cAMP-elevating compounds are active on leukemic cells primed with Retinoic acid for only 8-16 h (86).

The active form of Vitamin D_3, 1 alpha, 25 dihydroxyvitamin D_3, and vitamin D analogues may also prove of clinical utility in inducing myeloid leukemic cell differentiation. Abe et al. (1) theorized that since the active form of vitamin D_3 causes multinucleate osteoclasts to appear in bone-resorbing surfaces and since osteoclasts are thought to be derived from monocytes and macrophages, then the murine myeloid leukemia cell line M1 would be a good model to test whether vitamin D can induce this cell line to differentiate into macrophages. The degree of leukemic cell differentiation induced by 12 nM of 1 alpha, 25-dihydroxyvitamin D_3 was comparable to that induced by 1 nM dexamethasone, the most potent known stimulator of M1 differentiation, and unlike the action of Retinoic acid, differentiation-induction included development of phagocytic ability receptor expression and locomotive activities. In addition, the vitamin markedly inhibited cell growth in a time-dependent manner; we have recently shown vitamin D_3 (dihydroxycholecalciferol) was also potent in inducing differentiation of the human promyelocytic cell line HL-60 and the murine myelomonocytic leukemic cell line WEHI-3. In both instances (Figs. 3 and 4), differentiation was observed to both neutrophils and macrophages and was associated with significant inhibition of leukemic cell cloning, and this was seen at vitamin concentrations of 0.01-0.1 ug/ml. Comparable dose of calciferol significantly enhanced normal myelopoiesis, synergizing with CSF and causing a 2 - 2.5 augmentation of colony numbers (Figs. 3 and 4). Myelopoietic stimulation by vitamin D in vitro has been reported by Salahuddin et al. (108), who described a method for the routine long-term growth (greater than three months) of normal immature human myeloid cells in liquid suspension culture. The technique employs cell-separated cord blood leukocytes and special growth conditions including hydrocortisone and an obligatory requirement for vitamin D. The augmentation of normal myelopoiesis and inhibition

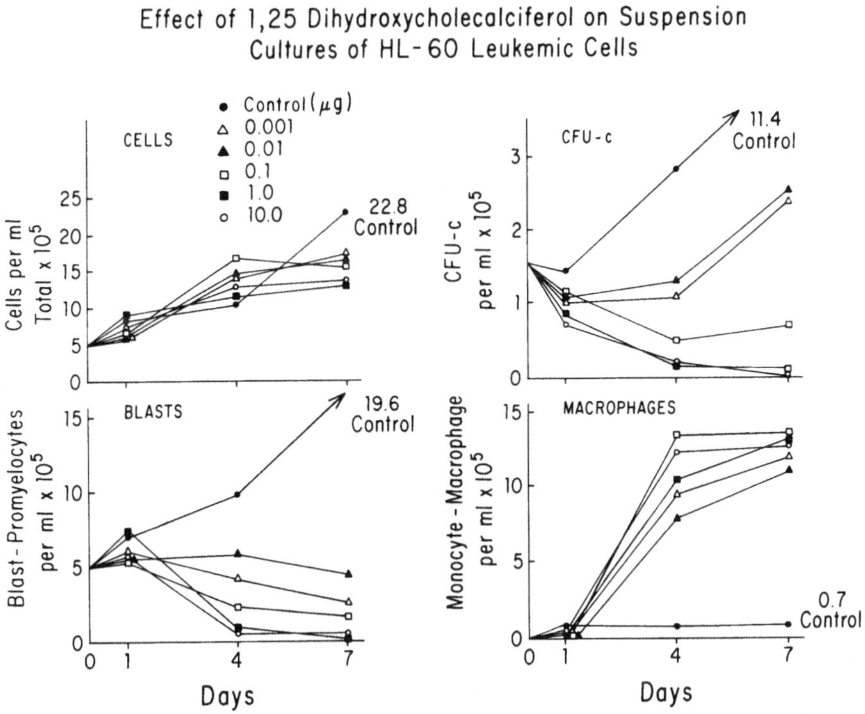

FIG. 3 - 10 ml suspension cultures of HL-60 D^+ leukemic cells at a concentration of 5 x 10^5 cells/ml were exposed to 0.001-10.0 μg of dihydroxycholecalciferol. At intervals of 1, 4, and 7 days cultures were assayed for recloning capacity in agar (CFU-c) and morphology.

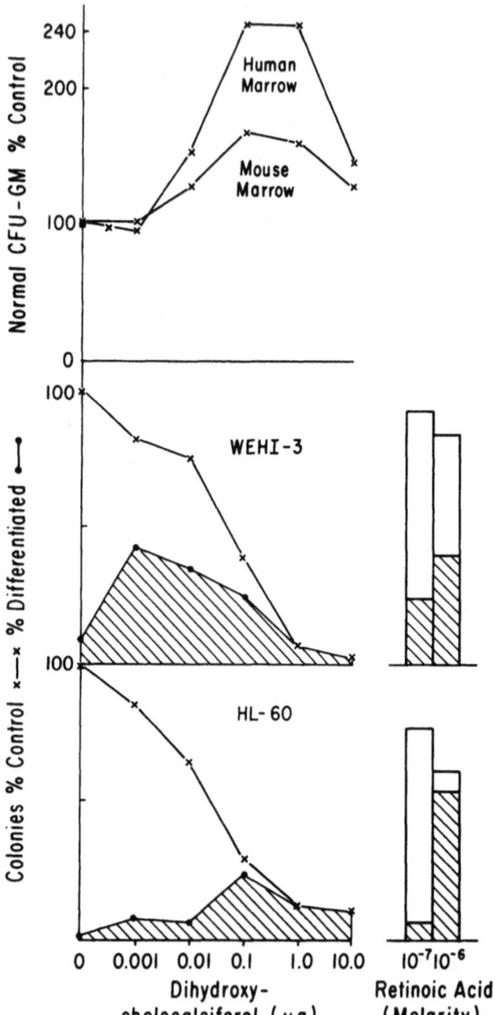

FIG. 4 - Influence of dihydroxycholecalciferol and 13-cis Retinoic acid in 1 ml agar cultures of a) 10^5 normal bone marrow stimulated by GCT-conditioned medium as a CSF source; b) 7.5 x 10^4 $B6D2F_1$ mouse bone marrow stimulated by L cell CM as a CSF source; c) 300 WEHI-3B(D^+) cells; d) 1000 HL-60 D^+ leukemic cells. Cultures were scored at 7-11 days for colony incidence and percent of diffuse/differentiated colonies (hatched areas).

of myeloid leukemic cell proliferation with induction of differentiation seen at comparable in vitro concentrations of vitamin D_3 suggest that in vivo studies may be warranted, particularly since calciferol induces differentiation of leukemic cells refractory to Retinoic acid (e.g., M1) and may have significantly fewer side effects at comparable dose levels.

T Cell-Mediated Regulation of Myeloid and Erythroid Progenitor Cell Proliferation

Control of hematopoietic cell proliferation. Analysis of the antigenic profiles of hematopoietic stem cells and their progeny indicates that human granulocyte-macrophage progenitor cells (CFU-GM), erythroid progenitor cells (BFU-e), and multipotential colony-forming cells (CFU-GEMM) express Ia-like HLA-DR antigen on their surface. The pattern of Ia-antigen expression on myeloid cells, their heterogenous expression on myeloid precursors (54, 78, 103), and their disappearance with progressive differentiation (54, 103, 126) suggest that these antigens are probably involved in the cellular interactions which regulate hemopoietic cell proliferation (78, 126). We have recently demonstrated that certain monoclonal mouse antihuman HLA-DR antibodies recognize normal CFU-GM, BFU-e, and CFU-GEMM preferentially during S-phase of the cell cycle and that Ia-antigen expression defines and characterizes a state of progenitor cell responsiveness to humoral regulation by prostaglandin E (PGE) and acidic isoferritins (AIF) (9, 67, 89). In support of this hypothesis we have shown that: a) in vitro human CFU-GM, BFU-e, and CFU-GEMM Ia-antigen expression is transient, being lost within 3-6 h at 37°C, and loss of antigen expression occurs coincident with loss of progenitor cell responsiveness to inhibition by prostaglandin E and acidic isoferritin (9, 67, 89); b) in patients with chronic myeloid leukemia (CML), CFU-GM Ia-antigen expression is absent or greatly diminished and correlates with hyporesponsiveness of leukemic colony-forming cells to normal growth inhibition (94, 95); c) a suspension preculture assay has been developed which demonstrates that prostaglandin E has the capacity to modulate CFU-GM, BFU-e, and CFU-GEMM responsiveness to regulatory control by prostaglandin E and acidic isoferritin as a consequence of modulation of Ia-antigen expression and cell cycle (89, 90); d) suspension preculture of CFU-GM from patients with CML with prostaglandin E results in the induction of a normal pattern of Ia-antigen expression on Philadelphia (PH1) chromosome-positive CFU-GM and their progeny and restoration of normal responsiveness of these CFU-GM to inhibition by prostaglandin E and acidic isoferritin in agar culture (95).

These studies provide evidence for a direct regulatory association between

Ia-antigen expression and control of myeloid progenitor cell differentiation and suggest a new role for prostaglandin E in the modulation of progenitor cell cycle, antigen expression, and growth regulation. For CFU-GM the mechanisms of action of prostaglandin E appears twofold: a) to induce differentiation of new Ia^{+} S-phase regulatory responsive CFU-GM from a noncycling, Ia^{-}H prostaglandin E and acidic isoferritin insensitive cell compartment; and b) to restore antigen expression to S-phase CFU-GM which have shed Ia-antigen (89, 90). The capacity of prostaglandin E to mediate these effects occurs in a plateau fashion between 10^{-6} to 10^{-10}M and to a lesser but significant degree at 10^{-12} to 10^{-14}M (89).

Cellular and humoral interactions in the control of hemopoietic cell proliferation. In a liquid preculture assay system it can be shown that prostaglandin E modulates Ia-antigen expression on CFU-GM, BFU-e, and CFU-GEMM. Prostaglandin E-induced Ia-antigen re-expression directly coincides with modulation (restoration) of progenitor cell responsiveness to inhibition by prostaglandin E and acidic isoferritin when these cells are subsequently cultured in semisolid matrix assay systems (89, 90, 94, 95). We have investigated cellular and humoral interactions in the regulation of CFU-GM, BFU-e, and CFU-GEMM proliferation particularly as they relate to cell cycle, modulation of Ia-antigen expression, and sensitivity to growth regulation. These studies indicate that T cells operate in regulatory networks which control the proliferation of CFU-GM and BFU-e. These networks are critical in the context of hemopoietic reconstitution following bone marrow transplantation and in the development of new methodologies to modify donor cells prior to transplantation particularly across HLA-DR barriers.

Modulation of CFU-GM cell cycle, Ia-antigen expression, and regulatory response by prostaglandin E in suspension culture requires marrow T lymphocytes. The capacity of prostaglandin E to modulate CFU-GM cell cycle, Ia-antigen expression, and regulatory sensitivity in suspension culture is dependent upon the presence of marrow T lymphocytes. Treatment of marrow cells with monoclonal anti-T lymphocyte antibodies indicates that the required cell has the phenotype: OKT3+, OKT4-, OKT8+, Leu 1+, Leu 4+, Leu 3a-, 3b-, Leu 2a+, 2b+, HLA-DR-, and Lyt3 (SRBC)+. This phenotype is consistent with a population of marrow T cytotoxic/ suppressor cells (Table 1). Removal of this population of cells by treatment with the appropriate cytotoxic antibody plus complement (C') or pulse exposure with antibody alone prevents the ability of prostaglandin E to mediate CFU-GM Ia-antigen expression and restoration of sensitivity to prostaglandin E and acidic isoferritin. Furthermore, the ability of prostaglandin E to augment the cycling rate of CFU-GM is also prevented by removal of marrow T cells (Table 2). In all cases, removal of T cells was without effect on primary cloning efficiency of CFU-GM tested prior to suspension culture.

TABLE 1 - Phenotypic analysis of T cell population required for PGE-mediated CFU-GM Ia-antigen re-expression.

Treatment prior to suspension culture	Present during suspension culture	CFU-GM (colonies + clusters)		
			% Inhibition	
		%Ia$^+$	+PGE(10^{-7}M)	+AIF(10^{-10}M)
C'	Media	0 ± 0	1 ± 1	2 ± 1
	+10^{-8}M PGE	41 ± 2	40 ± 1	41 ± 3
OKT4+C'	Media	4 ± 2	6 ± 3	6 ± 3
	+10^{-8}M PGE	39 ± 2	40 ± 2	43 ± 1
OKT8	Media	1 ± 2	3 ± 1	4 ± 1
	+10^{-8}M PGE	3 ± 1	4 ± 0	4 ± 1
OKT8+C'	Media	-1 ± 2	-1 ± 1	-1 ± 0
	+10^{-8}M PGE	1 ± 0	-3 ± 1	2 ± 0
Leu4	Media	0 ± 0	0 ± 1	0 ± 1
	+10^{-8}M PGE	2 ± 1	-3 ± 0	-2 ± 1
Leu4+C'	Media	2 ± 0	0 ± 0	0 ± 0
	+10^{-8}M PGE	-8 ± 2	3 ± 1	2 ± 1
Leu 2a	Media	3 ± 2	6 ± 1	2 ± 0
	+10^{-8}M PGE	1 ± 1	2 ± 1	0 ± 0
Leu 3a	Media	2 ± 1	2 ± 0	3 ± 1
	+10^{-8}M PGE	33 ± 3	32 ± 1	36 ± 2

- Prior to suspension culture: 38 ± 2% Ia$^+$; 37 ± 1% I-PGE; 36 ± 2% I-AIF.
- anti-Ia-antibody NEI-011 used at 1/100 final dilution.
- OKT4, OKT8 antibodies used at 1/100 final dilution.
- Leu4, Leu2a, Leu3a used at 1/50 final dilution.

TABLE 2 - The effect of PGE on cell cycle rate following OKT8+ cell depletion.

Treatment prior to suspension culture	Present during suspension culture	% CFU-GM in S-phase
Media	Media	46 ± 2%
	$+10^{-8}$M PGE_1	75 ± 3%
OKT8+C'	Media	51 ± 3%
	$+10^{-8}$M PGE_1	45 ± 3%

OKT8 antibody used at a final dilution of 1/100.

The ability of antibody alone to block the effects of prostaglandin E suggests a mechanism involving these receptors on the required T cell population. However, this effect prevents the use of these antibodies for positive cell selection. The anti-sheep erythrocyte antibody Lyt-3 in the presence of C' recognizes the required T lymphocyte population, but without C' does not block the effects of prostaglandin E. We have used this antibody positively to select total marrow T cells by affinity cell chromatography on plastic (panning). Following positive selection, the Lyt-3+ cells were pulsed with monoclonal antibodies which define T cell subsets prior to re-addition to T cell-depleted marrow populations. These studies confirmed the requirement for OKT8+ cells in prostaglandin E-mediated modulation of CFU-GM Ia-antigen expression and growth sensitivity.

The requirement for T8 cells in order to observe prostaglandin E-mediated modulation of CFU-GM Ia-antigen and growth sensitivity could be substituted by media conditioned by peripheral blood or marrow T cells. Conditioned media was prepared from positively selected blood and marrow T cells and added to T-depleted marrow cells during suspension preculture with and without prostaglandin E. Only media conditioned by OKT8+ cells interacted with prostaglandin E to mediate CFU-GM Ia-antigen re-expression and restoration of sensitivity to prostaglandin E and acidic isoferritin. This factor was found to be produced constitutively by marrow T8 cells, whereas peripheral blood T8 cells required mitogen activation. In all cases adherent cells were required for T cell production of this factor. Specificity analysis of this factor indicates that it is not IL-1,

IL-2, alpha or gamma interferon, or GM-CSF.

Biochemical purification of this factor from peripheral blood lymphocytes has proceeded using the purification schema for IL-2 (122). Briefly, peripheral blood-conditioned media was subjected to ammonium sulfate precipitation, DEAE ion exchange chromatography, gel filtration on ACA, and chromatography on blue agarose and red agarose. On red agarose, the activity was recovered in the 0.3M NaCl fraction and cleanly separated from the bulk of IL-2. The T8-derived factor appears to be a hydrophobic protein of MW = 12,000-14,000 daltons. On reverse-phase HPLC the activity was recovered in the 38-40% isopropanol fraction on a C:18 column. The HPLC data are preliminary and further purification is currently under way.

Augmentation of BFU-e proliferation. Involvement of Ia^+ BFU-e and a role for T lymphocytes. Several studies have shown that the addition of prostaglandin E to primary methycellulose cultures augments the total number of BFU-e which can be detected (5, 104). We now show that the ability of prostaglandin E to augment total BFU-e proliferation is restricted to a subpopulation of BFU-e which expresses HLA-DR antigen and is dependent upon T cells. Positive selection of T lymphocytes by rosetting with SRBC, treatment of selected cells with anti-Ia-antibody plus C', and re-addition to T-depleted marrow cells also treated with and without anti-Ia + C' indicate that T cells are required for prostaglandin E-mediated augmentation of BFU-e proliferation and that the effect of prostaglandin E is restricted to Ia^+ BFU-e and not mediated via an effect on Ia^+ T cells. Preliminary evidence indicates that the required T lymphocyte bears the OKT3+, OKT4-, OKT8 positive phenotype.

Hematopoietic Microenvironment

Characterization of human bone marrow fibroblast colony-forming cells (CFU-F) and their progeny. We have developed a liquid culture system to clone and to characterize human bone marrow fibroblast colony-forming cells (CFU-F). The linear relationship between the number of cells plated and the number of colonies formed suggests that fibroblast colonies originate in a single cell. Bone marrow CFU-F were adherent and non-phagocytic. The majority (90% ± 2%) were less dense than 1.070 g/ml. Velocity sedimentation separation demonstrated a heterogeneous CFU-F sedimentation rate, with a modal sedimentation of 4.95 ± 0.15 mm/hr. Analysis of CFU-F proliferative status by the thymidine suicide technique indicated that this cell was noncycling in individuals with undisturbed bone marrow function. Some of the more distinctive products of fibroblasts, other stromal cells, and hematopoietic colony-forming cells were used as positive and negative markers for CFU-F and the cells derived from them in vitro. Complement-mediated cytotoxicity using anti-Ia- and anti-factor-VIII-related antigen antisera did not inhibit fibroblast colony formation. Immunofluorescent staining was used to characterize the cells derived from CFU-F in vitro. No staining was observed after incubation of subconfluent cultures with anti-Ia- and anti-factor-VIII-related antigen antisera. A positive immunofluorescent staining was obtained when isolated antibodies against three of the main proteins of bone marrow matrix (type I collagen, type III collagen, and fibronectin) were used. Ultrastructural analysis showed that CFU-F progeny, in contrast to endothelial cells, did not contain Weibel-Palade bodies. These data support the conclusion that the colonies described in this study are of fibroblastic nature.

Reappraisal of the CFU-F assay: determination of optimal culture conditions. Although all the assays for CFU-F described in the literature consist of a liquid culture system with bovine serum as source of fibroblast growth factors, there have not been well standardized criteria for defining the concentration of serum, frequency of medium renewal, time of incubation, and colony size. Table 3 shows the results of a series of experiments in which one or more factors were modified in order to assess their effect on CFU-F growth. Alpha medium appeared to be the best medium for CFU-F culture. In contrast, alpha medium supplemented with nucleosides, McCoy's 5A medium, RPMI, and Medium 199 were less effective. Addition of 10^{-6}-10^{-7} hydrocortisone to marrow cells cultured in alpha medium and bovine serum resulted in lower fibroblast colony formation. A similar phenomenon occurred when the growth medium for long-term human bone marrow culture was employed. Comparison of bovine, horse, and human sera as source of fibroblast growth factors indicated that all of them support CFU-F growth, although bovine serum was the most effective. There were, however, differences between batches of calf sera. Inactivation of serum at 56°C for 30 min. generally did not increase or decrease CFU-F plating efficiency, although in some instances it could be enhanced. Dialysis of serum had no effect on CFU-F growth. Incubation of cultures at 33°C markedly decreased (60-80%) CFU-F colony formation. Addition of irradiated bone marrow cells to the cultures in alpha medium did not modify CFU-F plating efficiency. In conclusion, these data demonstrate that alpha medium and fetal calf serum, which are employed in our CFU-F assay, provide the optimal conditions for the clonal culture of bone marrow fibroblasts in a liquid system.

TABLE 3 - Factors affecting the human CFU-F assay.

Factor Tested	Number of Colonies (% control)	Factor Tested	Number of Colonies (% control)
A) Medium		D) Serum	
- α	100	- Bovine	100
- α + Ribonucleosides	97	- Horse	89
- α + 10^{-6}M Hydrocortisone	90	- Human	70
- α + 10^{-7}M Hydrocortisone	94		
- Gartner's	24	C) Serum Batch	
- McCoy's	26	- Batch I	100
- RPMI	37	- Batch II	50
- 199	34	- Batch III	102
		- Batch IV	137
B) Temperature		- Batch V	122
- 37°C	100		
- 33°C	10	D) Serum heat-inactivation and dialysis	
		- Non-heat-inactivated I	100
C) Feeder Cells		- Heat-inactivated I	68
- Irradiated cells alone	0	- Non-heat-inactivated II	100
- Cultures without feeder cells	100	- Heat-inactivated II	200
- Cultures with feeder cells	102	- Heat-inactivated & dialyzed II	252

Control cultures contained alpha medium supplemented with 20% heat-inactivated fetal calf serum. The growth medium was totally renewed at days 4 and 7. The cultures were ended at day 10. A colony is defined as a cell aggregate containing 40 cells or more. Results shown are from a representative experiment.

Characteristics of bone marrow fibroblast colony-forming cells (CFU-F) and their progeny in patients with myeloproliferative disorders. Chronic myeloproliferative disorders (MPD) are clonal diseases of the pluripotent hematopoietic stem cell frequently associated with myelofibrosis (MF). There is only indirect evidence indicating that the increased deposition of collagen in bone marrow matrix is a secondary phenomenon. A liquid culture system for cloning and growing bone marrow fibroblasts has permitted us to approach more directly the understanding of the pathogenesis of myelofibrosis by comparing the biophysical, growth, and functional characteristics of fibroblasts from normals, MPD patients without MF, and those with MF. In patients with MF, marrow fibroblast colony (CFU-F) formation could not be studied; fibroblasts were grown from marrow explants. CFU-F from normals and MPD patients exhibited similar cell density distribution and similar cell sedimentation rates. These similarities contrasted sharply with the differences seen when the erythroid and granulocyte-macrophage progenitors were studied by the same methods. There was a marked light density shift and a rapidly sedimenting shift of MPD hematopoietic colony-forming cells. Marrow fibroblasts from MPD patients with and without MF displayed the same in vitro growth characteristics as fibroblasts from normals. Both types of fibroblasts exhibited anchorage and serum dependence and contact inhibition of growth. Marrow fibroblasts were also characterized for the presence and distribution of fibronectin and collagen types by immunofluorescent staining using monospecific antibodies. Extracellular matrix, membrane-, and cytoplasm-associated fibronectin, type I, type III, and type V collagen showed a similar staining pattern in both normal and myelofibrotic marrow fibroblasts. Plasminogen-dependent fibrinolytic activity elicited from normal and myelofibrotic marrow fibroblasts were equivalent. Chromosomal analysis of hematopoietic cells and marrow fibroblasts from Philadelphia chromosome-positive chronic myelocytic leukemia patients with and without MF showed that the Philadelphia chromosome was present only in hematopoietic cells. These studies taken together demonstrate that bone marrow collagen-producing cells from MPD patients with and without MF behave in vitro as do those from normals. These findings support the hypothesis that the marrow fibrosis observed in patients with MPD results from a reactive process rather than from a primary disorder affecting the marrow collagen-producing cells.

Immunocytochemical identification of cells comprising the adherent layer of long-term human bone marrow cultures. Employing specific antibodies directed against components known to be associated with fibroblasts, endothelial cells, and the monocyte-macrophage system, we have analyzed by immunofluorescence (IMF) methods the identity and the distribution of the cells composing the adherent layer of long-term human marrow cultures. IMF studies were performed in situ on the bottom of culture flasks containing the adherent layer. IMF staining of membrane- and cytoplasm-associated components was performed using both the direct and the indirect method. Recognition and differentiation of cell types were done by using double labeling procedures with fluorescein and rhodamine conjugated antibodies. Analysis revealed that the adherent layer of long-term human marrow cultures was comprised of fibroblasts adipocytes, macrophages, and endothelial cells (Table 4). Fibroblasts formed a discontinuous monolayer over which laid macrophages and adipocytes. Macrophages were also found attached to the bottom of flasks.

Derivation of lipid-containing cells from monocytic and fibroblastic cells of human bone marrow. Lipid-containing cells (LCC) constitute an integral component of bone marrow. This stromal cell population includes two subtypes: the classical adipocytic cell derived from perisinal adventitial cells and the lipid-laden macrophages. The exact nature of LCC contained in the adherent layer of long-term human bone marrow cultures has not been defined. Adherent layers were established culturing normal bone marrow buffy coat cells in McCoy's 5A medium supplemented

TABLE 4 - Immunocytochemical identification of human bone marrow stromal cells in vitro.

	Endothelial Cells	Adipocytes	Fibroblasts	Macrophages
Factor VIII-antigen	+	-	-	-
Type IV Collagen	+	-	-	-
Type V Collagen	+	-	+	-
Laminin	+	-	-	-
Fibronectin	+	-	+	±
Type I Collagen	-	-	+	-
Type III Collagen	-	-	+	-
Lysozyme	-	-	-	+
Monocyte 1	-	-	-	+
Monocyte 2	-	-	-	+
Ia-Antigen	-	-	-	+

with horse serum (HoS), fetal calf serum (FCS), and 10^{-6}M hydrocortisone at 33°C. Oil Red-0 was used to evaluate lipid accumulation. At early stages of cultivation some mononuclear cells of the adherent layer showed some evidence of lipid accumulation. Subsequently, these cells progressively enlarged. However, with fibroblast overgrowth, only a few of such cells remained within or over the adherent layer. Electron microscopy showed that the lipid inclusions of these cells were of small and medium size. The monocytic nature of these cells was demonstrated by their staining with an anti-lysozyme, anti-Ia-antigen, and two monoclonal antibodies recognizing monocytes. When confluency was reached, a different type of LCC developed. At late stages of cultivation these cells were numerous and had few large-size lipid inclusions which almost completely occupied the cytoplasm. The latter LCC originated from cells having the morphological and antigenic characteristics of fibroblasts, as demonstrated by their staining with anti-type III collagen. Nevertheless, only a small proportion of fibroblastic cells had the capacity to undergo adipocyte conversion. This phenomenon was dependent on the presence of hydrocortisone in the culture medium as well as confluence and serum factors. Withdrawal of hydrocortisone resulted in lack of adipocyte conversion. In conclusion, we demonstrate here that two types of LCC can be derived from human bone marrow cells, one derived from cells exhibiting phenotypic characteristics of fibroblasts (adipocytes) and another from cells of the monocyte-macrophage system (MD-LCC).

In vitro culture of human monocyte-derived lipid-containing cells (MDLCC). The purpose of this work was to define the conditions for culturing MDLCC and to analyze the morphological, cytochemical, ultrastructural, antigenic, and functional changes occurring in these cells during their in vitro culture. Adherent low-density cells from normal bone marrow and peripheral blood were used as a source of monocytes. When marrow cells were used, fibroblasts were removed from the adherent layer by trypsinization. Lipid accumulation was monitored by staining with Oil Red-0. The culture conditions tested included several combinations of media, sera, and other supplements. Alpha medium supplemented with horse serum provided the best culture conditions. Horse serum at 20% final concentration was the best inducer of lipid accumulation (4+), followed by human serum (2 to 3+), and the combination of horse and fetal calf serum (2+). In the presence of horse serum, alpha medium (4+) was better than RPMI 1640 (2 to 3+) or McCoy's 5A medium (2+). Incubation at 37°C gave much better results than incubation at 33°C. Addition of insulin (1-10 ug/ml) or hydrocortisone (10^{-6}M) did not improve the adipogenic ability of horse serum. Sequential analysis of monocytic cells cultured in alpha medium 20% horse serum at 37°C revealed a series of changes. The cell size enlarged progressively up to 7-8 times (at day 21-28) the size at day 1 of culture. This change was associated with an increase in small and medium-size lipid granules, as well as acid phosphatase and nonspecific esterase activity. The number of lipid granules as shown by ultrastructural analysis was minimal at day 1 but subsequently increased, occupying a large part of cytoplasm by day 21. Concomitantly, there was an increase in the number of mitochondria, lysosomes, Golgi apparatus, and the RER. Moreover, the expression per cell of Fc receptors, Ia-antigens, and antigens recognized by monoclonal antibodies Mac 1 and Mac 2 was also increased. To evaluate the functional capacity of MDLCC, stimulatory and inhibitory activities for CFU-GM were assessed in culture supernatants. GM-CSA was detected during the first days of culture, declining rapidly later. In contrast, the activity of a factor (s) that enhanced the colony formation capacity of GM-CSA progressively increased.

GM-CSA-enhancing activity production by human monocyte-derived lipid-containing cells (MDLCC). This study was designed to investigate whether MDLCC exert any regulatory influence on hematopoiesis, particularly on the proliferation and differentiation of granulocyte-macrophage progenitors (CFU-GM). Alpha medium supplemented with 20% horse serum was conditioned for two days by MDLCC (MDLCC-CM) at several stages of cultivation. To test the effect on CFU-GM, MDLCC-CM was added to soft agar culture of normal nonadherent low-density human bone marrow cells containing unconditioned medium or GCT-conditioned medium as a source of GM-CSA. In the early stages of cultivation, GM-CSA could be detected in the MDLCC-CM, but it rapidly declined to undetectable levels at day 14. In contrast, an activity that enhanced the colony formation capacity of GCT-CM progressively increased reaching peak values at day 12-28. Subsequent experiments were done using day 21 CM, which had no detectable GM-CSA. The enhancing effect was noted on both day 7 and day 14 CFU-GM. The percent enhancement ranged from 50 to 150 with an average of 80 ± 5 ($x \pm$ sem). The same degree of enhancement was demonstrated by counting the total cell number per dish in similar cultures using methyl-cellulose instead of agar. Neither the enhancing activity nor its production were dependent on serum. Serum-free MDLCC-CM enhanced CFU-GM colony formation in a similar manner to serum-containing CM. MDLCC-CM enhanced colony formation by both granulocyte and monocyte progenitors; the distribution of granulocytic, monocytic, and mixed colonies was similar in CFU-GM cultures with and without MDLCC-CM. The enhancing effect was also seen when other sources of GM-CSA were used: medium conditioned by 5637 cell line, PHA-stimulated lymphocytes, and placental tissue. The enhancing activity contained in MDLCC-CM was heat-resistant (56°C and 75°C for 30 min.) and undialyzable (3,500 and 14,000 M.W. cutoff tubing). Furthermore, this enhancing activity appeared to be specific for CFU-GM; addition of MDLCC-CM to erythroid cultures (BFU-e) did not modify the number of erythroid bursts.

Studies on the hematopoietic microenvironment in acute leukemia. Previous studies have shown that acute leukemia (AL) is associated with quantitative and qualitative abnormalities of marrow microenvironmental cells (MMC). We report here our studies in 51 AL patients, 37 ALL, and 14 ANLL, using the marrow fibroblast colony-forming cell assay (CFU-F), the long-term marrow culture assay, and co-cultures of heterogeneous adherent layers (HAL) and fibroblasts derived from AL marrow with normal hemopoietic cells. The frequency of CFU-F in newly diagnosed patients was markedly decreased as compared to normals. During induction therapy there was an increase in CFU-F numbers. This increase was even higher during remission, particularly in patients off therapy. The frequency of CFU-F was inversely correlated with marrow cellularity, marrow blasts, and leukocyte counts. Cell extracts or medium conditioned by leukemic cells did not modify the plating efficiency of CFU-F from normal marrow. Long-term culture of AL marrows resulted, in the majority of patients, in the establishment of an HAL containing fibroblasts, adipocytes, endothelial cells, and few macrophages, as defined by immunocytochemical analysis. It was, however, necessary to inoculate a higher number of cells. There was a close correlation between the frequency of CFU-F and the number of cells required for establishing an HAL. Marrows with the lowest CFU-F frequency were unable to originate an HAL. Co-cultivation of passaged AL marrow fibroblasts with nonadherent low-density normal marrow cells in a liquid system demonstrated that AL marrow fibroblasts were capable of maintaining granulo-monopoiesis in vitro as normal fibroblasts did. Similar results were seen in two experiments in which normal hematopoietic cells were co-cultured with HAL derived from AL marrow. In conclusion, these studies show that the low frequency of CFU-F and other MMC in AL is due to a mere dilutional effect resulting from leukemic marrow infiltration. The relative increase of CFU-F frequency during induction therapy suggests that MMC, in contrast to hematopoietic and leukemic cells, are less sensitive to chemotherapy. No functional abnormalities of MMC could be shown by co-culturing AL MMC with normal marrow cells.

CONCLUSION

Significant advances in the therapy of ANLL have occurred over the past two decades. Thus, the frequency of complete clinical remission of these diseases by chemotherapy has exceeded 50%. Despite this improvement, further advances in the rate of remission induction have been slow and the duration of remission for the average patient has not been significantly improved. These clinical findings have prompted the consideration of alternative chemotherapeutic approaches to the treatment of leukemia. One possibility would be a therapy based on the induction of differentiation of the leukemia cells to end-stage forms that are no longer capable of division alone or in combination with marrow transplantation. For patients with ANLL transplanted in late remission or relapse, leukemic relapse post-transplantation remains a dominant problem. Thus of 29 patients transplanted for ANLL in tertiary remission or relapse, 14 patients died early of infectious complications, and of 15 patients surviving, 11 ultimately relapsed with their diseases. Including ALL in tertiary or greater remission or relapse in relatively chemotherapy refractory patients, recurrence of disease is in excess of 60%. Thus, better antileukemic approaches must be devised to address the problem of leukemic relapse in these high-risk patient groups.

The induction of leukemic cells to mature cells with little or no proliferative potential may represent an effective alternative or adjunct to a cytoreductive therapeutic modality. The dosages of agents employed as inducers of differentiation are probably lower than required for an effective cytoreductive therapy and may well synergize or complement the action of more conventional agents. Anthrocyclines have a major role in treatment of acute leukemias and lymphomas and have proven to be potent inducers of differentiation of HL-60 leukemic cells in vitro (110) and in vivo (111). Differences in the ability of various compounds to induce differentiation of myeloid leukemia cell lines or primary human myeloid leukemia can be detected in vitro. This may also apply to the effectiveness of various compounds in inducing differentiation of leukemic cells from different leukemic patients, either individually or in combination with other agents. Actinomycin-D (52) has proved to be a particularly effective agent in induction of myeloid leukemic cell differentiation and, at low concentrations, sensitizes "undifferentiated" leukemic cells to the differentiation-inducing action of various biological-response modifiers (52).

REFERENCES

(1) Abe, E.; Miyaura, C.; Sakagami, H.; Takeda, M.; Konno, K.; Yamazaki, T.; Yoshiki, S.; and Suda, T. 1981. Proc. Natl. Acad. Sci. USA 78(8): 4990-4994.

(2) Akagawa, K.S., and Tokunaga, T. 1980. Microbiol. Immunol. 24(10): 1005-1101.

(3) Allen, T.D. 1978. In Lord, The Second Symposium of the British Society for Cell Biology on Stem Cells and Tissue Homeostasis, eds. C. Potten and D. Cole, pp. 217-240. Cambridge, England: Cambridge University Press.

(4) Anderson, L.C.; Nilsson, K.; and Gahmberg, C.G. 1979. Intl. J. Cancer 23: 143.

(5) Arce, J.M.; Naughton, B.A.; Kolks, G.A.; et al. 1981. Prostaglandin 21: 367-377.

(6) Bernstein, S.E. 1970. Am. J. Surgery 119: 448-451.

(7) Bodel, P. 1978. J. Exp. Med. 147: 1503.

(8) Breitman, T.R.; Selonick, S.E.; Keene, B.R.; Richardson, E.; and Collins, S.J. 1980. Proc. Natl. Acad. Sci. USA 77: 2936-2940.

(9) Broxmeyer, H.E.; Grossbard, E.; Jacobsen, N.; and Moore, M.A.S. 1979. N. Engl. J. Med. 301: 346-351.

(10) Broxmeyer, H., and Ralph, P. 1977. Cancer Res. 37: 3578.

(11) Buick, R.N.; Till, J.E.; and McCulloch, E.A. 1977. Lancet 1: 862.

(12) Burgess, A.W., and Metcalf, D. 1980. Blood 56: 947.

(13) Castro-Malaspina, H.; Ebell, W.; and Wang, S.Y. 1984. Human Bone Marrow Fibroblast Colony-Forming Units (CFU-F). In Myelofibrosis and the Biology of Connective Tissue, eds. P. Berk and H. Castro-Malaspina, pp. 209-236. New York: Alan Liss, Inc.

(14) Castro-Malaspina, H.; Gay, R.E.; Jhanwar, S.C.; Hamilton, J.A.; Chiarieri, D.R.; Meyers, P.A.; Gay, S.; and Moore, M.A.S. 1982. Blood 59: 1046-1054.

(15) Castro-Malaspina, H.; Gay, R.E.; Resnick, G.; Kapoor, N.; Meyers, P.; Chiarieri, D.; McKenzie, S.; Broxmeyer, H.E., and Moore, M.A.S.

1980. Blood 59: 289-301.

(16) Collins, S.J.; Gallo, R.C.; and Gallagher, R.E. 1977. Nature 207: 347.

(17) Collins, S.J.; Ruscetti, F.W.; Gallagher, R.E.; and Gallo, R.C. 1979. J. Exp. Med. 149: 969.

(18) Creusot, F.; Schneiderman, N.; Herzog, D.; Acs, G.; and Christman, J.K. 1982. Biol. Cell 45(2): 96.

(19) Delmonte, L.; O'Reilly, R.J.; and Kirkpatrick, D. 1982. Transplantation 34: 100-103.

(20) Dexter, T.M.; Allen, T.D.; and Lajtha, L.G. 1977. J. Cell Physiol. 91: 335-344.

(21) Dexter, T.M., and Moore, M.A.S. 1977. Nature 269: 412-414.

(22) Dexter, T.M., and Testa, M.G. 1976. Methods in Cell Biology, ed. D.M. Prescott, vol. 14, pp. 387-405. New York: Academic Press.

(23) Dinsmore, R.E.; Strauss, D.J.; Pollock, M.S.; Garret, T.J.; Young, C.W.; Clarkson, B.D.; and Dupont, B. 1980. Blood 55: 831-834.

(24) Douer, D., and Koeffler, H.P. 1982. J. Clin. Invest. 69(2): 277-283.

(25) Douer, D., and Koeffler, H.P. 1982. Exp. Cell Res. 138: 193-197.

(26) Egorin, M.; Fox, B.; Spiegel, J.; Gutierrez, P.; Friedman, R.; and Bachur, N. 1982. Am. Ass. Cancer Res. Abstract 696.

(27) Elias, L.; Wogenrich, F.J.; Wallace, J.M.; and Longmire, J. 1980. Leuk. Res. 4(3): 301-303, 305-307.

(28) Falk, A., and Sachs, L. 1980. It. J. Cancer 26: 595-601.

(29) Fauser, A.A.; Kanz, L.; and Katz, R. 1982. Blood 60(Suppl.1): 144a.

(30) Fauser, A.A., and Messner, H.A. 1978. Blood 52: 1243.

(31) Fauser, A.A., and Messner, H.A. 1979. Blood 53: 1023.

(32) Fauser, A.A.; Neumann, H.A.; Bross, K.G.; et al. 1982. Blood 60: 1317.

(33) Fibach, E.; Hayashi, M.; and Sachs, L. 1973. Proc. Natl. Acad. Sci. USA 70: 343-346.

(34) Fogh, J. 1977. Natl. Cancer Inst. 58: 209-214.

(35) Fogh, J.; Trempe, L.; and Fogh, H., eds. 1975. New York: Plenum Press.

(36) Folkman, J., and Haudenschild, C.C. 1982. In Pathobiology of the Endothelial Cell, eds. H.L. Nossel and H.J. Vogel, pp. 79-93. New York: Academic Press.

(37) Folkman, J.; Haudenschild, C.C.; and Zetter, B.R. 1979. Proc. Natl. Acad. Sci USA 76: 5217-5221.

(38) Friedenstein, A.J.; Ivanov-Smolenski, A.A.; Chajlakjan, R.K.; Gorskaya, U.F.; Kuralesova, A.I.; Latzinik, N.W.; and Gerasimow, U.W. 1978. Exp. Hematol. 6: 440-444.

(39) Friend, C.; Scher, W.; Holland, J.G.; and Sato, T. 1971. Proc. Natl. Acad. Sci. USA 68: 378-383.

(40) Gallagher, R.; Collins, S.; Trujillo, J.; McCreedie, K.; Ahern, M.; Tsai, S.; Metzgar, R.; Aulakh, G.; Ting, R.; Ruscetti, F.; and Gallor, R. 1979. Blood 54: 713-720.

(41) Gallo, R.C.; Breitman, T.R.; and Ruscetti, F.W. 1982. In Maturation Factors in Cancer, ed. M.A.S. Moore, pp. 255-271. New York: Raven Press.

(42) Gartner, S., and Kaplan, H.S. 1980. Proc. Natl. Acad. Sci. USA 77: 4756-4759.

(43) Gatti, R.A.; Meuwissen, H.J.; Allen, H.D.; Hong, R.; and Good, R.A. 1968. Lancet 2: 1366-1369.

(44) Golde, D.W.; Hocking, W.G.; Quan, S.G.; Sparkes, R.S.; and Gale, R.P. 1980. Brit. J. Haemat. 44: 183-187.

(45) Goldman, R.; Faccninetti, T.; Bach, D.; Raz, A.; and Shinitsky, N. 1978. Biochim. Biophys. Acta 512: 254.

(46) Hayashi, M.; Okabe, J.; and Hozumi, M. 1979. Gann 70(2): 235-238.

(47) Nidekazu, N.; Kazuhisa, T.; Miyano, K.; Yamane, T.; and Sato, J. 1982. Cancer Res. 42: 3858-3863.

(48) Hirano, T.; Kuritani, T.; Kishimoto, T.; and Yamamura, Y. 1977. J. Immunol. 119: 1235-1241.

(49) Hong, R.; Gatti, R.A.; and Good, R.A. 1968. Lancet 2: 288-389.

(50) Honma, Y.; Takenaga, K.; Kasukabe, T.; and Hozumi, M. 1981. Biochem. Biophys. Res., Comm. 95: 507-512.

(51) Housset, M.; Daniel, M.T.; and Degos, L. 1982. Brit. J. Haemat. 51: 125-129.

(52) Hozumi, M. 1982. In Cancer Biology Reviews, eds. J.J. Marchalonis, M.G. Hanna, and I.J. Fiedler, vol. 3, p. 153. New York: Marcel Dekker.

(53) Hozumi, M. 1983. Adv. Cancer Res. 38: 121.

(54) Janassy, G.; Francis, G.E.; Capillano, D.; Goldstone, A.H.; and Greaves, M.F. 1978. Nature 276: 176-178.

(55) Jetten, A.M. 1981. Ann. NY Acad. Sci. 119: 200-217.

(56) Johnson, R.; et al. 1979. Int. J. Rad. Oncol. Biol. Phys. 5: 1605.

(57) Kapoor, N.; Kirkpatrick, D.; Blaese, R.M.; Oleske, J.; Hilgartner, M.H.; Chaganti, R.S.K.; Good, R.A.; and O'Reilly, R.J. 1981. Blood 57: 692-696.

(58) Keating, A.; Singer, J.W.; Killen, P.D.; Striker, G.E.; Salo, A.C.; Sanders, J.; Thomas, E.D.; Torning, D.; and Fialkow, P.J. 1982. Nature 298: 280-283.

(59) Kessel, D. 1979. Mol. Pharmacol. 16: 306.

(60) Koeffler, H.P., and Golde, D.W. 1978. Science 200: 1153.

(61) Kraft, N.; Bradley, R.; Becker, G.; and Atkins, R.C. 1980. 4th International Congress on Immunology, vol. 11, pp. 1-14.

(62) Kubanek, B.; Heit, W.; and Rich, I.N. 1981. Exp. Hematol. 9(Suppl.): 59.

(63) Kurland, J.I.; Pelus, L.M.; Ralph, P.; Bockman, R.S.; and Moore, M.A.S. 1979. Proc. Natl. Acad. Sci. USA 76: 2326.

(64) Lachman, L.B.; Hocker, M.P.; Blyden, G.T.; and Handschumacher, T. 1977. Cell Immunol. 34: 416-419.

(65) Lambertsen, R.H., and Weiss, L. 1983. Am. J. Anat. 166: 369-392.

(66) Lotem, J.; Lipton, J.H.; and Sachs, L. 1980. Intl. J. Cancer 25: 763-771.

(67) Lu, L.; Broxmeyer, H.E.; Meyers, P.A.; and Moore, M.A.S. 1983. Blood 61: 250-256.

(68) Maeda, M.; Horiuchi, M.; Numa, S.; and Ichikawa, Y. 1977. Gann 68: 435-447.

(69) Maciag, T.; Cerumdolo, J.; Ilsley, S.; Kelley, P.R.; and Forand, R. 1979. Proc. Natl. Acad. Sci. USA 76: 5674-5678.

(70) Messner, J.A.; Izaguirre, C.A.; and Jamal, N. 1981. Blood 58: 402.

(71) Metcalf, D. 1979. Intl. J. Cancer 24(5): 616-623.

(72) Metcalf, D. 1980. Intl. J. Cancer 25: 225-233.

(73) Metcalf, D. 1982. J. Cell Physiol. 1(Suppl.): 175-183.

(74) Metcalf, D., and Moore, M.A.S. 1970. J. Natl. Cancer Inst. 44: 801.

(75) Metcalf, D.; Moore, M.A.S.; and Warner, N. 1969. Natl. Cancer Inst. 43: 983-1001.

(76) Metcalf, D.; Parker, J.; Chester, H.M.; and Kincade, P.W. 1974. J. Cell Physiol. 84: 275.

(77) Mittwoch, V. 1974. In Human Chromosome Methodology, ed. J.J. Yunis, pp. 73-93. New York: Academic Press.

(78) Moore, M.A.S.; Broxmeyer, H.E.; Sheridan, A.P.C.; Jacobsen, N.; and Winchester, R.J. 1980. Blood 55: 682-690.

(79) Moore, M.A.S., and Sheridan, A.P.C. 1979. Blood Cells 5: 297-311.

(80) Moore, M.A.S., and Sheridan, A.P.C. 1982. In Maturation Factors in Cancer, ed. M.A.S. Moore, pp. 361-376. New York: Raven Press.

(81) Moore, M.A.S.; Spitzer, G.; Williams, N.; Metcalf, D.; and Buckley, J. 1974. Blood 44: 1-11.

(82) Nagata, K.; Ooguro, K.; Saito, M.; Kuboyama, M.; and Ogasa, K. 1977. Gann 68(6): 757-764.

(83) Nicola, N.A.; Burgess, W.W.; and Metcalf, D. 1979. J. Biol. Chem. 254: 5290.

(84) Nicola, N.A., and Metcalf, D. 1981. J. Cell. Physiol. 109(2): 253-264.

(85) Olsson, I., and Olofsson, T. 1981. Exp. Cell Res. 131: 225-230.

(86) Olsson, I.; Olofsson, T.; and Mauritzon, N. 1981. J. Nat. C.I. 67: 1225-1230.

(87) O'Reilly, R.J.; Dupont, B.; Pahwah, S.; Gaines, E.; Smithwick, E.M.; Pawah, R.; Schwartz, S.; Hansen, J.A.; Siegal, F.P.; Sorell, M.; Svegaard, A.; Jersild, C.; Thompsen, M.; Platz, P.; L'Esperance, P.; and Good, R.A. 1977. N. Engl. J. Med. 297: 1131-1318.

(88) Paige, C.J.; Kincade, P.W.; and Ralph, P. 1978. J. Immunol. 121: 641.

(89) Pelus, L.M. 1982. J. Clin. Invest. 20: 568.

(90) Pelus, L.M. 1983. Exp. Hematol. 10: 219-231.

(91) Pelus, L.M.; Broxmeyer, H.E.; Clarkson, B.D.; and Moore, M.A.S. 1980a. Cancer Res. 40: 2512.

(92) Pelus, L.M.; Broxmeyer, H.E.; Clarkson, B.D.; and Moore, M.A.S. 1980b. Cancer Res. 40: 2523.

(93) Pelus L.M.; Broxmeyer, H.E.; DeSouse, M.; and Moore, M.A.S. 1981. J. Immunol. 126: 1016.

(94) Pelus, L.M.; Gold, E.; Salenta, S.; and Coleman, M. 1983. Blood 62: 158-165.

(95) Pelus, L.M.; Saletan, S.; Silver, R.; and Moore, M.A.S. 1982. Blood 59: 284.

(96) Perussia, B.; Lebman, D.; Ip, S.H.; Rovera, G.; and Trinchieri, G. 1981. Blood 58(4): 836-843.

(97) Pollack, M.S.; Mauer, D.; Callaway, C.; and Mattes, M.J. 1983. In Topics in Histocompatibility, eds. E.R. Heise and J.A. Hansen. Am. Assoc. Clin. Histocomp. 3: 37-50.

(98) Pollack, M.S.; Mauer, D.; Levine, L.S.; New, M.I.; Pang, S.; Duchon, M.A.; Owens, R.P.; Merkatz, I.R.; Nitowsky, H.M.; Sachs, G.; and Dupont, B. 1979. Transplantation Proc. 11(4): 1726-1728.

(99) Ralph, P.; Broxmeyer, H.E.; Moore, M.A.S.; and Nakoinz, I. 1978. Cancer Res. 38: 1414-1419.

(100) Ralph, P.; Moore, M.A.S.; and Nilsson, K.J. 1976. Exp. Med. 143: 1528-1533.

(101) Ralph, P.; Punjabi, C.J.; Welte, K.; Litcofsky, P.B.; Ho, M.K.; Moore, M.A.S.; and Springer, T.A. 1983. Blood 62: 1169-1175.

(102) Ralph, P.; Williams, N.; Moore, M.A.S.; and Litcofsky, P.B. 1982. Cell Immunol. 71: 215-223.

(103) Robinson, J.; Lieff, D.; Delia, D.; Edwards, P.A.W.; and Greaves, M. 1981. Nature 289: 68-71.

(104) Rossi, G.B.; Migliaccio, A.R.; Migliaccio, G.; et al. 1980. Blood 56: 74-79.

(105) Rovera, G.; O'Brien, T.G.; and Diamond, L. 1979. Science 204: 868.

(106) Rubin, P.; Landman, S.; Mayer, E.; Keller, B.; and Ciccio, S. 1973. Cancer 32: 699.

(107) Sachs, L. 1978. Nature 274: 535-539.

(108) Salahuddin, S.Z.; Markham, P.D.; Ruscetti, F.W.; and Gallo, R.C. 1981. Blood 58(5): 931-937.

(109) Schaeffer, W.I. 1979. In Vitro 15: 649-653.

(110) Schwartz, E.; Brown, A.; Nierenburg, M.; Marsh, T.; and Sartorelli, A. 1982. Proc. Am. Assoc. Cancer Res. 23: 173.

(111) Schwartz, E., and Sartorelli, A. 1982. Cancer Res. 42: 2651.

(112) Springer, T.G.; Galfre, D.S.; Secher, S.; and Milstein, C. 1979. Eur. J. Immunol. 9: 301.

(113) Takeda, K.; Minowada, J.; and Bloch, A. 1982. Cancer Res. 42: 5152.

(114) Takenaga, K.; Honma, Y.; and Hozumi, M. 1981. Cancer Lett.

13: 1.

(115) Trentin, J.J. 1976. In Stem Cells of Renewing Cell Populations, ed. D.G. Osmond, pp. 255-264. New York, London: Academic Press.

(116) Trentin, J.J. 1980. In Regulation of Hematopoiesis, ed. A.S. Gordon, vol. 1, pp. 161-168. New York: Appleton-Century-Crofts.

(117) Tsuchita, S.; Yamabe, M.; Yamaguchi, Y.; Kobayashi, Y.; Konno, T.; and Tada, K. 1980. Intl. J. Cancer 26: 171.

(118) Uchida, I.A., and Lin, C.C. 1974. In Human Chromosome Methodology, ed. J.J. Yunis, pp. 47-58. New York: Academic Press.

(119) Warner, N.; Moore, M.A.S.; and Metcalf, D. 1969. J. Natl. Cancer Inst. 43: 963.

(120) Weiden, P.L.; Zuckerman, N.; Hansen, J.A.; Sale, G.E.; Remlinger, K.; Beck, T.M.; and Buckner, C.D. 1981. Blood 57: 328-332.

(121) Weiss, B., and Sachs, L. 1978. Proc. Natl. Acad. Sci. USA 75(3): 1374-1378.

(122) Welte, K.; Wang, C.Y.; Mertelsmann, R.; et al. 1982. J. Exp. Med. 156: 454.

(123) Williams, N.; Eger, R.R.; Moore, M.A.S.; and Mendelsohn, N. 1978. Differentiation 11: 59.

(124) Williams, N.; Jackson, H.; Ralph, P.; and Nakoinz, I. 1981. Blood 57: 157-163.

(125) Wilson, F.D.; Greenberg, B.R.; Konrad, P.N.; Klein, A.K.; and Walling, P.A. 1978. Transplantation 25: 87-88.

(126) Winchester, R.J.; Ross, G.D.; Jarowski, C.I.; Wang, C.Y.; Halper, J.; and Broxmeyer, H.E. 1977. Proc. Natl. Acad. Sci. USA 74: 4012-4016.

(127) Yamamoto, Y.; Tomida, M.; Hozumi, M.; Ayusawa, D.; Seno, T.; and Tamura, G. 1981. Cancer Res. 41(6): 2534-2539.

(128) Yung, Y.; Eger, G.; Tertian, G.; and Moore, M.A.S. 1981. J. Immunol. 127: 794.

Leukemia, ed. I.L. Weissman, pp. 69-82. Dahlem Konferenzen 1985. Berlin, Heidelberg, New York, Tokyo: Springer-Verlag.

Induction of B Cell Proliferation and Differentiation

W.E. Paul
Laboratory of Immunology, NIAID, National Institutes of Health
Bethesda, MD 20205, USA

Abstract. B lymphocyte activation, growth, and differentiation is an ordered process controlled by distinct stimuli acting at each step. Activation of resting B cells can be achieved by suitable cross-linkage of membrane receptors, by cognate interaction with helper T cells, and through nonspecific T cell-derived activating stimuli. Activated B cells will proliferate under the influence of growth factors, of which the best characterized is the B cell growth factor BSF-p1. The differentiation of such cells into cells capable of secreting immunoglobulin is controlled by a set of differentiation factors or "T cell replacing factors." Efforts to purify the various factors, to understand their mode of action, and to isolate their receptors will be a major theme of research on B cells during the next several years.

INTRODUCTION

B cells, one of the two major types of lymphocytes, are responsible for the secretion of antibodies, a key element in protective immune responses. An understanding of the stimuli which cause the activation, proliferation, and differentiation of B cells is critical to the delineation of the normal regulation of immunity. This is particularly so because physiologic immune responses depend upon the clonal expansion and differentiation into an immunoglobulin (Ig) secretory state of cells, initially present as a very small fraction of the total population, which bear receptors complementary to a foreign antigen. Furthermore, the normal regulatory events operating on this highly diverse family of cells must be understood as a prelude to considering the processes involved in the leukemic transformation of members of the B cell population. In this regard, it will be useful first to review the types of heterogeneity which are a feature of physiologic populations of B cells.

There are three distinct forms of heterogeneity which apply to B cells. These are: a) A heterogeneity based on developmental state. The B cell lineage(s) includes pre-B cells, immature B cells, mature B cells, and immunoglobulin-secreting cells. Furthermore, B cells appear to exist in two major subdivisions, $Lyb5^-$ and $Lyb5^+$ cells, which may represent distinct developmental lineages. b) A heterogeneity based on state of activation. B cells may be found in a resting state, as activated (G_1) cells, as cells undergoing proliferation, and as cells in various stages of differentiation to immunoglobulin secretion. c) A heterogeneity based on the structure and specificity of the membrane Ig (mIg) which acts as the antigen-binding receptors of these cells.

This high degree of diversity introduces serious complexities into efforts to analyze "cleanly" the steps in the response program of B cells. No entirely satisfactory resolution of this difficulty has been obtained, but several simplifying approaches have been employed which have led to important insights into the process of activation.

Among these approaches are: a) The separation of B cells according to their density and/or size; small, dense B cells are very highly enriched for resting (G_0) B cells and thus constitute a good cell population with which to examine early activation requirements. b) The use of activation systems which act on virtually all B cells in a population (i.e., anti-Ig antibodies, histocompatibility-restricted T cells, mitogenic lectins). c) The use of measurements such as entry into G_1 and S phases of the cell cycle and the enumeration of all Ig-secreting cells. These approaches, although valuable, have the disadvantage that they do not employ a normal "physiologic" stimulus (i.e., antigen) and that a residual cellular heterogeneity still exists in the test populations. Clearly, the use of purified antigen-specific B cells and of normally responsive long-term cell lines derived from them would represent important technical advances in the study of B cell activation.

ACTIVATION OF RESTING B CELLS

B cells prepared from spleen cell populations of normal mice can be activated from the G_0 state to enter and progress through the G_1 phase of the cell cycle by several distinct sets of stimuli. These include activation signals based on receptor cross-linkage, on "cognate" interaction with histocompatibility-restricted T cells, and on the direct action of T cells, or their secreted products, on resting B cells. In such studies of B cell activation, it is important to prepare highly purified cell populations and, particularly, to free the B cells of contaminating T cells and macrophages. This is essential to avoid difficulties stemming from indirect B cell activation, mediated through residual cells of other types present in the cultures.

Anti-immunoglobulin Antibodies As B Cell Activating Agents

Anti-IgM antibodies have been employed by several laboratories as polyclonal B cell activators on the assumption that, by binding to and crosslinking the mIg which acts as the B cell's receptor for antigen, they may mimic the action of multivalent antigens on B cells. Specifically, purified goat anti-mouse IgM antibodies and $F(ab)'_2$ fragments of rabbit anti-IgM antibodies have proved to be powerful stimulants of B cell activation. In serum-free media, anti-IgM antibodies, at concentrations of 1 to 10 ug/ml, cause virtually all resting B cells to enlarge and to synthesize RNA (7). Since enlargement is exhibited by all the cells and since it is detectable within the first two hours of culture, it appears certain that anti-IgM exerts its stimulatory activity on resting B cells. Recently, Cambier et al. have shown membrane depolarization of essentially all B cells within one hour of addition of anti-IgM to cultures of purifed B cells (16).

At high cell density (e.g., 5 x 10^5/0.2 ml well), anti-IgM antibodies can also stimulate B cells to enter the S phase of the cell cycle. This stimulation requires the use of substantially higher concentrations of anti-IgM (25-100 ug/ml). F(ab) fragments fail to cause DNA synthesis. Approximately half of the B cells which have entered the G_1 phase in response to anti-IgM enter S phase (7). B cells from mice with the xid-determined immunodeficiency enter G_1 normally in response to anti-IgM, but these cells fail to enter S phase. Since xid mice lack $Lyb5^+$ B cells, it has been concluded that anti-IgM antibodies cause both $Lyb5^-$ and $Lyb5^+$ B cells to enter G_1 but only $Lyb5^+$ cells to enter S. This conclusion has been supported by analysis of the phenotype of normal B cells which enter S phase in response to anti-IgM (20).

The first B cells which enter S phase in response to high concentrations of anti-IgM do so at about thirty hours after addition of antibody to the culture. Anti-IgM may be removed from culture approximately nine hours before B cells enter S phase without affecting that process, indicating that a late G_1 point exists after which the B cells have become independent of further signals received through their mIg receptors. Based on this, we have divided the G_1 phase into $G_{1\alpha}$ and $G_{1\beta}$, the former an anti-IgM dependent phase, the latter an anti-IgM independent phase (DeFranco and Paul, in preparation).

Recent results raise the possibility that $G_{1\alpha}$ may require subdivision. As has already been noted, anti-IgM is required only during $G_{1\alpha}$ and low concentrations of anti-IgM will cause resting B cells to enter $G_{1\alpha}$. Since low concentrations of anti-IgM are insufficient to cause B cells to enter S phase, it would appear that high anti-IgM concentrations must be required for the completion of the $G_{1\alpha}$ phase of the cell cycle. Direct experimentation indicates that, in populations of B cells activated with 1-2 ug/ml of anti-IgM, a high concentration of anti-IgM must be added approximately six hours before the cell becomes independent of the need for anti-IgM (i.e., six hours before the end of $G_{1\alpha}$). However, it remains possible that these high concentrations of anti-IgM act indirectly on small numbers of contaminating cells to cause in situ production of growth factors. Efforts to clarify this issue are still in progress.

Although low concentrations of anti-IgM fail to stimulate B cells to enter S phase, cells cultured with such concentrations of antibody can be caused to take up ^{3}H-thymidine by the addition of a soluble T cell-derived product designated B cell growth factor (now abbreviated BSF-p1) (10). BSF-p1 has a molecular weight of 15,000 daltons by sodium dodecyl sulfate-polyacrylamide gel electrophoresis; two charged species, one of pI 6.4, the other 7.4, can be resolved by isoelectric focusing (9). Both of these properties distinguish BSF-p1 from interleukin-2 (IL-2). Murine IL-2 has a molecular weight of 21,000-23,000 daltons and much more acidic pI's. BSF-p1 may also be separated from IL-2 by phenylsepharose chromatography and by trisglycinate gel electrophoresis. Efforts to purify BSF-p1 by high performance liquid chromatography and to obtain cDNA clones complementary to BSF-p1 mRNA are now in progress.

When highly purified B cells are cultured at low cell density (10^4 cells/ 0.2ml), in the absence of 2-mercaptoethanol, ^{3}H-thymidine uptake does not occur in response to anti-IgM antibodies and BSF-p1 unless a soluble macrophage product is added to the culture. Based on the co-purification of this material with interleukin-1 (IL-1) and the activity of highly purified mouse and human IL-1 preparations in responsiveness of B cells to anti-IgM and BSF-p1, it has been concluded that IL-1 itself plays a critical role in B cell activation mediated by receptor cross-linkage (12).

The nature of the stimuli deliverd by BSF-p1 and IL-1 to B cells, the time at which these agents are required, and the nature of the cellular receptors for them are unresolved issues now receiving considerable attention.

B cells treated with anti-IgM antibodies, BSF-p1, and IL-1 do not differentiate into Ig-secreting cells. Recent studies indicate that such cells will enter the Ig secretory state if provided with two additional soluble factors (17). These materials, which lead to Ig secretion, have been designated by some as "differentiation factors." Since their precise functional role is not yet clear, we have preferred the term "T cell replacing factor" (TRF) and have designated the two substances EL-4 TRF (EL-TRF) and B151K12-TRF (B15-TRF) based on the cell lines which produce them. B15-TRF is required relatively early in the B cell differentiation process; it was originally defined based on its differential action on B cells from normal mice and from DBA/2Ha mice. B cells from DBA/2Ha mice have been shown to fail to respond to B15-TRF because of a defective X-chromosomal gene, different from xid (23). The chemical properties of B15-TRF are currently under study by Takatsu, Hamaoka, and their colleagues.

EL-TRF is required much later in the process of B cell differentiation. It migrates on isoelectric focusing and on phenylsepharose chromatography similarly to IL-2. Although affinity chromatography-purified human IL-2 has failed to exhibit EL-TRF activity, the general issue of whether IL-2 acts upon B cells has not been fully resolved. IL-2 does not have BSF-like activity (10) nor can internally labelled IL-2 be demonstrated to bind to resting or activated B cells (Nakanishi et al., in preparation). The binding assay employed in this study has a lower limit of sensitivity of 300 to 500 affinity binding sites/cell. The possibility that some IL-2 binding sites do exist on B cells is raised by the capacity of monoclonal antibodies specific for the mouse IL-2 receptor to bind, although at very low density, to activated B cells (15). It remains to be established whether these molecules on B cells are IL-2 receptors and whether they play a role in any aspect of B cell responsiveness.

B cells from mice with the xid-determined immunodeficiency enter the G_1 phase of the cell cycle but not the S phase in response to anti-IgM; the addition of BSF-p1 does not cause these cells to enter S phase. Furthermore, highly purified xid B cells proliferate very poorly to lipopolysaccharide (LPS). The addition of BSF-p1 and separated fractions from EL-4 supernatant has only a limited effect on LPS-treated xid

B cells. However, if these cells are cultured with low concentrations of anti-IgM, LPS, and certain chromatographic fractions from EL-4 supernatants, they mount very substantial proliferative responses (Howard, unpublished observations). This implies that, under appropriate circumstances, xid (and, by inference, normal Lyb5$^-$) B cells can respond to stimuli flowing from receptor cross-linkage and are sensitive to soluble factors. Whether such activation can lead to Ig synthesis is still to be resolved.

A final question which should be considered in this section is to what extent anti-IgM stimulated B cell activation truly reflects antigen-dependent activation. Although this subject has not been extensively explored, initial studies with hapten-specific B cells purified from normal cell populations suggest that hapten conjugates of simple proteins, even if multivalent, do not cause resting B cells to become sensitive to BSF-p1 and IL-1 (18). By contrast, hapten conjugates of Ficoll, a semisynthetic cross-linked polysucrose, do cause the activation of resting B cells in the presence of growth factors (Howard et al., unpublished observations). It will remain for more detailed examination to determine what physiologic responses are analogous to anti-IgM mediated B cell activation.

Activation of Resting B Cells by "Cognate" Interaction with T Cells

Receptor cross-linkage by anti-immunoglobulin antibodies provides a mechanism for B cell activation by "natural" antigens which bear a repetitive epitope (e.g., bacterial polysaccharides, viruses). However, many antigens express only a single copy of any individual epitope and should not be able to activate resting B cells in this way because they could not cause such cross-linkage. An alternative way specifically to activate resting B cells which have bound "univalent" antigens to their membrane receptors would be for such antigens to be the "targets" of specific helper T cells. "Cognate" interactions between T cells and B cells implies that the T cells "have knowledge" of the B cells which they help, through the recognition on the B cell membrane of the antigens for which the T cells are specific. That is, cognate help implies that antigen forms a bridge between the interacting cells. Furthermore, the T cells which participate in cognate interactions have membrane receptors which display "co-specificity" for antigenic epitopes and for structures on major histocompatibility complex (MHC) gene products. These "co-recognized" MHC gene products are termed restriction elements. Helper T cells generally use class II MHC molecules as restriction elements. For physiologic responses, we postulate that cognate T cell-B cell interactions require that the T cells are specific for antigens which have bound to the B cell through its receptor and that the T cells co-recognize class II molecules expressed by the B cell. Generally, T cells recognize determinants (histotopes) on class II molecules which are polymorphic between distinct MHC haplotypes; thus, such T cells will usually help B cells expressing class II molecules similar to those expressed by the donor of the T cells and will fail to help allogeneic B cells.

Recent studies of B cell activation in cognate systems have employed either antigen-specific B cell responses or generalized B cell activation as their end points. The results obtained with these two systems have been different in certain important ways.

"Antigen-specific" Cognate T Cell-B Cell Interactions

Antigen-specific cognate interations involve the culture of purified B cells with a source of "MHC-restricted" helper T cells and, usually, with a source of antigen-presenting cells. Cognate responses in such systems generally require that the T cell be co-specific for a restriction element expressed on the B cell and that the T cell recognize an epitope on the same antigenic molecule for which the B cell is specific. Recent studies suggest that such "cognate" help is only observed when low concentrations of antigen are used (4) and that cognate help can act upon resting B cells (2). Several issues are unresolved in the analysis of B cell activation in antigen-specific cognate systems. Among these are the question of whether the binding of antigen to the receptor of the B cell plays a direct role in B cell activation or only functions indirectly by binding to the appropriate B cells, antigens for which the helper T cell is specific. Zubler and his colleagues (25) have recently developed evidence that receptor occupancy may play an important role in cognate activation. They have utilized an experimental system which allows separation of the antigen which binds to the B cell's receptor from the antigen, on the B cell surface, for which the helper T cell is specific. This was accomplished by using a T cell line specific for the H-Y antigen on male cells and using TNP-protein to elicit anti-TNP antibody responses. Zubler observed that in the absence of the TNP protein, little anti-TNP response was observed, suggesting that the TNP-protein directly delivered some type of "signal" to the B cell, since the delivery of the cognate T cell signal is independent of binding to the B cell receptor. It should be noted that in the very same cultures substantial T cell-dependent Ig synthesis occurred in the absence of TNP-protein, suggesting that many B cells may be activated by cognate interactions without receptor occupancy.

Cognate T Cell-B Cell Interactions in Which B Cells Are Activated Polyclonally

As alluded to in the last sentence of the previous section, it has also proved to be possible to study cognate interactions between T and B cells in situations in which the B cell does not bind antigen through its membrane receptors. Experiments of this type generally utilize T cell lines specific for minor histocompatibility antigens, thus allowing interaction between the cognate T cell and all members of the B cell population (5). Under such circumstances, activation of a very substantial fraction of the B cells occurs, leading both to ^{3}H-thymidine uptake and to production of immunoglobulin, as measured by the appearance of "reverse" plaque-forming cells (PFC). It has been suggested that such cognate activation actually does require a receptor-mediated signal and that the B cells activated in such cultures are those which have mIg's capable of binding to proteins in the culture medium such as the antigen for which the T cell is specific or for proteins in fetal calf serum. However, the high frequency of responding cells makes this very unlikely.

If we examine the disparate sets of results obtained in antigen-specific and polyclonal systems in terms of the stimuli required for B cell activation, proliferation, and differentiation, it seems to be valid to conclude that resting B cells can be activated in the course of cognate interactions without the need for receptor occupancy and/or cross-linkage. However, when antigens of suitable structure, capable of providing receptor-mediated stimulation, are present, B cells with receptors complementary to these antigens have a major advantage and expand (or differentiate) much more efficiently, leading to relative clonal expansion of such B cells. The advantage provided by antigen should be most evident when the degree of T cell "help" is limited.

Non-cognate, Polyclonal Activation of Resting B Cells by T Cells

In a series of recent studies, DeFranco, Ashwell, Schwartz, and I (DeFranco et al., submitted; Ashwell et al., submitted) examined the interaction between B cells and cloned T cell lines specific for pigeon cytochrome c. One such line (11.4) had the property that it could be activated by resting B10.A B cells in the presence of cytochrome c to cause those B10.A (I-A^k) B cells to proliferate and differentiate. This T cell line also was "allospecific" for B10.RIII (I-A^r) cells, and the mixture of 11.4 cells and resting B10.RIII cells led to the proliferation of the resting cells. If allogeneic (B10.S(9R)) [I-A^s] B cells were added to cultures containing 11.4 cells and cytochrome c, no proliferation or differentiation occurred. However, resting B10.S(9R) B cells became activated, proliferated, and differentiated into Ig secretory cells in the presence of 11.4 cells, cytochrome c, and lightly irradiated B10.A B cells. This implies that resting B cells may be activated, through "non-cognate" T cell-B cell interactions, if the T cells are themselves activated by cognate interactions. Furthermore, in such systems, virtually all the allogeneic B cells enter G_1, indicating that this activation of resting B cells is independent of receptor occupancy. Similar results have been obtained with several antigen-specific cloned T cell lines and with three of four antigen-specific T cell hybridomas. Thus, the activation of resting B cells may be achieved by non-cognate, receptor-independent signals delivered by T cells.

A striking finding obtained with 11.4 T cells is that, although irradiated B10.A B cells and cytochrome c stimulate them to activate B10.S(9R) B cells, irradiated B10.RIII B cells, for which 11.4 T cells are allospecific, do not cause 11.4 T cells to activate B10.S(9R) B cells. Thus, the very same T cell clone appears to engage in both cognate and non-cognate help, depending on the nature of the stimulus. One interpretation of these results is that the molecular mediator of T cell-B cell interactions is a nonspecific polyclonal activator capable of acting on any resting B cell. Cognate interactions are observed under conditions in which the "cloud" of activating factor around a given T cell is only sufficient to activate B cells in contact with the T cells. B cells which bear class II molecules and antigen for which the T cells are co-specific will be efficiently activated because T cells will be bound to the B cells through an antigen-bridge. By contrast, allogeneic, nonantigen-specific B cells will, on the average, be at a greater distance from the T cells, beyond the effective radius of the cloud of nonspecific factor. If the very same T cell clone can be more efficiently stimulated so that a cloud of much larger radius is produced, then non-cognate interactions should be observed. We may postulate that the difference in activation of 11.4 cells by B10.RIII B cells and B10.A B cells together with cytochrome c is quantitative. The former stimulus is sufficient only for local (cognate) activation of B cells, the latter, for distant (non-cognate) activation. Of course, the reader must be aware that although this mechanism could explain all cases of cognate activation of B cells, no direct evidence that it does explain all cases exists. Indeed, antigen-specific MHC-restricted soluble T cell factors (3, 14) and allogeneic effect factors (8) have been described which have properties consistent with molecular mediators of truly cognate interactions.

I stress the non-cognate aspect of the system described here because it appears to be a novel physiologic mechanism for activation of resting B cells. Furthermore, since it is difficult to distinguish T cell-B cell interactions based on specific factors from those based on nonspecific factors made locally, I will hereafter refer to cognate in quotes ("cognate") to cover both cases.

Are Additional T Cell Stimuli Required for "Cognate" B Cell Responses?
In general, "cognate" T cell-B cell interactions have been studied using intact helper T cells. This had made it quite difficult to examine when in the B cell activation program the "cognate" stimulus is required and whether additional stimuli are required for full responses of B cells, just as several factors acting in an ordered sequence appear to be required in anti-IgM mediated B cell responses. The difficulty imposed by using helper T cells in culture is that such cells, in addition to their "cognate" activation potential, may very well produce all other required factors in situ. Indeed, antigen-specific T cell lines produce many soluble factors including BSF-p1 and gamma-interferon. One approach to solving this problem which has been used by Roehm et al. (19) is to select antigen-specific T cell hybridomas which are unable to provide help in the absence of added soluble factors but which can provide such help when an appropriate soluble factor is provided. A second way to attack this problem would be to isolate in soluble form, if possible, the active principle involved in "cognate" interaction and to then determine what additional factors are needed for activation, proliferation, and differentiation and when these factors are needed.

LONG-TERM GROWTH OF B CELLS
As alluded to at the beginning of this paper, the approaches currently used to study B cell activation and subsequent stimulatory events each represent a compromise of some sort. Antigen-specific responses usually employ cell populations in which only a small fraction of the cells bear receptors specific for antigen. Assessment of responses thus requires the study of rare cells and, in most cases, requires indirect approaches. The use of polyclonal activators, even those which react with receptors, makes the assumption that such activation mimics the physiologic case. A potential solution would be to purify antigen-specific cells from normal populations; this has been used to some extent and has provided useful information, but it is difficult, expensive, and the yield of cells is very low. A routine technique to propagate antigen-reactive B cells in long-term culture and to clone these cells would meet many of the requirements needed for an ideal model for the study of B cell activation. Of course, even such a model has the deficiency that B cells which are replicating

over extended periods of time may not faithfully reflect normal resting B cells in their activation requirements.

Several groups have reported some success in propagating B cells in long-term culture ((1, 6, 11, 21); Maizel et al., personal communication), but none of the reports has yet described a simple technique for the growth of antigen-specific cells in large numbers.

Success has been achieved in propagating B cells for from three months to one year by initially stimulating these cells with LPS, anti-Ig on insoluble matrices, or lectins such as ConA or PHA. After suitable periods, growth-promoting factors were added to the cultures and the cells were thereafter propagated with growth factors only. In most instances, the growth-promoting factors required for long-term stimulation were not well-defined. Indeed, a principal difficulty in this approach is that no suitable assays for evaluating growth factors for propagation of B cell lines are available. In our own experience (11, 21), the inability to determine in advance which batches of factor would support long-term growth and which would not proved to be a major difficulty. Furthermore, we have found that BSF-p1 by itself is insufficient to maintain B cell growth beyond the first few rounds of division. A major goal, which should become achievable with our increasing understanding of B cell growth control, will be the use of purified preparations of growth-promoting factors which, acting together, should allow longer-term B cell growth. Among the factors which we believe deserve extensive investigation, in addition to BSF-p1, are a) B15-TRF, which appears to have proliferogenic activity for resting B cell populations; b) a high molecular weight B cell growth factor, detected in studies of proliferation of LPS blasts (13); and c) a material designated BCFG-II, which acts upon B cells treated with dextran sulfate (22).

Another approach, which has been quite successful in propagating B cells in long-term culture, is that introduced by Whitlock and Witte (24). They have utilized monolayers of cells which grow out of bone marrow cultures, in relatively low density cultures, to act as feeder cells for pre-B cells from bone marrow. Pre-B cells and B cells grow on such monolayers and can be successfully propagated and expanded without the need for additional factors or for agents which can cross-link receptors. Witte and his colleagues have succeeded in cloning both pre-B cells and B cells from such cultures (Witte, personal communication). Thus far, methods to develop antigen-specific lines from these cultures have not yet been reported, nor is the nature of the growth-promoting factors made by the monolayer known.

CONCLUSIONS

The study of B cell activation is currently an active and rapidly progressing field. The recognition that the various steps in the B cell activation program are dependent upon external growth and differentiation stimuli has led to an intense study of the factors regulating each step. Furthermore, our recognition that B cells may be activated in several distinct ways leads to the obvious question as to whether each mode of activation results in cells which then require distinct stimuli at subsequent steps, or whether cells of a given activated state are sensitive to the same stimuli, no matter how they have arrived at that state.

A fruitful area for study will be the identification of the growth factor receptors and a delineation of how growth factor-receptor interaction generates signals within the cells. An obvious question to flow from this study will be to develop both agonists and antagonists for these receptors, in order to obtain efficient means to regulate B cell growth in physiologic situations and to control growth of transformed B cells which continue to express growth factor receptors.

REFERENCES

(1) Aldo-Benson, M., and Scheiderer, L. 1983. Long term growth of lines of murine dinitrophenyl-specific B lymphocyte in vitro. J. Exp. Med. 157: 342.

(2) Andersson, J.; Schreier, M.H.; and Melchers, F. 1980. T-cell dependent B cell stimulation is H-2 restricted and antigen dependent only at the resting B cell level. Proc. Natl. Acad. Sci. USA 77: 1612.

(3) Apte, R.N.; Eshar, Z.; Lowy, I.; Zinger, H.; and Mozes, E. 1981. Characterization of a poly(L-tyr, L-glu)-poly(D, L-Ala)-poly(L-lys)-specific helper factor derived from a T cell hybridoma. Eur. J. Immunol. 11: 931.

(4) Asano, Y.; Shigeta, M.; Fathman, C.G.; Singer, A.; and Hodes, R.J. 1982. Role of the major histocompatibility complex in T cell activation of B cell subpopulations. A single monoclonal T helper cell activates different B cell subpopulations by distinct pathways. J. Exp. Med. 156: 350.

(5) Augustin, A.A., and Coutinho, A. 1980. Specific T helper cells that activate B cells polyclonally. In vitro enrichment and cooperative

function. J. Exp. Med. 151: 587-601.

(6) Braun, J. 1983. Spontaneous in vitro occurrence and long-term culture of murine B lymphoblast cell lines. J. Immunol. 130: 2113.

(7) DeFranco, A.; Raveche, E.; Asofsky, R.; and Paul, W.E. 1982. Frequency of B lymphocytes responsive to anti-immunoglobulin. J. Exp. Med. 155: 1523-1536.

(8) Delovitch, T.L., and Phillips, M.L. 1982. The biological and biochemical basis of allogeneic effect factor (AEF) activity: relationship to T cell alloreactivity. Immunobiol. 161: 51.

(9) Farrar, J.J.; Howard, M.; Fuller-Farrar, J.; and Paul, W.E. 1983. Biochemical and physicochemical characterization of mouse B-cell growth factor: a lymphokine distinct from interleukin-2. J. Immunol. 131: 1838.

(10) Howard, M.; Farrar, J.; Hilfiker, M.; Johnson, B.; Takatsu, K.; et al. 1982. Identification of a T-cell derived B-cell growth factor distinct from interleukin 2. J. Exp. Med. 155: 914-923.

(11) Howard, M.; Kessler, S.; Chused, T.; and Paul, W.E. 1981. Long-term culture of normal mouse B lymphocytes. Proc. Natl. Acad. Sci. USA 78: 5788-5792.

(12) Howard, M.; Mizel, S.B.; Lachman, L.; Ansel, J.; Johnson, B.; and Paul, W.E. 1983. Role of interleukin 1 in anti-immunoglobulin-induced B cell proliferation. J. Exp. Med. 157: 1529-1543.

(13) Lernhardt, W.; Corbel, C.; Wall, R.; and Melchers, F. 1982. T cell hybridomas which produce B lymphocyte replication factors only. Nature 300: 355.

(14) Lonai, P.; Puri, J.; Bitton, S.; Benneriah, Y.; Givol, D.; and Hammerling, G. 1981. H-2-restricted helper factor secreted by cloned hybridoma cells. J. Exp. Med. 154: 942.

(15) Malek, T.R.; Robb, R.J.; and Shevach, E.M. 1983. Identification and initial characterization of a rat monoclonal antibody reactive with the murine interleukin 2 receptor ligand complex. Proc. Natl. Acad. Sci. USA 80: 5694.

(16) Monroe, J.G., and Cambier, J.C. 1983. B cell activation. I. Anti-immunoglobulin-induced receptor cross-linking results in a decrease in plasma membrane potential of murine B lymphocytes. J. Exp. Med. 157: 2073.

(17) Nakanishi, K.; Howard, M.; Muraguchi, A.; Farrar, J.; Takatsu, K.; Hamaoka, T.; and Paul, W.E. 1983. Soluble factors involved in B cell differentiation: identification of two distinct T cell replacing factors (TRFs). J. Immunol. 130: 2219-2224.

(18) Noelle, R.J.; Snow, E.C.; Uhr, J.W.; and Vitetta, E.S. 1983. T cell activities which regulate T cell-dependent, antigen-driven B cell growth and differentiation. Fed. Proc. 42: 833.

(19) Roehm, N.; Marrack, P.; and Kappler, J. 1983. Helper signals in B cell responses. Fed. Proc. 42: 692.

(20) Sieckmann, D.G.; Habbersett, R.; Scher, I.; and Paul, W.E. 1981. Activation of mouse lymphocytes by anti-immunoglobulin. III. Analysis of responding B lymphocytes by flow cytometry and cell sorting. J. Immunol. 127: 205-211.

(21) Sredni, B.; Sieckmann, D.; Kumagai, S.; House, S.; Green, I.; et al. 1981. Long-term culture and cloning of nontransformed human B lymphocytes. J. Exp. Med. 154: 1500-1516.

(22) Swain, S.; Howard, M.; Kappler, J.; Marrack, P.; Watson, J.; Booth, R.; and Dutton, R. 1983. Evidence for two distinct classes of murine B cell growth factors which have activities in different functional assays. J. Exp. Med. 158: 822.

(23) Takatsu, K.; Tanaka, K.; Tominaga, A.; Kumahara, Y.; and Hamaoka, T. 1980. Antigen-induced T cell-replacing factor (TRF). III. Establishment of T cell hybrid clone continuously producing TRF and functional analysis of released TRF. J. Immunol. 125: 2646-2653.

(24) Whitlock, C., and Witte, O. 1982. Long-term culture of B lymphocytes and their precursors from murine bone marrow. Proc. Natl. Acad. Sci. USA 79: 3608-3612.

(25) Zubler, R.H., and Kanagawa, O. 1982. Requirement for three signals in B cell responses. II. Analysis of antigen- and Ia-restricted T helper cell-B cell interaction. J. Exp. Med. 156: 415-429.

Leukemia, ed. I.L. Weissman, pp. 83-94. Dahlem Konferenzen 1985. Berlin, Heidelberg, New York, Tokyo: Springer-Verlag.

Lymphoid Tumor Stem Cells and Their Regulation

R.G. Lynch
Dept. of Pathology, University of Iowa College of Medicine
Iowa City, IA 52242, USA

INTRODUCTION

The objective of this paper is to review what is known about lymphoid tumor stem cells and their regulation. As will be discussed in some detail below, a great deal of what is known comes by inference from studies that were not concerned with lymphoid tumor stem cells, but typically addressed an aspect of differentiation in lymphoid tumors.

While many studies of stem cells in non-lymphoid tumors have been conducted over the past ten years, tumor stem cells are still operationally defined entities. It has been shown for many tumors that in vitro and in vivo cloning techniques can identify tumor cells that: a) have an extensive proliferative capacity and b) produce progeny that differentiate into cells that express "luxury" functions coincident with a diminished proliferative capacity. The frequency of such cells in a tumor is very small, usually on the order of 10^{-3} or less. It is not clear whether the low frequency is a reflection of the conditions of assay or an accurate assessment of the tumor stem cell population. The in vitro cloning assays have provided a means to identify one potentially important, functional subpopulation that is present in many tumors. Whether other cells in the tumor are part of its proliferative compartment but fail to be detected with the assays remains an open question.

As with most neoplasms, lymphoid tumors express considerable cytologic heterogeneity. This feature has long been known to pathologists and has been used as a criterion to classify lymphomas as well as an index to predict their clinical behavior. While tumor cell heterogeneity was initially appreciated on morphological grounds, it is now clear that cellular subpopulations in a tumor differ in their biochemical, functional, proliferative, and invasive properties (25). One of the first pieces of experimental evidence that implied the existence of a stem cell population in tumors came from studies by Pierce and his colleagues (28). They used autoradiography to visualize short-term ^{3}H-thymidine incorporation into murine teratocarcinomas and human skin cancers and observed labeling of a minor fraction of the tumor cell population. By morphological criteria the labeled cells were poorly differentiated, while the unlabeled cells conspicuously expressed highly differentiated functions such as keratin production. Subsequent studies in other laboratories began to construct a rather convincing argument that subpopulations of cells in tumors had different degrees of growth potential.

The development of in vitro and in vivo colony-forming assays provided methods capable of some degree of quantitation of tumor stem cells. Until recently, these assays, which quantitate an operationally defined tumor stem cell, had been used primarily to evaluate pharmacological and physical agents for potential use in the treatment of cancer (34). In the past five years an increasing number of studies have begun to use cloning methods to address the regulation of tumor stem cells. The majority of these studies have dealt with non-lymphoid hematological malignancies in experimental animals and humans. The use of colony assays to study the regulation of lymphoid tumor stem cells has received little attention. Thus, in the first two years (1981, 1982) of a new journal devoted to studies of stem cells, only three of 174 papers and abstracts that appeared dealt with lymphoid tumor stem cells (23). In part, the emphasis on non-lymphoid hematological neoplasms can be accounted for by a sizeable preexisting fund of information about the growth factors that support the in vitro growth of non-lymphoid hematopoietic cells. It has been only very recently that certain lymphoid cell growth factors have become readily available. Paradoxically, while lymphoid cells of the B lineage express several well characterized molecular markers that would prove useful in the study of neoplastic B cell growth and differentiation, most of what is known about lymphoid cell growth factors relates to T cells. Factors that influence B cell growth and differentiation are known to exist, are the subjects of intensive study in a number of laboratories, and are likely to prove useful in establishing the conditions to routinely support neoplastic B cell growth in vitro.

Two major problems have hampered the development of information about lymphoid tumor stem cells, and both problems relate to their detection: a) Molecular markers specific for lymphoid tumor stem cells have not yet been identified. Were they to be found and monoclonal antibodies developed, it would be possible to select for stem cells by flow cytometry. b) The cloning assays used to detect and quantitate lymphoid tumor stem cells have certain limitations. Both the in vitro and in vivo colony-forming assays are functional assays whose efficiencies are unknown. The in vivo assays typically involve injecting graded numbers of tumor cells intravenously and counting macroscopic tumor colonies in the spleen or another organ after an incubation period of one to three weeks (8). This approach is limited by the unknown efficiency of targeting of stem cells to the indicator organ and the failure to detect those tumor cells that may have considerable proliferative capacity but do not form macroscopic tumors. In most studies it is assumed, not proven, that each colony originated from a single tumor cell. The use of long-passaged in vitro lines of lymphoid tumor cells to study tumor stem cells is also limited because it is never clear what the relationship is between the apparently rare in vivo tumor stem cells and the highly clonogenic tumor cells that have been selected for their ability to grow in vitro.

In summary, little has been done thus far to attempt directly to visualize regulatory influences on lymphoid tumor stem cells. However, as discussed below, an abundance of experimental data has established that the growth and differentiation of lymphoid tumors can be immunologically regulated. These findings indicate that further study of the cellular subpopulations in lymphoid tumors is clearly warranted and is likely to generate useful information about the role(s) of tumor stem cells in the interesting regulatory effects that have been observed with many lymphoid tumors.

INTRA-TUMOR HETEROGENEITY IN LYMPHOID TUMORS

As discussed above, morphological heterogeneity within lymphoid tumors has long been recognized. In spite of this, it is not at all uncommon to read still that lymphoid tumors consist of cells "frozen" at a fixed point in lymphoid cell differentiation.

Three main factors have been identified that account for the intra-tumor heterogeneity of lymphoid tumors: a) variation due to cell cycle, b) development of sub-clones, and c) heterogeneity due to intra-tumor differentiation.

Variation Due to Cell Cycle
Studies with synchronized tumor cells and with cells isolated by velocity sedimentation or flow cytometry have convincingly shown that the expression of many surface antigens varies according to the stage of the cell cycle.

Development of Sub-clones
The earliest studied example of this is the work by Coffino and Scharff (6) with established culture lines of murine myeloma cells. They showed that parental myeloma cells that synthesized and secreted intact (H & L) immunoglobulin molecules spontaneously generated (L) light chain-producing variants at a frequency as high as 10^{-3}. Other investigations have reported spontaneous variants that produce truncated (36), recombinant (3), or a different class of heavy chain (29), and other variants have been identified that show altered expression of allotypic and idiotypic markers as well as antigen-binding properties. Studies by Leibson et al. (18) have shown that the heterogeneity in some myeloma cell lines results from stable variants that differ in their degree of expression of surface membrane and secreted immunoglobulin. The spontaneous development of stable sub-clones emphasizes the need to frequently reclone cell lines, especially if they are used in studies of lymphoma cell regulation.

Heterogeneity Due to Intra-tumor Differentiation
Relative to the subject of this paper, the most important basis for intra-tumor heterogeneity is that which results from the "spontaneous" differentiation of progeny derived from lymphoid tumor stem cells. It is now well established that the intra-tumor heterogeneity seen in chronic myeloid leukemia and in other malignant myeloproliferative disorders in humans is due to differentiation within the clone (11). In chronic myeloid leukemia, it is now generally accepted that the differentiated leukemic cells have a diminished growth potential and that the most highly differentiated leukemic cells no longer divide. While it has not been definitely established that lymphoid tumors contain stem cells whose progeny continuously differentiate into more specialized, presumably less "malignant" cells, there is abundant indirect evidence in support of this concept. If this were formally proven, it would likely have important practical implications.

SUMMARY OF STUDIES THAT DEMONSTRATE THE FUNCTIONAL PLASTICITY OF LYMPHOID TUMORS

Most of the studies that have addressed the intra-tumor heterogeneity of lymphoid tumors have studied B cell neoplasms. Spontaneous and experimentally induced alterations in the phenotypic properties of lymphoid tumor cells have been described in lymphomas of pre-B and mature B cells, and in plasmacytomas and hybridomas (reviewed in (1)). There are a number of examples in which a human with a B cell tumor appears to develop a second B cell tumor. In the past this was usually considered to reflect a chance event or an individual with an increased risk of developing lymphoid neoplasms. It is now definitely established that in some instances the second neoplasm is actually the original neoplastic clone expressing a strikingly different phenotype. Examples include individuals with chronic lymphocytic leukemia who develop lymphoblastic lymphoma (Richter's Syndrome). The phenotypic changes are striking. Chronic lymphocytic leukemia cells are small, IgM-producing, nonsecreting tumor cells that produce an indolent disease. This leukemia appears to have an extremely small growth fraction. In Richter's Syndrome, the clone takes on the appearance of large lymphoblasts, the proliferation of tumor cells is markedly increased, and clinically the disease is more aggressive and patient survival is short (12). Karyotypic analysis has established that the rapidly proliferating lymphoblasts in Richter's Syndrome are members of the same clone as the small lymphocytes that dominate the indolent phase of this disease (24). Thus the dimorphism of Richter's Syndrome is analogous to the situation in chronic myeloid leukemia in which blast crisis develops (see Greaves and Fialkow, both this volume).

Another example of a similar process is the development of multiple myeloma in patients with chronic lymphocytic leukemia. While this event is uncommon, it demonstrates that a clone of neoplastic B cells may show a stable phenotype for ten or more years and then begin to differentiate into malignant antibody-secreting cells. The phenotypic changes that accompany this process are striking. In some instances, differentiation to malignant antibody-secreting cells is accompanied by a heavy chain class switch but preservation of expression of the previous V_H and light chain genes (7). The cytologic features of the clone are changed, the anatomic distribution of the malignant cells is strikingly changed, and the malignant plasmacytes induce the changes in host macrophages that lead to the severe skeletal demineralization and the severe polyclonal B cell immunodeficiency that is characteristic of multiple myeloma. Thus, the development of myeloma from chronic lymphocytic leukemia is not simply a matter of malignant B lymphocytes beginning to secrete immunoglobulin, it involves changes in gene expression, surface membrane markers, cellular migration, cell cycle progression, and other basic processes.

The two examples of clonal progression that on occasion occur in chronic lymphocytic leukemia demonstrate that neoplastic lymphoid cells are not "frozen" at a fixed stage of B cell differentiation. While the striking clinical examples cited are unusual, the potential of malignant B cells for further differentiation is common and considerable. Fu et al. (13) and Robert et al. (30) have shown that neoplastic B lymphocytes in chronic lymphocytic leukemia can be induced with mitogens and T cell-derived factors to differentiate into immunoglobulin-secreting plasma cells. Similar approaches have been used by several groups to demonstrate that BCL_1, a spontaneous BALB/c tumor with the phenotypic features of a virgin mature B lymphocyte, can also be induced to differentiate and alter its proliferative properties (15). LPS has been shown to induce a pre-B cell lymphoma to take on the phenotypic features of a mature B cell (27). The list of examples continues to grow.

Collectively, while the spontaneous and induced alterations in tumor phenotype just discussed do not directly address the subject of lymphoid tumor stem cells, they do point out that neoplastic lymphoid cells have many more features in common with normal lymphoid cells than was previously assumed. A thorough review of this topic was recently published by Abbas (1). Since the growth and differentiation of normal lymphoid cells is a highly regulated process, and since, as discussed above, lymphoid tumors recapitulate many developmental features of normal lymphoid cells, the possibility that normal immunoregulatory processes might be capable of regulating malignant lymphoid cells immediately comes to mind.

STUDIES THAT HAVE SUCCESSFULLY USED IMMUNOREGULATORY STRATEGIES TO MANIPULATE LYMPHOID TUMOR GROWTH AND DIFFERENTIATION

Over the past ten years, a number of investigators have reported that murine lymphomas, plasmacytomas, and hybridomas are responsive to normal immunoregulatory signals (reviewed in (1)). In many instances, the regulatory effect observed was prevention or cessation of tumor cell growth. While not all of these studies directly measured tumor stem cells, in three well characterized systems the data strongly argued that plasmacytoma stem cells were being specifically regulated (8, 16, 32).

The original studies of this type were reported in 1972 by Lynch et al. (19). They established that immunization of BALB/c mice with purified myeloma protein protected the mice from subsequent subcutaneous challenge with otherwise lethal numbers of myeloma cells. The protective immunity was specific for the idiotype of the immunizing myeloma protein. Thus mice immunized with M315 or M460 failed to develop tumors when challenged with MOPC-315 or MOPC-460, respectively. Even though M315 and M460 are both IgA, anti-TNP immunoglobulins, they have dissimilar idiotypes and fail to cross-protect.

In subsequent studies, Daley et al. (8) used a spleen colony assay to quantitate the protective immunity and observed that idiotype-immune mice prevented spleen colonization by myeloma cells. While it is not valid to assume that the spleen colony-forming assay detects <u>the</u> myeloma stem cell, this assay clearly detects <u>a</u> myeloma stem cell. This cell has a relatively unlimited growth potential when compared to most of the cells in the myeloma. It is clear from the data in Table 1 that idiotype-immune mice have a great capacity to prevent spleen colonization by myeloma cells.

The mechanism that mediates idiotype-specific tumor immunity is still incompletely defined. It clearly involves a T cell, is sensitive to post-immunization thymectomy (9), and the effect appears to be <u>cytostatic</u> rather than <u>cytotoxic</u> (discussed in (20)). The finding that an immunoglobulin idiotype could function as a tumor-specific transplantation antigen has been confirmed for a large number of plasmacytomas (10, 21) and for murine lymphomas (14, 37).

In addition, there have been several reports in which antigen-specific regulatory effects have been successfully employed to influence the growth and differentiation of antigen-binding myelomas (32) and hybridomas (5). Furthermore, myeloma cells can be regulated by allotype-specific (4) and isotype-specific (2) regulatory T cells. Collectively, these findings establish the general principle that tumors of the immune system are frequently responsive to immunoregulatory signals. It is clear from some of the studies (31) that the effects on tumor cell growth are distinct from the effects on tumor cell differentiation. Whether the effects on growth always involve tumor stem cells remains to be examined.

In an interesting study by Kans et al. (16), it was shown that mice neonatally suppressed for the expression of an idiotype inhibited the proliferation and maturation of myeloma cells that expressed the suppressed idiotype. These findings are of particular interest because the neonatal suppression was established by injection of anti-idiotypic antibody, but the myeloma suppression appeared to be T cell-dependent. This sequence has been observed in the anti-idiotypic suppression of anti-arsenate antibody

TABLE 1 - Idiotype-specific transplantation resistance as measured by the spleen plasmacytoma colony-forming assay.

Experiment	Immunogen[a] 200 μg	Immunizations	MOPC-315[S] cells injected IV	PCFU-s per spleen ± S.E.	P value[b]
1	None	-	$4x10^4$	33.6 ± 2.7	-
	RA-460	6	$4x10^4$	49.5 ± 7.6	0.075
	RA-315	6	$4x10^4$	0.1 ± 0.1	0.001
	None	-	$8x10^4$	75.6 ± 9.0	-
	RA-460	6	$8x10^4$	64.4 ± 11.7	0.44
	RA-315	6	$8x10^4$	0.7 ± 0.3	0.001
2	None	-	$3.5x10^4$	25.0 ± 4.3	-
	BSA	6	$3.5x10^4$	37.4 ± 4.0	0.55
	RA-315	6	$3.5x10^4$	0.1 ± 0.1	0.001
	None	-	$7x10^4$	57.3 ± 6.0	-
	BSA	6	$7x10^4$	77.0 ± 7.0	0.06
	RA-315	6	$7x10^4$	0.1 ± 0.1	0.001
3	H γ G	3	$6.8x10^4$	77.8 ± 6.8	-
	RA-315	3	$6.8x10^4$	2.5 ± 1.1	0.02

[a] All immunized mice were injected at weekly intervals, the indicated number of times, with 200 μg of immunogen. The first injection was administered in CFA, the second in IFA, and all subsequent injections in PBS. Each group within each experiment consisted of six to ten mice.

[b] The one-tailed Student's t-test was performed to evaluate the statistical significance of the differences between various immunized experimental groups and the appropriate unimmunized control group.

responses (26) and in other defined systems. The mechanism whereby an injected anti-idiotypic antibody leads to establishment of a T cell-dependent anti-idiotypic response that persists long after the anti-idiotypic antibody has been cleared is perplexing but could be relevant to the findings reported by Miller et al. (22). They observed regression and stable remission of a B cell lymphoma in a patient given several courses of treatment with a monoclonal antibody specific for the idiotype of the lymphoma immunoglobulin. While it is premature to conclude anything from the treatment of a single patient, further studies are clearly warranted since the murine studies have convincingly established that immunoregulatory circuits can be induced and directed to malignant lymphoid cells and influence their growth and differentiation in a highly specific, and often striking, fashion.

A major limitation in our understanding of the biology of lymphoid neoplasms derives from the narrow time window during which a malignant clone is accessible for study. For example, it has been estimated by Salmon and Durie (35) that multiple myeloma in humans is not detected clinically until the malignant clone has reached a size of approximately 10^{12} cells. Since myeloma is a monoclonal neoplasm, if one ignores tumor cell death, the initial malignant cell has undergone at least forty generations of growth before the disease is detected. It has been estimated that at the time of demise of the patient the clonal size is about 6 - 8 x 10^{12}. Thus, most of what we know about human myeloma has come from studies of the last three generations of clonal evolution. Obviously there exists a great need for information about the processes that take place during the eclipse period between transformation of the single B cell and the appearance of overt clinical disease. While myeloma is usually considered a neoplasm of plasma cells, studies in the murine model (33) and in humans (17) have identified clonal members with features of earlier lymphoid cells. These cells could be important elements in the potential for growth exhibited by the malignant clone.

In spite of the complexity and the lack of information about the early events in the development of lymphoid neoplasms, it appears likely that recent developments in cell culture methods and recombinant DNA technology will provide the tools to make progress towards understanding lymphoid tumor cell heterogeneity in precise biological terms.

REFERENCES

(1) Abbas, A.K. Immunologic regulation of lymphoid tumor cells: model systems for lymphocyte function. Adv. Immunol. 32: 301-368.

(2) Binion, S.B.; Hoover, R.G.; and Lynch, R.G. 1983. Induction of Fc receptors on murine T lymphoma cells. Fed. Proc. 42: 1341.

(3) Birshtein, B.K.; Preud'homme, J.-L.; and Scharff, M.D. 1974. Mutations in mouse myeloma cells. In The Immune System: Genes, Receptors, Signals, eds. E.E. Sercarz, A.R. Williamson, and C.F. Fox, pp. 339-351. New York: Academic Press.

(4) Bosma, M.J., and Bosma, G.C. 1977. Prevention of IgG_{2A} production as a result of allotype-specific interaction between T and B cells. J. Exp. Med. 145: 743.

(5) Boyd, A.W., and Schrader, J.W. 1980. Mechanism of effector-cell blockade. I. Antigen-induced suppression of Ig synthesis in a hybridoma cell line, and correlation with cell-associated antigen. J. Exp. Med. 151: 1436-1451.

(6) Coffino, P., and Scharff, M. 1971. Rate of somatic mutation in immunoglobulin production by mouse myeloma cells. Proc. Natl. Acad. Sci. USA 68: 219.

(7) Cryer, P.E., and Kissane, J. 1975. Multiple malignancies: chronic lymphocytic leukemia, malignant melanoma, multiple myeloma and acute myelomonocytic leukemia. Am. J. Med. 58: 408-416.

(8) Daley, M.J.; Bridges, S.H.; and Lynch, R.G. 1978. Plasmacytoma spleen colonization: a sensitive quantitative in vivo assay for idiotype-specific immune suppression of MOPC-315. J. Immunol. Meth. 24: 47-56.

(9) Daley, M.J.; Gebel, H.M.; and Lynch, R.G. 1978. Idiotype-specific transplantation resistance to MOPC-315: abrogation by post-immunization thymectomy. J. Immunol. 120: 1620.

(10) Eisen, H.M.; Sakato, N.; and Hall, S.J. 1975. Myeloma proteins as tumor specific antigens. Transpl. Proc. 7: 309.

(11) Fialkow, P.J. 1980. Clonal and stem cell origin of blood cell neoplasms. Cont. Hemat./Oncol. 1: 1-46.

(12) Foucar, K., and Rydell, R.E. 1980. Richter's Syndrome in chronic lymphocytic leukemia. Cancer 46: 118-134.

(13) Fu, S.M.; Chiorazzi, N.; and Kunkel, H.G. 1979. Differentiative capacity and other properties of the leukemia cells of chronic lymphocytic leukemia. Immunol. Rev. 48: 23-44.

(14) Haughton, G.; Lanier, L.L.; Babcock, G.F.; and Lynes, M.A. 1978. Antigen-induced murine B cell lymphomas. II. Exploitation of the surface idiotype as tumor specific antigen. J. Immunol. 121: 2358.

(15) Isakson, P.C.; Puré, E.; Uhr, J.W.; and Vitetta, E.S. 1981. Induction of proliferation and differentiation of neoplastic B cells. In B Lymphocytes in the Immune Response: Functional, Developmental and Interactive Properties, eds. N. Klinman, D.E. Mosier, I. Scher, and E.S. Vitetta, pp. 501-504. New York: Elsevier/North-Holland.

(16) Kans, J.; D'Ottavio, R.; and Köhler, H. 1981. Mechanism of neonatal idiotype suppression. III. Delayed maturation of plasmacytoma stem

cells in neonatally suppressed hosts. J. Immunol. 127: 509.

(17) Kubagawa, H.; Vogler, L.B.; Capra, J.D.; Conrad, M.E.; Lawton, A.R.; and Cooper, M.D. 1979. Studies on the clonal origin of multiple myeloma: Use of individually-specific (idiotype) antibodies to trace the oncogenic event to its earliest point of expression in B-cell differentiation. J. Exp. Med. 150: 792.

(18) Leibson, P.J.; Loken, M.R.; Panem, S.; and Schreiber, H. 1979. Clonal evolution of myeloma cells leads to quantitative changes in immunoglobulin secretion and surface antigen expression. Proc. Natl. Acad. Sci. USA 76: 2937-2941.

(19) Lynch, R.G.; Graff, R.; Sirisinha, S.; Simms, E.S.; and Eisen, H.N. 1972. Myeloma proteins as tumor specific transplantation antigens. Proc. Natl. Acad. Sci. USA 69: 1540.

(20) Lynch, R.G., and Milburn, G.L. 1984. Murine plasmacytoma MOPC-315 as a tool for the analysis of network regulation: M315 idiotopes are inducers and targets of immunoregulatory signals. In Idiotypic Networks in Immunology, eds. M.I. Greene and A. Nisonoff, pp. 229-313. New York: Plenum Publishing Corporation.

(21) Meinke, G.C.; McConakey, P.J.; and Spiegelberg, H.L. 1974. Suppression of plasmacytoma growth in mice by immunization with myeloma proteins. Fed. Proc. 33: 792.

(22) Miller, R.A.; Maloney, D.G.; Warnke, R.; and Levy, R. 1982. Treatment of B-cell lymphoma with monoclonal anti-idiotype antibody. New Eng. J. Med. 306: 517-522.

(23) Murphy, M.J., Jr., ed. 1981, 1982. Stem Cells: The International Journal of Cellular Differentiation and Proliferation. Volumes 1 and 2. Basel: Karger Medical and Scientific Publishers.

(24) Nowell, P.; Finan, J.; Glover, D.; and Guerry, D. 1981. Cytogenetic evidence for the clonal nature of Richter's syndrome. Blood 58: 183.

(25) Owens, A.H.; Coffey, D.S.; and Baylin, S.B. 1982. Tumor Cell Heterogeneity: Origins and Implications. New York: Academic Press.

(26) Owen, F.L.; Ju, S.-T.; and Nisonoff, A. 1977. Presence on idiotype-specific suppressor T cells of receptors that interact with molecules bearing the idiotype. J. Exp. Med. 149: 1559.

(27) Paige, C.J.; Kincade, P.W.; and Ralph, P. 1978. Murine B cell

leukemia line with inducible surface immunoglobulin expression. J. Immunol. 121: 641-647.

(28) Pierce, G.B., and Cox, W.F. 1978. Neoplasms as caricatures of tissue renewal. In Cell Differentiation and Neoplasia, ed. G.F. Saunders, pp. 57-66. New York: Raven Press.

(29) Radbruch, A.; Liesegang, B.; and Rajéwsky, K. 1980. Isolation of variants of mouse myeloma X63 that express changed immunoglobulin class. Proc. Natl. Acad. Sci. USA 77: 2909-2913.

(30) Robert, K.-H.; Gahrton, G.; Möller, E.; and Nilsson, B. 1980. Clinical significance of mitogen-induced responses in lymphocytes from patients with chronic lymphocytic leukemia. Acta Med. Scand. 207: 97-103.

(31) Rohrer, J.W.; Gershon, R.K.; Lynch, R.G.; and Kemp, J.D. 1984. Two T cells regulate B cell growth and differentiation. J. Cell. Mol. Immunol. 1: 50-62.

(32) Rohrer, J.W., and Lynch, R.G. 1979. Immunoregulation of localized and disseminated murine myeloma: antigen-specific regulation of MOPC-315 stem cell proliferation and secretory cell differentiation. J. Immunol. 123: 1083-1087.

(33) Rohrer, J.W.; Vasa, K.; and Lynch, R.G. 1977. Myeloma cell immunoglobulin expression during in vivo growth in diffusion chambers: Evidence for repetitive cycles of differentiation. J. Immunol. 119: 861.

(34) Salmon, S.E. 1982. In vitro cloning and chemosensitivity of human myeloma stem cells. Clin. Hemat. 2: 47-63.

(35) Salmon, S.E., and Durie, B.G.M. 1975. Cellular kinetics in multiple myeloma. Arch. Int. Med. 135: 131.

(36) Sonenshein, G.; Siekevitz, M.; Siebert, G.; and Gefter, M. 1978. Control of immunoglobulin secretion in the murine plasmacytoma line MOPC-315. J. Exp. Med. 148: 301.

(37) Suzai, S.; Palmer, D.W.; Talal, N.; and Witz, I.P. 1974. Protective and cellular immune responses to idiotypic determinants on cells from a spontaneous lymphoma of NZB/NZW$_{F1}$ mice. J. Exp. Med. 140: 1547.

Leukemia, ed. I.L. Weissman, pp. 95-110. Dahlem Konferenzen 1985. Berlin, Heidelberg, New York, Tokyo: Springer-Verlag.

Phenotypic Heterogeneity and the Origins of Lymphoid Malignancy in Man: Biological and Clinical Implications

M.F. Greaves
Leukemia Research Fund Center, Institute for Cancer Research
London SW3 6JB, England

Abstract. The phenotypic heterogeneity of human leukemia can best be analyzed within the framework of normal hematopoietic differentiation and proliferation. Leukemia phenotypes (excluding chromosome changes) appear to be minimally deviated replicas of normal ones. Uncoupling of proliferation from differentiation in acute leukemia results in the stabilization of progenitor cell phenotypes that would ordinarily be very transient. The phenotypic abnormality of leukemia/lymphoma may therefore be considered simply as an alteration in the time-frame of expression of normal gene products.

INTRODUCTION

It is now possible to type or classify human lymphoid malignancies in considerable detail using immunological, enzymatic, and karyotypic assays. In this paper I would like to summarize these data and their implications with respect to both the biology of these diseases and their future diagnosis and treatment. To facilitate discussion I have structured this discussion in the form of a series of four propositions. The data I have taken to support these view are largely taken from the work of my own group, and I have not attempted to review or incorporate all the many similar studies by other laboratories.

HETEROGENEITY OF PHENOTYPE

Leukemia and lymphoma cell populations show marked phenotypic heterogeneity from patient to patient and also within a single patient. This diversity reflects a) the target cell origin of individual cases; b) the level of apparent maturation arrest, its stringency plus the proliferative activity of the dominant clone (at the time of study); c) the overall conservation or fidelity of "normal" phenotypic features in leukemia and lymphoma; and d) the existence of abnormal phenotypic traits which may have a direct or causal significance (e.g., chromosome translocations) and others which may be acquired or accumulate especially with malignant progression and treatment. These may be clinically significant (i.e., correlates of prognosis) but have little or no direct, causal significance for leukemogenesis (e.g., drug resistance).

The evidence for points a) to c) have been discussed several times in the past (see (3, 12, 14, 16, 18)); there seems little doubt that these generalizations are correct. On this basis one can draw up a "phenotypic map" of lymphoid malignancy in humans (Fig. 1; (20)). Note that whilst such a map relates leukemia type to its nearest normal counterpart, it does not immediately identify the "target" cell (see below). Some leukemias or lymphomas have been difficult to fit into any such map. These include hairy cell leukemias, which have, in most cases at least, a predominant B cell phenotype including rearranged immunoglobulin genes (27), and Hodgkin's disease in which lymphocytes are usually involved but where the diagnostic cell type - the Reed Sternberg (R-S) cell - is of uncertain lineage origin (51).

The selective association of particular chromosomal abnormalities with these different lymphoid subtypes is also of considerable significance and interest (25, 46). The conclusions currently drawn from these observations, namely, that these rearrangements result in altered c-oncogene expression (i.e., either altered regulation or qualitatively and functionally altered product), seem very plausible. From the point of view of the present discussion, the important implication is that different genes can confer selective growth advantages on lymphoid cells according to stage of differentiation (Fig. 1). This possibility is endorsed by detection of transforming cellular sequences of human lymphoid leukemias assayed in the NIH3T3 transfection assay (5, 34), although similar assays also detect some "common" genes that are less cell type-restricted (e.g., N-, H-, or K-ras, (6)).

Different lymphoid leukemia/lymphoma, subtypes may have other very specific etiological associations which link leukemogenic events and differentiation status. Thus, Epstein Barr Virus (EBV), when found in leukemia/lymphoma, is invariably associated with what appears to be a particular mature B cell subset whereas Human T cell leukemia (retro-)

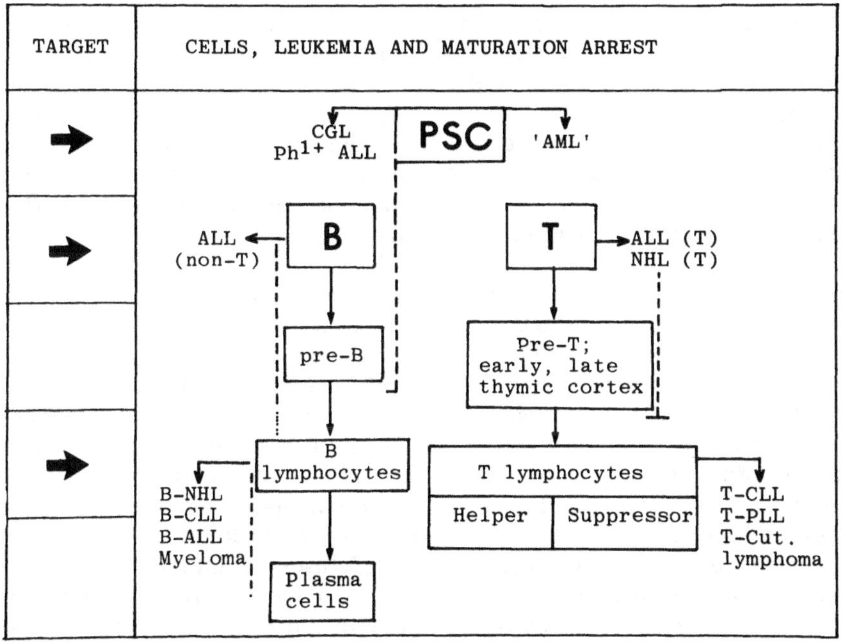

FIG. 1 - Target cells and maturation arrest in lymphoid malignancy.
➡ Major "target" cell population + postulated level of clonogenic population.
- - - - Maturation competence of major leukemic population in vivo. Taken from (17).

CGL, Chronic Granulocytic Leukemia; ALL, Acute Lymphoblastic Leukemia; AML, Acute Myeloblastic Leukemia; NHL, Non-Hodgkin Lymphoma; CLL, Chronic Lymphocytic Leukemia; PLL, Prolymphocytic Leukemia; ATL, Adult T Cell Leukemia (Human T Leukemia Virus-associated); PSC, Pluripotential Stem Cell; Ph^{1+}, Philadelphia Chromosome Positive.

virus (HTLV), the recently discovered retrovirus (44, 57), is integrated as a provirus in mature T cells of the $T4^{+}$ $T8^{-}$ "helper/inducer" antigenic subset in clinically distinct leukemias common in Japan and the Caribbean region.

There are some dissenting voices in these analyses. Thus McCulloch and colleagues (49) argue that differentiation programs are profoundly disturbed or scrambled in acute leukemia with co-expression of lineage markers indicating phenotypic infidelity with respect to the normal. In lymphoid leukemias this interpretation rests primarily on the observation of monoclonal immunoglobulin and spectrin in the same cell. It is difficult to know what to make of these observations since such "double" marked cells are said not to exist in normal tissue, and yet it is widely recognized that spectrin-like molecules (cross-reacting immunologically via their α-chain epitopes) are not at all erythroid-specific and can be identified in many cell types including lymphoid cells (40).

It is worth noting that the "phenotypic map" of leukemias and lymphomas reveals an interesting correlation between disease subtype, age association, and differentiation status (15). Thus lymphoid malignancies of children, at least in the developed countries, largely correspond to transformation of T or B cell precursors whilst in adults malignancies of mature, immunocompetent lymphocytes are the general rule. This generalization is paralleled in other cancers (e.g., childhood neural, connective tissue, and muscle tumors versus adult epithelial carcinomas (40)) and can most simply be interpreted as reflecting the cell types most "at risk" for oncogenic events at the gene level (15). Thus in fetuses and infants the progenitor populations would be most at risk due to the proliferative demands of lymphoid ontogeny. In contrast, in adults the long life span plus proliferative potential of immunocompetent, mature lymphoid populations (mostly memory cells) would provide a risk factor in association perhaps with disturbed regulatory controls of immune responses and/or repetitive carcinogenic insults over a prolonged period.

Phenotypic features which help subclassify lymphoid malignancies include immunoglobulin gene expression (26), differentiation-linked, cell surface antigens defined by monoclonal antibodies (reviewed in (16, 30)), enzymes, e.g., terminal deoxynucleotidyl transferase (2), and enzymes involved in nucleotide metabolism such as adenosine deaminase, PNP (purine nucleoside phosphorylase), 5' nucleotidase (53). The intriguing possibility of using selective expression of mRNA species identified from cDNA libraries has also been recently proposed (56).

On the basis of composite phenotypes observed, acute lymphoblastic leukemia can be divided into pre-T (or thymic) and pre-B subclasses (15, 17), both of which express the nuclear enzyme marker, TdT. Furthermore, within these two major subclasses it is possible to categorize broadly further subsets representing likely differentiation sequences or compartments. Thus the majority of T-ALL correspond to the earliest or most immature thymic cells (20, 43); the normal equivalent cell is represented by large, proliferating cells residing in the subcapsular region of the outer thymic cortex, representing no more than 1-2% of the total lymphocytes in a pediatric thymus (43, 54). The common or consistent phenotype of these cells is: T13$^+$, DR$^-$, Ig$^-$, TdT$^+$ (90% are also T1$^+$, T11$^+$). ALL corresponding to B cell precursors can be similarly divided according to expression of cell surface antigens and μ heavy chain genes (15, 17). Thus the least mature group would appear to be those that are DR$^+$, TdT$^+$, μ^-, cALL$^-$ (= "null ALL"), compared with the "common ALL" subclass that are DR$^+$, TdT$^+$, cALL$^+$, and μ^+ (in one third of the cases). These are overlapping rather than distinct subgroups both biologically and clinically (see below).

These differentiation-linked subdivisions have more recently been endorsed by molecular analyses of immunoglobulin heavy and light chain rearrangements (8, 26-29). To date, all ALL with a non-T phenotype have had rearranged μ genes (8, 26). Studies of normal B cell ontogeny (29) indicate a programmed sequence of Ig heavy and light chain gene rearrangements. Both Abelson virus-induced leukemias in mice and pre-B ALL in humans can involve clones corresponding to each of any of these stages of Ig gene "differentiation." These stages also show the anticipated correlation with other markers. Thus whilst most common ALL have rearranged light as well as heavy chains, not only rearranged heavy chain genes but germ line light chain genes are often found in null (cALLA$^-$) ALL (26).

Rearranged Ig genes are generally not observed in T-ALL, although a few T-ALL cell lines show changes in a single allele (8, 28). Rather more frequent Ig gene rearrangements (but probably restricted to D-J) have been observed in murine T cell leukemias (32). As would be expected, all mature B cell leukemias/lymphomas investigated have had rearranged Ig genes.

It is important to note that myeloid leukemias do not have rearranged Ig genes with one very interesting exception (7). When Philadelphia chromosome positive chronic granulocytic leukemia evolves into blast crisis, rearranged μ genes are observed exclusively in those cases in which a lymphoid pre-B (i.e., ALL-like) phenotype dominates (13). In this study granulocytic and pre-B lymphoid cells were available from the same clone which permitted two clear conclusions: a) the rearrangements were acquired and not constitutive polymorphisms, and b) the common lymphoid-myeloid stem cell which gave rise to these leukemias has a germ line Ig gene configuration of its μ gene.

FIDELITY OR PRESERVATION OF PHENOTYPE IN LYMPHOID MALIGNANCY HAS IMPLICATIONS FOR MECHANISMS OF LEUKEMOGENESIS

The overall fidelity of phenotype observed in lymphoid leukemia is imperfect, i.e., the malignant cells are not precise replicas of normal. Thus, some apparent asynchrony of gene expression compared to that postulated for normal cells can be identified (12). Also, with malignant progression and intense selection (e.g., in relapses and during establishment and continued culture of cell lines), additional phenotypic abnormalities may accrue. It is nevertheless very striking that no unequivocally leukemia-, lymphoma-specific antigens have been detected (14, 16), and in most patients presenting with a disseminated and lethal lymphoid malignancy the phenotype is essentially normal apart from the chromosomal changes (cf. "minimal deviation" concept of Potter (42)). You could argue that this is just what is expected and the subtle qualitative or quantitative alterations in proteins critically linked to leukemogenesis are simply not detected by the narrow observation "window" employed by immunologists to look at these cells. This may well be the case, but one can argue a different viewpoint. This is that perhaps in some leukemias and other cancers little or no true phenotypic alteration at all occurs outside of rearrangements in the genome itself and regulation of the oncogene-coded protein. The argument is that all the "information" required for leukemic cell "behavior" in vivo is intrinsic to the normal genome and even transiently expressed by normal, proliferating stem cells (11). What then happens in leukemogenesis is that genetic alterations effectively uncouple proliferation from differentiation (9, 10, 48) with the result that a normally rare and transient progenitor cell phenotype is stabilized (i.e., in relative maturation arrest) (10, 18). At this stage, no phenotypic abnormalities need be postulated to exist, although they could occur later with progression or relapse of disease and selection for altered sensitivity to growth factors. The corollary or prediction of this simple hypothesis is that some cellular oncogene products implicated in leukemia/lymphoma, e.g., c-myc in Burkitt's lymphoma (25), will be qualitatively or quantitatively altered in a manner which neutralizes or bars the effects of negative or down regulation. No greatly enhanced expression is required, but expression will simply be retained in an "on-mode," at relatively normal levels, compared to equivalent, normal dividing cells. In terms of phenotypic consequences, then, it might be necessary and sufficient simply to alter the time-frame of expression of an essentially normal phenotype (18). This conjures up in my mind a picture of leukemia similar to that portrayed to Alice by the Queen in Lewis Carroll's Alice Through the Looking Glass:

> "Now, here, you see, it takes all the running you can do, to keep in the same place."

I doubt if this explanation holds true for all or even most leukemias, but it may be a plausible hypothesis to hold for some leukemias, particularly in the early stages of progression (which can nevertheless still be clinically malignant!).

"TARGET" CELL POPULATIONS CANNOT BE DIRECTLY IDENTIFIED IN HUMAN LEUKEMIA BUT MAY BE INFERRED BY CLONAL AND PHENOTYPIC ANALYSIS. TARGET CELLS FOR LYMPHOID MALIGNANCY EXIST AT THREE DIFFERENT STAGES OF DIFFERENTIATION. THIS IS AN UNUSUAL OR UNIQUE FEATURE OF THIS TYPE OF CANCER.

Molecular biologists have recently highlighted the multistep nature of leukemogenesis (5, 33, 47) - something which hematologists, physicians, pathologists, and epidemiologists have in one sense taken for granted for some time. Given that an unknown number of selective "oncogene" events may precede the clinical detection of overt disease, it clearly is not possible to define accurately the "target" cell population. Indeed, there may not even be a discrete "target" population if successive essential steps occur in different but related cells. Despite this necessary reservation, it is possible to pinpoint the likely developmental level at which rare, clonal events may have occurred in various types of lymphoid malignancy.

All the data I am aware of are compatible with the view, discussed in detail elsewhere (17), that three distinct target cell populations exist for lymphoid malignancy: a) pluripotential stem cells for CGL which later evolves into "lymphoid blast crisis" or may occasionally commence (clinically) as Ph^1-positive ALL and later change to CGL (13); b) committed progenitors restricted to the T or B cell pathway in thymic (pre-T) or "common/null" (pre-B) ALL; c) mature, immunocompetent T or B lymphocytes providing, in adults, the target populations for the great majority of chronic leukemias, lymphomas, and myelomas.

The monoclonality of Ig light chain expression in B cell leukemias, lymphomas, and myelomas establishes that by the time these neoplasms are detected they have expanded from a single clone of mature B cells.

Similarly, the pattern of rearrangements of Ig genes observed when DNA from ALL cells are probed in Southern blots (8, 26) indicates monoclonality with respect to a B cell progenitor, i.e., only one or two rearrangements of parental alleles are observed. A word of caution here, however. The rearrangements observed in CGL in lymphoid blast crisis are also clearly indicative of clonal selection occurring at the level of a single committed B cell progenitor (8). However, we know in this case from enzymatic and karyotypic analysis (reviewed in (7, 13)) that the early oncogenic events in CGL occur at the level of multipotential progenitor. The conclusion we draw from this is that lymphoid blast crisis occurs as a consequence of a late(r) event at the level of a B cell committed progenitor which is, however, a member of the multilineage clonal progeny of the (Ph^1-positive) stem cell transformed by an earlier event (8). How then do we know that all lymphoid leukemias are not initiated subclinically at the stem cell level with subsequent events in more mature cell populations giving rise to overt disease and distinct cellular populations? The answer is that we do not know for sure, and indeed it has been argued that this is the origin of myeloma (31). I suspect that CGL is unique as a pluripotential leukemia and that all other lymphoid malignancies are clonally selected by events at the two more restricted levels of differentiation listed above. The reason for this view are as follows:

1 - Limited glucose 6 PD analyses in lymphoid leukemia (ALL and B-CLL) indicate monoclonality of lymphocytes and polyclonality of other cell lineages (i.e., in contrast to CGL) ((7), and Fialkow, personal communication).

2 - In contrast to CGL, where the pluri- or multipotential stem origin of early transformation events permits subsequent drastic intraclonal shifts in phenotype between lymphoid and myeloid characteristics, other lymphoid malignancies show a marked restraint in phenotypic shift (12). Thus pre-T and pre-B ALL's very rarely, if ever, evolve into myeloid leukemias. Moreover, pre-T and pre-B ALL, although showing some phenotypic changes in relapse, never in our experience shift between the B and T lineage categories. Similarly, by analogy with CGL in "myeloid" blast crisis, mature lymphoid malignancies have never been recorded to evolve intraclonally into pre-B or pre-T ALL. Such phenotypic shifts would be expected, by analogy with CGL, with at least modest frequency if these categories of leukemia originated in earlier developmental compartments and have a clinical course prolonged enough for these changes to occur.

3 - The widely divergent clinical response to Ph^1 CGL in "pre-B" blast crisis and Ph^1-negative ALL are best explained by differences in the transformed, target cell population involved (13).

It is probably relatively rare for malignant tumors of any sort to arise in mature cells. Most cancers probably originate in tissue stem cells (40). Mature T and B cells may provide unique "targets" in this respect due to their longevity and proliferative potential.

THE DEVELOPMENTAL LEVELS OF TARGET/TRANSFORMED CELLS, CLONOGENIC CELLS, AND BULK DISEASE PLUS THE OVERALL FIDELITY OF PHENOTYPES HAVE IMPORTANT CLINICAL IMPLICATIONS

Since the heterogeneity of immunological and enzymatic phenotypes is correlated in a consistent and relatively stable manner to biological subsets of cells, this provides us with new handles on discriminating diagnosis and therapy. It does not necessarily follow that biological heterogeneity as discussed above will correlate with clinical heterogeneity, particularly since the latter variable is itself dependent upon treatment regimes applied. However, there is ample evidence that the phenotypic subgroups detected in lymphoid malignancy are prognostically relevant and therefore of diagnostic value.

Thus pre-B and pre-T ALL have markedly different prognoses with almost all regimes of chemotherapy and irradiation, the former being curable at relatively high frequency (50-75%), the latter being much more intractable with a low "cure" rate (25%) (19, 39). The explanation for these correlations resides primarily, though not entirely, in the association between differentiation or lineage status and growth rate which is high in most T-ALL and low or modest in most pre-B ALL (19, 39). Immunological phenotype, white cell count, growth fraction, and karyotype together constitute a diagnostic set for identifying high versus low risk patients and hence allocation of appropriate therapy. Immunological phenotypes are also of value in identifying those acute leukemias which are considered "undifferentiated or AUL (Acute Undifferentiated Leukemia)," or in whom a distinction between myeloid and lymphoid is not possible.

Similarly, in blast crisis of CGL, an immunological phenotype is a predictor of a response to "ALL"-type therapy including steroid (24, 37). Herein lies an interesting and revealing fact. Pre-B ALL and pre-B CGL in blast crisis both respond well to steroid therapy; they do so almost certainly because these cells maintain the normal steroid sensitivity of lymphocyte precursors. However, the former is "cured" at high frequency whilst the latter is incurable by conventional treatment. The explanation for this paradox lies in the distinction between drug sensitivity of bulk disease in maturation arrest and the clonogenic or potentially clonogenic population (13). Pluripotential stem cells are relatively steroid-resistant and in the transformed state could only be entirely eliminated by therapeutic regimes which ablate normal stem cell pools to lethal levels. Hence, despite transient remission induced by steroids, CGL invariably relapses (unless the patient is successfully transplanted) whereas in pre-B ALL the clonogenic population presumably exists with the same steroid-sensitive B cell compartment as the majority of the clonal progeny typed by cell markers and can therefore be eliminated. Long-term remission or cure is then possible in ALL, provided steroid or drug-resistant mutants have not arisen prior to the commencement of therapy - which, unfortunately, is almost certainly what does occur in the more rapidly evolving T-ALL (19). The developmental level of the "target" or clonogenic populations in leukemia therefore has a major impact on overall therapeutic response.

Despite the plethora of histopathological classifications that are still applied to the non-Hodgkin lymphomas, prognostic subclasses can be fairly consistently defined, and the overall correlation with immunological subtypes is quite good (1, 21, 23, 50). It is interesting, however, that as in ALL, growth rate or fraction of different cell types may be a more significant parameter than differentiation phenotype per se. Thus, we observed that high expression of the cell surface receptor for transferrin, detected by monoclonal antibody OKT9, was strongly associated with subgroups of poor prognosis (22).

Immunological phenotypes in conjunction with kinetic parameters (e.g., DNA content measured by flow cytofluorimetry or detected by transferrin receptors) and karyotype now provide the basis for a routine laboratory analysis of leukemias and lymphomas. These data are currently incorporated into therapeutic schemes structured both as randomized trials and single protocol strategies.

More significantly perhaps, the consistent phenotypes detectable in lymphoid malignancy have provided the impetus for exploring the possibility of immunotherapy with monoclonal antibodies, directed not at the elusive tumor-specific determinants (which I do not believe exist!) but at cell-type or clonally restricted surface determinants correlated with maturation stage or proliferation status (e.g., 37, 45, 52)).

The success of these new ventures will depend upon the identification of monoclonal antibodies or cocktails of antibodies (35) which comprehensively and consistently "cover" the potential antigenic heterogeneity of the clonogenic fractions of disease (14) and efficiently remove these cells (e.g., magnetic or affinity filtration of autologous marrow in vitro) or deliver a lethal hit (e.g., with complement, toxins, or isotopes) in vivo or in vitro (4).

Finally, the associations now emerging between lymphoid subset, karyotypic changes, specific oncogene involvement, and disease diversity have an obvious implication for epidemiological studies of lymphoid malignancy. The association between HTLV and T cell leukemia in Japan emerged in part because of the ability of immunologists there to identify T cells unequivocally. In the past, epidemiological investigations of leukemia have not involved subtyping, and few if any interesting geographic or ethnic associations have emerged (except perhaps for the relative scarcity of B-CLL and B cell follicular lymphoma in Japan and SE Asia). Important associations may, however, emerge as lymphoid subset identification is taken into account (36).

REFERENCES

(1) Bloomfield, C.D.; Gajl-Peczalska, K.J.; Frizzera, G.; Kersey, J.H.; and Goldman, A.I. 1979. Clinical utility of lymphocyte surface markers combined with the Lukes-Collins histologic classification in adult lymphoma. N. Eng. J. Med. 301: 512-518.

(2) Bollum, F. 1979. Terminal deoxynucleotidyl transferase as a hemopoietic cell marker. Blood 54: 1203-1215.

(3) Brouet, J.C., and Seligmann, M. 1978. Immunological classification of acute lymphoblastic leukemias. Cancer 42: 817-827.

(4) Crumpton, M.C., and Davies, A.J.S. 1983. Cancer Surveys, vol. 3. Oxford University Press.

(5) Diamond, A.; Cooper, G.M.; Ritz, J.; and Lane, M-A. 1983. Identification and molecular cloning of the human Blym transforming gene activated in Burkitt's lymphomas. Nature 305: 112-116.

(6) Eva, A.; Tronick, S.R.; Gol, R.A.; Pierce, J.H.; and Aaronson, S.A. 1983. Transforming genes of human hematopoietic tumors: Frequent

detection of ras-related oncogenes whose activation appears to be independent of tumor phenotype. Proc. Natl. Acad. Sci. USA 80: 4926-4930.

(7) Fialkow, P. 1982. Cell lineages in hematopoietic neoplasia studied with glucose-6-phosphate dehydrogenase cell markers. J. Cell. Physiol. Suppl. 1: 37-43.

(8) Ford, A.M.; Molgaard, H.V.; Greaves, M.F.; and Gould, H.J. 1983. Immunoglobulin gene organisation and expression in haemopoietic stem cell leukaemia. EMBO J. 2: 997-1001.

(9) Greaves, M.F. 1979. Cell surface characteristics of human leukaemic cells. In Essays in Biochemistry, eds. P.N. Campbell and R.D. Marshall, vol. 15, pp. 78-124. London: Academic Press.

(10) Greaves, M.F. 1979. Tumour markers, phenotypes and maturation arrest in malignancy: A cell selection hypothesis. In Tumour Markers, eds. E. Boelsma and P. Rümke, pp. 201-211. New York: A.R. Liss, Inc.

(11) Greaves, M.F. 1982. Leukaemogenesis and differentiation: A commentary on recent progress and ideas. Cancer Surveys 1(2): 189-204.

(12) Greaves, M.F. 1982. 'Target' cells, cellular phenotypes and lineage fidelity in human leukaemia. J. Cell. Physiol. Suppl. 1: 113-126.

(13) Greaves, M.F. 1982. 'Target' cells, differentiation and clonal evolution in chronic granulocytic leukaemia: A 'model' for understanding the biology of malignancy. In Chronic Granulocytic Leukaemia, ed. M.T. Shaw, pp. 15-47. London: Praeger Publ.

(14) Greaves, M.F. 1982. 'Target' structures and 'target' cells for cancer therapy with monoclonal antibodies: Finding the candidates. Cancer Surveys 1(3): 451-466.

(15) Greaves, M.F.; Delia, D.; Katz, F.; Schneider, C.; Sutherland, R.; and Newman, R. 1983. Biological diversity of acute lymphoblastic leukaemia. In Leukaemia Research: Advances in Cell Biology and Treatment, eds. S. Murphy and J. Gilbert, pp. 97-116. Amsterdam: Elsevier, North Holland.

(16) Greaves, M.F.; Delia, D.; Newman, R.A.; and Vodinelich, L. 1982. Analysis of leukaemic cells with monoclonal antibodies. In Monoclonal Antibodies in Clinical Medicine, eds. A.J. McMichael and J.W. Fabre, pp. 129-165. London: Academic Press.

(17) Greaves, M.F.; Delia, D.; Robinson, J.; Sutherland, R.; and Newman, R. 1981. Exploitation of monoclonal antibodies: A 'Who's who' of haemopoietic malignancy. Blood Cells 7: 257-280.

(18) Greaves, M.F., and Janossy, G. 1978. Patterns of gene expression and the cellular origins of human leukaemias. Biochim. Biophys. Acta 516: 193-230.

(19) Greaves, M.F.; Janossy, G.; Peto, J.; and Kay, H. 1981. Immunologically defined subclasses of acute lymphoblastic leukaemia in children: their relationship to presentation features and prognosis. Br. J. Haematol. 48: 179-197.

(20) Greaves, M.F.; Rao, J.; Hariri, G.; Verbi, W.; Catovsky, D.; Kung, P.; and Goldstein, G. 1981. Phenotypic heterogeneity and cellular origins of T cell malignancies. Leukemia Res. 5: 281-299.

(21) Habeshaw, J.A.; Bailey, D.; Stansfeld, A.G.; and Greaves, M.F. 1e cellular content of non Hodgkin lymphomas. A comprehensive anhenotypialysis using monoclonal antibodies and other surface marker techniques. Brit. J. Cancer 47: 327-351.

(22) Habeshaw, J.A.; Lister, T.A.; Stansfeld, A.G.; and Greaves, M.F. 1983. Correlation of transferrin receptor expression with histological class and outcome in non Hodgkin lymphoma. Lancet i: 498-500.

(23) Jaffe, E.S.; Braylan, R.C.; Nanba, K.; Frank, M.M.; and Berard, C.W. 1977. Functional markers, a new perspective on malignant lymphomas. Cancer Treat. Rep. 61: 953.

(24) Janossy, G.; Woodruff, R.K.; Pippard, M.J.; Prentice, G.; Hoffbrand, A.V.; Paxton, A.; Lister, T.A.; Bunch, C.; and Greaves, M.F. 1979. Relation of 'lymphoid' phenotype and response to chemotherapy incorporating vincristine-prednisolone in the acute phase of Ph^1 positive leukaemia. Cancer 43: 426-434.

(25) Kelin, G. 1982. The role of specific chromosomal translocations and trisomies in the origin of some murine and human tumours of lymphoid origin. Cancer Surveys 1(2): 299-308.

(26) Korsmeyer, S.J.; Arnold, A.; Bakhshi, A.; Ravetch, J.V.; Siebenlist, U.; Hieter, P.A.; Sharrow, S.O.; LeBien, T.W.; Kersey, J.H.; Poplack, D.G.; Leder, P.; and Waldmann, T.A. 1983. Immunoglobulin gene rearrangement and cell surface antigen expression in acute lymphocytic leukemias of T cell and B cell precursor origins. J. Clin. Invest. 71: 301-313.

(27) Korsmeyer, S.J.; Greene, W.C.; Cossman, J.; Hsu, S-M.; Jensen, J.P.; Neckers, L.M.; Marshall, S.L.; Bakhshi, A.; Depper, J.M.; Leonard, W.J.; Jaffe, E.S.; and Waldmann, T.A. 1983. Rearrangement and expression of immunoglobulin genes and expression of Tac antigen in hairy cell leukemia. Proc. Natl. Acad. Sci. USA 80: 4522-4526.

(28) Korsmeyer, S.J.; Hieter, P.A.; Ravetch, J.V.; Poplack, D.G.; Waldmann, T.A.; and Leder, P. 1981. Developmental hierarchy of immunoglobulin gene rearrangements in human leukemic pre-B cells. Proc. Natl. Acad. Sci. USA 78: 7096-7100.

(29) Korsmeyer, S.J.; Hieter, P.A.; Sharrow, S.O.; Goldman, C.K.; Leder, P.; and Waldmann, T.A. 1982. Normal human B cells display ordered light-chain gene rearrangements and deletions. J. Exp. Med. 156: 975-985.

(30) Knapp, W., ed. 1981. Leukemia Markers. New York: Academic Press.

(31) Kubagawa, H.; Vogler, L.B.; Capra, J.D.; Conrad, M.E.; Lawton, A.R.; and Cooper, M.D. 1979. Studies on the clonal origin of multiple myeloma: Use of individually specific (idiotype) antibodies to trace the oncogenic event to its earliest point of expression in B-cell differentiation. J. Exp. Med. 150: 792-807.

(32) Kurosawa, Y.; von Boehmer, H.; Haas, W.; Sakano, H.; Trauneker, H.; and Tonegawa, S. 1981. Identification of immunoglobulin heavy chain genes and their rearrangement in T lymphocytes. Nature 290: 565-570.

(33) Land, H.; Parada, L.F.; and Weinberg, R.A. 1983. Tumorigenic conversion of primary embryo fibroblasts requires at least two cooperating oncogenes. Nature 304: 596-601.

(34) Lane, M-A.; Sainten, A.; and Cooper, G.M. 1982. Stage-specific transforming genes of human and mouse B- and T-lymphocyte neoplasms. Cell 28: 873-880.

(35) LeBien, T.W.; Ash, R.C.; Zanjani, E.D.; and Kersey, J.H. 1983. In vitro cytodestruction of leukemic cells in human bone marrow using a cocktail of monoclonal antibodies. In Modern Trends in Human Leukemia V, eds. R. Neth, R.C. Gallo, M.F. Greaves, M.A.S. Moore, and K. Winkler, pp. 112-116. Berlin, Heidelberg: Springer-Verlag.

(36) Magrath, I., and Ramot, B., eds. 1983. The Influence of the Environment on Leukemia and Lymphoma Subtypes. New York: Raven Press.

(37) Marks, S.M.; Baltimore, D.; and McCaffrey, R. 1978. Terminal transferase as a predictor of initial responsiveness to vincristine-prednisone in blastic chronic myelogenous leukemia. N. Eng. J. Med. 298: 812-814.

(38) Miller, R.A.; Maloney, D.G.; Warnke, R.; and Levy, R. 1982. Treatment of B-cell lymphoma with monoclonal anti-idiotype antibody. N. Eng. J. Med. 306: 517-522.

(39) Murphy, S., and Gilbert, J., eds. 1983. Leukaemia Research: Advances in Cell Biology and Treatment. Amsterdam: Elsevier, North Holland.

(40) Nelson, W.J.; Colaco, C.A.L.S.; and Lazarides, E. 1983. Involvement of spectrin in cell-surface receptor capping in lymphocytes. Proc. Natl. Acad. Sci. USA 80: 1625-1630.

(41) Pierce, G.B.; Shikes, R.; and Fink, L.M. 1978. Cancer: A Problem of Developmental Biology. New Jersey: Prentice Hall Inc.

(42) Potter, V.R. 1978. Phenotypic diversity in experimental heptomas: The concept of partially blocked ontogeny. Br. J. Cancer 38: 1-23.

(43) Reinherz, E.L.; Kung, P.C.; Goldstein, G.; Levey, R.H.; and Schlossman, S.F. 1980. Discrete stages of human intrathymic differentiation: Analysis of normal thymocytes and leukemic lymphoblasts of T lineage. Proc. Natl. Acad. Sci. USA 77: 1588-1592.

(44) Reitz, M.S.; Poiesz, B.J.; Ruscetti, F.W.; and Gallo, R.C. 1981. Characterization and distribution of nucleic acid sequences of a novel type C retrovirus isolated from neoplastic human T lymphocytes. Proc. Natl. Acad. Sci. USA 78: 1887-1891.

(45) Ritz, J.; Sallan, S.E.; Bast, R.C.; Lipton, J.M.; Clavell, L.A.; Feeney, M.; Hercend, T.; Nathan, D.G.; and Schlossman, S.F. 1982. Autologous bone marrow transplantation in cALLA positive acute lymphoblastic leukaemia following in vitro treatment with J5 monoclonal antibody and complement. Lancet ii: 60-63.

(46) Rowley, J.D. 1983. Human oncogene locations and chromosome aberrations. Nature 301: 290-291.

(47) Ruley, H.E. 1983. Adenovirus early region 1A enables viral and cellular transforming genes to transform primary cells is culture. Nature 304: 602-606.

(48) Sachs, L. 1980. Constitutive uncoupling of pathways of gene expression that control growth and differentiation in myeloid leukemia: A model for the origin and progression of malignancy. Proc. Natl. Acad. Sci. USA 77: 6152-6156.

(49) Smith, L.J.; Curtis, J.E.; Messner, H.A.; Senn, J.S.; Furthmayr, H.; and McCulloch, E.A. 1983. Lineage fidelity in acute leukemia. Blood 61: 1138-1145.

(50) Stein, H.; Bonk, A.; Tolksdorf, G.; Lennert, K.; Rodt, H.; and Gerdes, J. 1980. Immunohistological analysis of the organization of normal lymphoid tissue and non-Hodgkin's lymphomas. J. Histochem. Cytochem. 28: 746-760.

(51) Stein, H.; Gerdes, J.; Schwab, U.; Lemke, H.; Mason, D.Y.; Ziegler, A.; Schienle, W.; and Diehl, V. 1982. Identification of Hodgkin and Sternberg-Reed cells as a unique cell type derived from a newly-detected small-cell population. Int. J. Cancer 30: 445-459.

(52) Sutherland, R.; Delia, D.; Schneider, C.; Newman, R.; Kemshead, J.; and Greaves, M. 1981. Ubiquitous, cell surface glycoprotein on tumour cells is proliferation-associated receptor for transferrin. Proc. Natl. Acad. Sci. USA 78: 4515-4519.

(53) Sylwestrowicz, T.A.; Ma, D.D.F.; Murphy, P.P.; Prentice, H.G.; Hoffbrand, A.V.; and Greaves, M.F. 1982. 5' nucleotidase, adenosine deaminase and purine nucleoside phosphorylase activities in acute leukaemia. Leukemia Res. 4: 475-482.

(54) Tidman, N.; Janossy, G.; Bodger, M.; Granger, S.; Kung, P.C.; and Goldstein, G. 1981. Delineation of human thymocyte differentiation pathways utilizing double-staining techniques with monoclonal antibodies. Clin. Exp. Immunol. 45: 457-467.

(55) Trowbridge, I.S., and Domingo, D.L. 1982. Prospects for the clinical use of cytotoxic monoclonal antibody conjugates in the treatment of cancer. Cancer Surveys 1(3): 543-556.

(56) Wiedemann, L.M.; Burns, J.H.; and Birnie, G.D. 1983. Differences among the polyadenylated RNA sequences of human leucocyte populations: an approach to the objective classification of human leukaemias. EMBO 2: 9-13.

(57) Yoshida, M.; Miyoshi, I.; and Hinuma, Y. 1982. Isolation and characterization of retrovirus from cell lines of human adult T-cell leukemia and its implication in the disease. Proc. Natl. Acad. Sci. USA 79: 2031-2035.

Leukemia, ed. I.L. Weissman, pp. 111-130. Dahlem Konferenzen 1985. Berlin, Heidelberg, New York, Tokyo: Springer-Verlag.

Differentiation of T Lymphocytes

J.J.T. Owen
Dept. of Anatomy, University of Birmingham
Birmingham B15 2TJ, England

Abstract. Differentiation of T cells from stem cells to mature, functional subsets is discussed. Arguments concerning the level of maturation achieved by pre-T cells and the absolute necessity of intrathymic processing are evaluated. Emphasis is placed on the crucial role of the thymus in T cell differentiation, and recently acquired information about the heterogeneous thymic stromal cell types should provide a sound basis for further work on intrathymic events. The use of phenotypic markers and functional studies to analyze T cell lineage relationships is discussed in the context of some of the conflicting data available.

INTRODUCTION

It is now more than twenty years since the crucial role of the thymus in the maturation of the immune response was first demonstrated. The severe immune deficiency which results from neonatal thymectomy, but not from adult thymectomy, of rodents illustrates the importance of the thymus in early development. Subsequently, it was shown that the thymus produces its effect by exporting lymphocytes (later named T lymphocytes) to other developing lymphoid organs where they participate in immune responses. The lymphocytes of the thymus are derived from stem cells which migrate into the organ from the blood. Hence, the thymus imports stem cells, matures them into T cells which then seed to peripheral lymphoid organs (reviewed in (40)). These results have been confirmed in subsequent studies using a variety of methods in a number of vertebrate species. However, some key questions remain unanswered, and I will attempt to evaluate the various propositions which relate to them.

IS PASSAGE OF CELLS THROUGH THE THYMUS OBLIGATORY FOR T CELL MATURATION? IN VITRO VERSUS IN VIVO DATA

The idea of an extra thymic pathway of T cell maturation has been mooted on a number of occasions. One of the major pillars supporting such arguments is the detection of cells with some of the morphological and functional characteristics of T lymphocytes in nude mice which lack a lymphoid thymus. These cells carry the Thy-1 and other T cell antigens and they are capable of developing into cytolytic cells in culture. Their frequency and antigenic phenotype varies with age and pathogenic status of nude mice (51). Few Thy-1^+ cells are found in the lymphoid organs of SPF nude mice less than six weeks old; thereafter, their number increases but is always substantially lower than that of T cells in normal mice. A curious feature of most Thy-1^+ cells in the spleens of young nude mice is that they are also TL^+ - in normal mice, TL^+ cells are found only in the thymic cortex. In addition, like normal cortical thymocytes, these cells are Lyt-123^+. In older nude mice, the proportion of Thy-1^+ cells which are TL^+ declines, while the number which are Qa-1^+ increases, and there is evidence of diversification into Lyt-1^+ and Lyt-23^+ subsets.

Superficially, these results suggest that nude mice have a T cell differentiation pathway which follows the pattern of changes of surface antigen expression seen in T cells of normal mice. However, the greatest obstacle to accepting these results as evidence of an extra thymic pathway is the lack of T cell function in nude mice. Although in vitro, Thy-1^+ cells of nude mice are capable of developing into cytolytic cells, killing of target cells has been reported to be nonspecific (11), antigen-specific but not MHC-restricted (18), antigen-specific and MHC-restricted (1, 38), and sometimes specific (42)! The variability of results obtained in similar assay systems hardly encourages confidence in the conclusions or, for that matter, in the methods as performed here where low functional activity requires the presence of IL-2 (interleukin 2). However, the most serious criticism of the notion that Thy-1^+ cells in nude mice are T lymphocytes is that in vivo they are unable to alleviate the gross T cell-associated immune deficiency of nude mice, whereas injection of as few as 10^6 normal syngeneic thymocytes can restore immunity (29). Nor can the argument that they merely lack the ability to produce IL-2 (if this is true) be easily sustained, since injection of IL-2 into nude mice does not restore immunity - although this might be explained by the fact that IL-2 has a serum half-life of only 3.7 minutes after IV injection (12)! Likewise, the significance of Thy-1^+ cytolytic cells generated in thymectomized, irradiated chimeras transplanted with bone marrow depleted of Thy-1^+ cells (14) and of cytolytic cells grown in spleen and bone marrow colonies (9) must be questioned, since generation of cytotoxicity is not limited to T cells and in neither case has an in vivo T cell role for these cells been demonstrated.

Earlier arguments for a thymic-independent pathway of T cell maturation based on the failure of intrauterine thymectomy to prevent the genesis of T cells in fetal sheep are easily dismissed on the basis that thymic lymphopoiesis had proceeded for at least thirty days prior to thymectomy, allowing ample time for migration of thymus-processed cells to the periphery (28). However, what these experiments may tell us is that the initial waves of lymphocytes to migrate from thymus to peripheral lymphoid organs have considerable stem cell capabilities. The fact that thymectomy of rodents, if delayed beyond the first few days of life, has a much reduced effect on the maturation of T cell responses in vivo (as reviewed in (41)) also argues for the notion that sufficient T cells migrate from the thymus in early life to provide a repertoire which is adequate for the development and maintenance of an efficient immune system. Interestingly, the inability of thymic hormones to restore immunity in athymic animals has drawn proponents of thymic hormones to the conclusion that these act on post-thymic T cells (2, 57). However, the lack of effect of thymectomy delayed beyond the neonatal period suggests that if thymic hormones are necessary for the maturation of post-thymic T cells, they must act over a short period of time. Alternatively, they may act intrathymically.

In conclusion, despite many in vitro studies claiming to demonstrate a thymic-independent pathway of T cell maturation, in vivo data collected in the 1960s which show the drastic effect of neonatal thymectomy on immunogenesis (later confirmed in athymic nude mice), together with the ability of thymic grafts or small numbers of thymus-derived cells to alleviate these effects, argue for the necessity of intrathymic processing in the T cell maturation pathway. Although the development of cells expressing T cell antigens in nude mice might indicate that a retarded extra thymic pathway is possible, the support provided for this idea by in vitro studies is questionable because of the uncertainty of their functional significance.

ARE PRE-T CELLS ALREADY MATURED ALONG THE T CELL PATHWAY BEFORE THEY MIGRATE TO THE THYMUS? INDUCIBLE PHENOTYPIC CHANGES, REPERTOIRE DEVELOPMENT, AND SPARSE SEEDING OF THE THYMUS

In recent years, a number of papers have claimed that pre-T cells are already partially mature prior to migration to the thymus. Many of these claims have been based upon observations that some cells in hemopoietic tissues can be induced in vitro to express surface antigens characteristic of the T cell lineage (30, 37). Treatment with thymic hormones or with a variety of agents which elevate intracellular cyclic AMP produces this effect. However, it is questionable whether these results can be accepted as evidence for pre-T cell maturation since in no instance has direct proof of the ability of the cells in question to migrate to and to proliferate in the thymus been shown. In one study an attempt was made to demonstrate the capacity of inducible spleen cells to repopulate the thymus of irradiated mice (30). Although treatment with antibody to the induced surface antigen (Thy-1) in the presence of complement was said to reduce the effectiveness of induced spleen cells, certain aspects of the study may be questioned. First, it is not clear why spleen cells (as opposed to the more usual source of thymic stem cells - bone marrow) were used. Second, thymic repopulation was measured by the percentage of cells carrying donor-type TL antigen. Although this percentage was reduced in animals injected with induced and antibody-treated spleen cells, no overall effect on the total recovery of thymus lymphocytes was found. This is difficult to understand if the number of stem cells in the donor inoculum was reduced by Thy-1 induction and subsequent antibody treatment. Questions may also be asked about the recent claim that Tpre, an alloantigen encoded in the IgT-C region of chromosome 12, is expressed on mouse pre-T cells (47). Anti Tpre, but not anti Thy-1, antibody plus complement reduced the ability of marrow cells to repopulate the irradiated thymus. However, considerable variations in thymic recovery between individual mice may be noted in the data, and evidence is presented elsewhere in the same paper (47) that $Tpre^+$ marrow cells are also $Thy\text{-}1^+$, thus contradicting the earlier results.

In another approach to this question, Morrissey et al. attempted to demonstrate that pre-T cells generate antigen recognition receptors prior to entry to the thymus (44). Strain A thymus was transplanted into (A x B)F_1 mice, which were then irradiated and repopulated with stain A bone marrow cells. Cells repopulating the thymic graft were shown to be of donor A marrow origin and were tolerant to host B determinants. Since the authors could not detect stain B MHC determinants in thymus cell suspensions, they argued that pre-T cells must have been exposed to these antigens pre-thymically and hence possess antiallogeneic MHC receptors through which they can be rendered specifically tolerant. However, the authors did not exclude the possibility that F_1 cells (for example, dendritic cell precursors, as discussed later) might migrate into the grafted thymus and contribute to the thymic stroma. Thymus grafts are known to undergo a period of initial necrosis followed by regeneration (13) which might accelerate dendritic cell turnover. Although dendritic cells are potent stimulators of alloreactivity in fully mature T cells, the presentation of host cell antigens on medullary dendritic cells might provide a potent mechanism for inducing tolerance in immature T cells as they approach maturation at the corticomedullary junction. Using a different experimental design, Besedovsky et al. claimed that tolerance to alloantigens can be induced in pre-T cells (7). Here, BALB/c nude mice, which had been grafted with allogeneic thymus, were shown to accept BALB/c skin grafts. The authors reasoned that since the alloantigens of the thymus graft could not have induced tolerance to BALB/c grafts, lack of self-reactivity must be due to mechanisms operating at the pre-T cell level (they provided evidence that post-thymic cells are not rendered tolerant). However, again this argument overlooks the possibility that syngeneic BALB/c antigens might be present within the thymic graft on migrant dendritic cells and, of course, on the host-derived lymphocytes which populate the graft. If tolerance does operate at the pre-T cell level, a possible mechanism has recently been suggested by Muraoka and Miller (45). Cells in fetal liver or in lymphoid colonies grown from fetal liver can suppress the development of cytotoxic activity in mixed lymphocyte reactions. The suppression has specificity since it is only found when the suppressors (named "veto cells") are of the same haplotype as either responder or target. Veto cells are Thy-1^- in fetal liver, but are Thy-1^+ in bone marrow. The authors suggest that veto cells might maintain self-tolerance.

Other considerations reduce the likelihood of pre-T cell repertoire development. Although it has been commonly assumed that there is considerable inflow of stem cells to the thymus throughout the life span of an individual, chromosome marker experiments, which first demonstrated inflow of stem cells to the thymus, also indicated that the inflow of cells was slow (16). These observations were confirmed in later experiments in which the thymus of irradiated mice was repopulated with mixtures of two syngeneic but chromosomally distinguishable bone marrow populations (62). Individual thymic lobes varied considerably in the proportions of cells derived from each marrow type and probability analysis suggested that as few as ten stem cells were responsible for thymic repopulation. An intermittent inflow of stem cells has been demonstrated during avian embryogenesis (34), but the number of stem cells entering the thymus in each migratory phase is not known. We have been able to colonize mouse embryonic thymus rudiments, previously depleted of lymphoid cells by culture in the presence of deoxyguanosine (49), with very small numbers of lymphoblastic cells removed from 13-day embryonic thymus. As few as five cells will recolonize an alymphoid thymus and during a period of culture will generate many thymus lymphocytes. If few stem cells colonize the thymus, generation of the repertoire at a pre-thymic level without further expansion intrathymically would greatly limit the diversity of T cells.

In conclusion, direct evidence for maturation of pre-T cells prior to migration to the thymus is lacking. Relatively few stem cells may colonize the thymic stroma - the implication of this notion is that intrathymic processing is required for T cell diversification.

COMPONENTS OF THE THYMIC STROMA: ARE THERE DISTINCT MICROENVIRONMENTS WITHIN THE THYMUS?

The conclusions reached in the preceding sections focus on the importance of the thymic stroma in T cell maturation. Surprisingly, after so many years of study, the developmental origins of thymic stromal cells are still uncertain. There is little doubt that a major component of the stroma derives from pharyngeal epithelium. However, conflicting results on the relative roles of ectoderm and endoderm have been reported. On the one hand, it has been claimed that avian pharyngeal endoderm, when separated from ectoderm and cultured with mesenchyme, will form a thymus, thereby ruling out the intervention of ectoderm in thymic differentiation (34). On the other hand, it has been shown that extirpation of pharyngeal ectoderm during avian development results in the formation of embryos with small thymic remnants (22). This observation is particularly interesting in view of comparative studies of thymic morphogenesis in nude and normal mice where the failure of ectoderm to contribute to thymic development is said to be the basis for the thymic defect in nude mice (10). Could the endodermal remnant found in avian embryos following extirpation of ectoderm be the counterpart of the nude mouse thymic remnant? There is less doubt about the importance of pharyngeal mesenchyme in thymic histogenesis, both in providing necessary inductive interactions with epithelium and in contributing directly to the thymic stroma. It has recently been realized that bone marrow-derived dendritic cells also occupy fixed positions within the thymic medulla (4, 52).

The possibility that the thymus might direct the major histocompatibility complex (MHC) restriction pattern of T cells (66) as well as induce unresponsiveness to self-MHC antigens (20) has heightened interest in the expression of MHC antigens on thymic stromal cells on the basis that they might act positively or negatively to select differentiating T cells. Both class I and class II MHC antigens are expressed on thymic stromal cells, but the pattern of expression is complex and it has been suggested that distinct MHC microenvironments for T cell maturation exist (60). Before discussing this further, it is useful to define the distinction between cortex and medulla since they are the most obvious histological areas. Although traditionally the cortex is identified as the outer part of each lobule and the medulla as its center, in practice these regions are recognized by the density of lymphoid cells they contain. The cortex is packed with lymphocytes and the cortical stromal cells possess thin wafer-like cytoplasmic processes which envelope lymphocytes. The medulla is more sparsely populated by lymphocytes and so the stromal cells are more compact and obvious.

Examination of frozen sections labeled with the appropriate antibodies shows that class II (Ia) antigens are distributed throughout both cortical and medullary stromal cells. However, analysis of radiation chimeras indicates that, whereas cortical epithelial cells express Ia antigen of host type, medullary Ia^+ cells are of donor marrow origin (4, 52). These marrow-derived cells are probably antigen-presenting, dendritic cells as described in other studies (6). The dendritic cells could account for all Ia positivity of the medulla, i.e., the medullary epithelial cells might be Ia^-. In this context, it is of interest to note that the epithelial cells of the nude mouse thymic remnant and the cells which line cysts developing in cultures of normal embryonic thymus are Ia^- (48). These observations suggest the possibility that, like the Ia^- nude thymus, some of the medullary epithelial cells are derived from endoderm and that it is the cortical epithelial cells, which are strongly Ia^+, which are derived from ectoderm. Caution, however, is required in using Ia expression as a marker of cell lineage since Ia expression in some other tissues is now known to be highly variable, depending in some instances on immune stimulation (3).

In frozen sections of thymus, class I antigens are strongly expressed in medullary regions but are weakly expressed or absent in cortical areas (60). However, medullary dendritic cells show strong class I antigen expression (17), and they may account for much of the intensity of medullary staining. Cortical epithelial cells do show class I antigen expression when studied as unfixed cells growing out as monolayers from thymic fragments (48). The epithelial cells of the nude mouse thymus, although lacking class II antigens, express class I MHC antigens (48).

Thus, a complex picture emerges in which there seems to be a marked distinction between cortex and medulla. Cortex, which is thickly populated by lymphocytes, is made up of a network of epithelial cells which express class I and class II MHC antigens - the latter much more strongly. We have noted that these cells also stain strongly with antibodies to prekeratin filaments. The medulla, which is sparsely populated by lymphocytes, contains epithelial cells, some of which are Ia^-. However, the medulla also contains a network of marrow-derived dendritic cells, many of which express class II as well as class I antigens. Recently, thymic stromal cells have been described which bind a monoclonal antibody (antibody A2 B5) to a ganglioside (24). We have noted the presence of these cells in both the medulla and cortex of the embryonic mouse thymus. They are probably Ia^- and also fail to react with antibody to prekeratin filaments. They are present in the nude mouse thymus and seem to represent yet another stromal cell type. There is some evidence that they may be involved in the synthesis of thymic hormones (24), which, if correct, is interesting in view of their presence in nude mice.

Of course, the crucial question is, what is the functional significance of these observations? Cortical lymphocytes are generated by the proliferation of precursor cells situated in the outer cortex, and as they mature they pass to the corticomedullary junction from where at least some migrate to peripheral organs - many others, however, probably die in the cortex. The association between cortical lymphocytes and epithelial cells is an intimate one - witness the thymic nurse cells which are closely associated with clusters of maturing lymphocytes (33). Ia antigen is expressed on thymic epithelial cells from an early stage of gestation when lymphopoiesis is beginning in the absence of expression on other fetal organs. It is tempting to draw the inference that Ia expression on cortical epithelial cells in some way directs the MHC restriction pattern of the differentiating T cells. However, direct evidence for this is lacking, although a recent report indicates that injection of anti-Ia antibodies into neonatal mice can interfere with the development of MHC restriction of helper T cells (31). This was said to be associated with reduced Ia expression, although the latter was measured very indirectly by assessing Ia antigen passively acquired by thymocytes. The significance of medullary stromal cells, especially of the dendritic cell population, is even more puzzling. Medullary lymphocytes are thought to be a population of mature cells with a slow turnover. However, the persistence of medullary lymphocytes within the thymus was based on experiments in which resting cells were activated with phytohemaglutinin to allow chromosome marker analysis - hence, only a sample of PHA-responsive cells was examined (15). The turnover of medullary lymphocytes as a whole may be greater than previously thought. Could the dendritic cells be involved in tolerance induction? What is the significance of the cells with membrane gangliosides?

In conclusion, progress is being made in unraveling the complex mixture of cell types which constitute the thymic stroma. Interesting differences have been noted in the expression of MHC antigens on stromal cells. Studies on human thymus have produced a broadly similar picture of results (26). Recently, a monoclonal antibody against human T cell leukemia virus p 19 has been found to react with thymic epithelial cells (23). The cells which label are those which contain thymic hormones although they are not infected with virus. In this context, it has been claimed that thymic epithelium is responsible for the induction of preleukemic changes in leukemic susceptible mice (65). Although it is tempting to speculate that MHC antigens expressed on stromal cells influence the development of the T cell repertoire as originally proposed (27), direct evidence in support of this view is still lacking.

T LYMPHOCYTE DIFFERENTIATION PATHWAYS: EVIDENCE DERIVED FROM STUDIES USING PHENOTYPIC MARKERS

There is a conspicuous absence of surface markers which might be used to study the stem cells which migrate into the thymus. Studies both in ontogeny (59) and in the initial phases of marrow repopulation of the irradiated thymus (35) have shown that these cells do not express any of the classic T cell surface antigens (Thy-1, TL, Lyt-123, etc.). A rabbit antiserum against the neutral glycolipid asialo GM_1 has been found to react with the "blast" cells of the early embryonic thymus, and this reaction is lost as Thy-1 and other antigens appear (21). In addition, rabbit antisera to macromolecular insoluble cold globulin reacts with lymphoblasts of the early embryonic thymus, as well as with mature T cells (5). The usefulness of these markers for studies on thymic stem cells has yet to be evaluated.

Within a short interval after entry into the thymus, the lymphoblasts begin to express various T lineage markers. Examination of frozen sections (59) and of cell suspensions (39) indicates that cell heterogeneity, as measured by cell membrane antigen expression, is present within the embryonic thymus from an early stage. Lyt-1 expression precedes that of Lyt-2 and Mathieson et al. have interpreted this result as evidence for independent lineages of Lyt-1^+23^- and Lyt-123^+ cells (39); the implication being that cells with the "helper" phenotype, Lyt-1^+23^-, differentiate separately from the bulk of "immature" cortical thymocytes which are Lyt-123^+. The idea of separate lineages for cortical thymocytes (high Thy-1^+, Lyt-123^+, TL^+) and medullary thymocytes (low Thy-1^+, Lyt-1^+23^-, or Lyt-1^-23^+, TL^-) is not new. A dual pathway has been proposed on a number of occasions (reviewed in (55)). However, evidence for this view has never been entirely convincing. Lyt-1^+23^- cells of the early embryonic thymus do not have helper function. They may be cells in the process of developing Lyt-2 antigen, or they may be selectively expressing Lyt-1 during a particular phase of the cell cycle. Furthermore, Lyt^+ cells are generated from Lyt^- precursors continuously throughout ontogeny. Thus, up to 20% of Thy-1^+ cells in the 19-day embryo thymus are Lyt^-, and these cells are situated in the outer cortex (59) which is known to be the site of generation of cortical lymphocytes. Simple anatomical considerations suggest that this population, as it matures and progresses towards the medulla, gives rise to the medullary population as originally proposed (64). However, the difference between cortical and medullary phenotype is a sharp one and a transition between the two has never been directly demonstrated, either in vitro or in vivo. Many cortical lymphocytes are thought to die in situ (55), and this might explain the difficulty in demonstrating a precursor-product relationship between the few cortical cells which might develop a "mature" phenotype. IL-2, at one time thought to convert cortical thymocytes into mature cells, is now known not to do so (63). The cells which actually migrate from the thymus to peripheral organs have a "mature" phenotype and so conversion of cortical lymphocytes to "mature" cells (if it occurs) presumably takes place within the thymus (53). It should be noted that opposite conclusions have been drawn from experiments by Piguet et al., in which PNA (peanut agglutinin) binding was used as a marker of cortical phenotype (50). Because peripheral T cells of young mice are PNA^+, the authors claimed that they derive from the cortex. However, activated T cells are also PNA^+, and this is therefore not a suitable marker to resolve the question.

The use of other cell markers has not clarified the matter of lineage relationships. The nuclear enzyme terminal deoxynucleotidyl transferase (TdT) is not present in the lymphoblasts of the early human thymus but develops in the cortical lymphocyte population (26). The TdT^+ population is restricted to the cortex and very few positive cells are found in the medulla. Analysis of human thymus lymphocyte populations with monoclonal antibodies shows that T6 antigen is selectively expressed on cortical cells (? equivalent to the murine TL antigen); T4, T8, T10, and T11 antigens are found on cortical and medullary lymphocytes, and T1, T2, and T3 antigens are selectively expressed on medullary cells (26). It has been claimed that products of the IgT-C region of chromosome 12 are maturational markers for murine T cells. It is also suggested that these antigens might be allotypic determinants in constant regions of antigen-specific receptors (46). However, it is difficult to map these antigens onto other T lineage markers in order to produce a coherent picture of T cell differentiation. $Tthy^d$ is present on 35% of the thymocytes but is expressed equally on cortisone-sensitive (presumably cortical) thymocytes and cortisone-resistant (presumably medullary) thymocytes. Tsu^d and $Tind^d$ are expressed on medullary thymocytes, but only on antigen-activated peripheral lymphocytes. It is puzzling why these antigens should be expressed on medullary thymocytes of non-primed animals but only on primed peripheral cells.

In summary, the use of antigenic markers has provided evidence for the presence of major subpopulations of differentiating T cells. However, these markers have not provided a means of delineating cell lineages. The fidelity of markers as evidence of lineage has not always been proven, and it is perhaps instructive in this context that there is still some controversy about the use of Lyt markers as a means of identifying functional T cell subsets (25). Clearly, it is crucial in future work to try to clarify the relationship between cortical thymocytes and mature T cells.

T LYMPHOCYTE DIFFERENTIATION PATHWAYS: EVIDENCE DERIVED FROM FUNCTIONAL STUDIES

The literature on the development of the T cell repertoire is too extensive to cover adequately here. On the other hand, there are a limited number of important issues which I will attempt to highlight and I will summarize the various viewpoints. One of the issues which has attracted considerable attention is the important matter of the development of the T cell repertoire in terms of H-2 restriction during ontogeny. In the first place, there are two conflicting views about how H-2 restriction is brought about. One claims that the repertoire is selected by self-MHC antigens in the absence of foreign antigens; the other claims that restriction is a consequence of priming by foreign antigens (as discussed in (61)). Those who argue against selection by self-MHC antigens point to the presence of T cells restricted by allogeneic MHC antigens in the peripheral T cell pool, whereas this argument is countered by the claim that all allorestricted T cells are simply cross-reactive self-MHC restricted cells.

It is difficult to come to a reasoned conclusion on the basis of the experimental data available, especially since a substantial part of the data was obtained using limiting dilution assays for cytolytic T cells. The specificity of these assays has come under scrutiny, and difficulties are particularly evident in estimations of precursor frequency for minor H antigens (58) and haptens after in vitro priming (19). In both instances, a high proportion of clones show killing against various targets not expressing the antigens to which the responders were primed. The problem has been highlighted recently in studies where precursors of cytolytic T cells are activated with high efficiency so that virtually all respond. The clones derived from these cells were found to kill most targets nonspecifically without lectin mediation (56)! Obviously, further reevaluation is required before definite conclusions can be made, but these results do raise doubts about the experimental basis for many of the conclusions reached.

The point in their developmental pathway at which T cells acquire MHC-restricted specificity has also been a matter of controversy. Both the MHC phenotype of the thymus (66) and the MHC phenotype of the extrathymic environment have been implicated in the process. A consensus of conclusions seems to point to the importance of the thymus in this respect, but opinions differ as to whether epithelial cells or marrow-derived dendritic cells of the thymus are involved. The problem is perhaps best illustrated by two recent papers. In both studies, irradiation bone marrow chimeras of $F_1 \rightarrow P$ type is used to determine whether host thymic H-2 or donor marrow-derived dendritic cells determine the restriction specificity of chimeric T cells. The argument pivots on the claim that dendritic cells turn over slowly in the thymus after irradiation and hence the initial restriction pattern is thymic in type, but later when donor dendritic cells populate the thymus, the restriction pattern changes to donor-type. However, one study shows that the restriction pattern remains thymic (host) in type long after the establishment of chimerism and even when the T cells which had initially matured were eliminated and replenished by new cells (67). In the other study, increasing the dose of irradiation was found to accelerate the turnover of thymic dendritic cells from host to donor, and this was correlated with the acquisition of donor-type MHC restriction patterns (36).

Even allowing for the use of different assay systems (some measuring restriction by class I MHC antigens, others by class II) and the notion that MCH restriction is a quantitative phenomenon, it is difficult to reach a satisfactory conclusion. Returning to the simple anatomical considerations outlined in an earlier section, the substantial amounts of Ia antigens on cortical epithelial cells, some of which may be passively acquired by differentiating thymocytes (54), and the intimate relationship between epithelial cells and maturing lymphocytes argues for the role of cortical epithelial cells in Ia-linked restriction by a selection process. The kinetic pattern of cortical thymocyte production, involving extensive generation of new cells (most of which die within a few days), suggests that selection might operate at the level of survival of those few cells with receptors which match the cortical epithelial cell phenotype. Whilst there is some evidence to support this notion, unfortunately the studies mentioned previously (36) which indicate the exclusive role of thymic dendritic cells in restriction do, in fact, measure Ia-limited restriction, thus contradicting this idea!

Turning to another aspect of the development of the T cell repertoire in ontogeny, namely, the acquisition of tolerance to self-MHC antigens, the situation is no less confused. Arguments casting some doubt on the claims that tolerance is maintained at a pre-thymic level have been presented in earlier sections. Most remaining suggestions focus on the thymus as the site of tolerance induction. Thus thymocyte populations from recently reconstituted $P \rightarrow F_1$, $(A \rightarrow A \times B)$ chimeras are said not to contain precursors of cytolytic T cells reactive against either parental haplotype (32). This result suggests that the host thymus influences tolerance in the donor parental-type thymocytes. However, in chimeras of the type $F_1 \rightarrow P$ $(A \times B \rightarrow A)$, the reconstituted thymus contains cells which react to third parties but not to B, i.e., the haplotype expressed on the donor stem cells but not on the host thymus (32). This result can be explained if donor-derived dendritic cells which populate the host thymus induce tolerance. This idea is in line with discussions in earlier sections of this paper concerning tolerance in nude mice provided with allogeneic thymus grafts.

Another aspect of this problem is whether tolerance is produced by a clonal deletion or a suppressive mechanism. In a recent report by Good et al., embryonic thymic epithelial rudiments, removed prior to their population by migrant stem cells, were cultured with fetal liver fragments as a source of stem cells (20). The thymus cultures, when harvested, were examined in limiting dilution assays for cytolytic cell precursors to MHC antigens corresponding to the haplotypes of the fetal liver, thymus rudiment, and third party, respectively. The results showed deletion of precursors reactive against fetal liver donor and thymic epithelial host in the presence of precursors to third party antigens. The authors suggest that clonal deletion is responsible for these results. However, recent doubts about the specificity of responses in limiting dilution assays for primary responses have been mentioned earlier, and there is no shortage of other studies showing that tolerance to alloantigens is maintained by suppressor mechanisms (e.g., (8)).

In summary, although there are many doubts about the relative roles of the various thymic stromal components in influencing the ontogenetic development of the T cell repertoire and about the mechanisms that might operate here, recent progress in delineating these components offers promise for the future, also recent knowledge of T cell receptor should aid progress. Although it has been necessary to reconsider whether clonal selection operates in T cells (43), it is perhaps heartening after so much work to see that the evidence is still in favor of a qualified "yes"!

CONCLUSION

It is difficult to escape the conclusion that too much emphasis has been placed on the use of surface antigens (valuable though they have been in many situations) in tracing T cell lineages and identifying T cell types. Likewise, the unsatisfactory situation with regard to some in vitro assays for T cell function renders their usefulness in explaining in vivo phenomena problematical. Unfortunately, a situation has resulted in which it is possible to marshal a substantial number of studies in support of almost any viewpoint. However, emphasis here has been placed on the importance of intrathymic events and a promising start has been made to unraveling the interrelationships between the various stromal cell types and differentiating T cells.

REFERENCES

(1) Ando, I., and Hurme, M. 1981. Self-MHC-restricted cytotoxic T-cell responses without thymic influence. Nature 289: 494-495.

(2) Bach, J-F., and Goldstein, G. 1980. Newer concepts of thymic hormones. Thymus 2: 1-4.

(3) Barclay, A.N., and Mason, D.W. 1982. Induction of Ia antigen in rat epidermal cells and gut epithelium by immunological stimuli. J. Exp. Med. 156: 1665-1676.

(4) Barclay, A.N., and Mayrohofer, G. 1981. Bone marrow origin of Ia-positive cells in the medulla of the rat thymus. J. Exp. Med.

153: 1660-1671.

(5) Batuman, O.A.; Caro, J.; Schmidt, R.R.; and Hauptman, S.P. 1983. Macromolecular insoluble cold globulin (MICG): a marker for pluripotential hemopoietic stem cells. J. Immunol. 130: 1051-1055.

(6) Beller, D.I., and Unanue, E.R. 1980. I-A antigens and antigen-presenting function of thymic macrophages. J. Immunol. 124: 1443-1450.

(7) Besedovsky, H.O.; Del Rey, A.; and Sorkin, E. 1979. Role of prethymic cells in acquisition of self-tolerance. J. Exp. Med. 150: 1351-1358.

(8) Chen, B.P.P., and Splitter, G.A. 1983. Transplantation tolerance: Lyt-1^+2^- helper T cells require a second proliferative signal to overcome Lyt 1^-2^+ suppressor T cell activity. J. Immunol. 131: 57-63.

(9) Ching, L-M., and Miller, R.S. 1982. Development of cytotoxic T lymphocyte precursor cells in T cell colonies grown in vitro. J. Immunol. 129: 2345-2351.

(10) Cordier, A.C., and Heremans, J.F. 1975. Nude mouse embryo. Ectodermal nature of the primordial thymic defect. Scand. J. Immunol. 4: 193-196.

(11) Dennert, G., and Hyman, R. 1980. Functional Thy-1^+ cells in cultures of spleen cells from nu/nu mice. Eur. J. Immunol. 10: 583-589.

(12) Donohue, J.H., and Rosenberg, S.A. 1983. The fate of interleukin-2 after in vivo administration. J. Immunol. 130: 2203-2208.

(13) Dukor, P.; Miller, J.F.A.P.; House, W.; and Allman, V. 1965. Regeneration of thymus grafts. I. Histological and cytological aspects. Transplantation 3: 639-644.

(14) Duprez, V.; Hamilton, B.; and Burakoff, S.J. 1982. Generation of cytolytic T lymphocytes in thymectomized, irradiated and bone marrow-reconstituted mice. J. Exp. Med. 156: 844-859.

(15) Elliott, E.V. 1973. A persistent lymphoid cell population in the thymus. Nature New Biol. 242: 150-152.

(16) Ford, C.E.; Micklem, H.S.; Evans, E.P.; Gray, J.S.; and Ogden, D.A. 1966. The inflow of bone marrow cells to the thymus: studies with part-body irradiated mice injected with chromosome marked bone marrow and subjected to antigenic stimulation. Ann. NY Acad. Sci. 129: 283-296.

(17) Fukumoto, T.; McMaster, W.R.; and Williams, A.F. 1982. Mouse monoclonal antibodies against rat major histocompatibility antigens. Two Ia antigens and expression of Ia and class I antigens in rat thymus. Eur. J. Immunol. 12: 237-243.

(18) Gillis, S., and Watson, J. 1981. Interleukin-2 induction of hapten-specific cytolytic T cells in nude mice. J. Immunol. 126: 1245-1248.

(19) Good, M.F.; Boyd, A.W.; and Nossal, G.J.V. 1983. Analysis of true anti-hapten cytotoxic clones in limit dilution microcultures after correction for "anti-self" activity: precursor frequencies, Ly-2 and Thy-1 phenotype, specificity and statistical methods. J. Immunol. 130: 2046-2055.

(20) Good, M.F.; Pyke, K.W.; and Nossal, G.J.V. 1983. Functional clonal deletion of cytotoxic T-lymphocyte precursors in chimeric thymus produced in vitro from embryonic anlagen. Proc. Natl. Acad. Sci. USA 80: 3045-3049.

(21) Habu, G.; Kasai, M.; Nagai, Y.; Tamaoki, N.; Tada, T.; Herzenberg, L.A.; and Okumura, K. 1980. The glycolipid asialo G.M, as a new differentiation antigen of fetal thymocytes. J. Immunol. 125: 2284-2288.

(22) Hammond, W.S. 1954. Origins of thymus in the chick embryo. J. Morphol. 95: 501-515.

(23) Haynes, B.F.; Robert-Guroff, M.; Metzgar, R.S.; Franchini, G.; Kalyanaranan, V.S.; Palker, T.J.; and Gallo, R.C. 1983. Monoclonal antibody against human T cell leukaemia virus p 19 defines a human thymic epithelial antigen acquired during ontogeny. J. Exp. Med. 157: 907-920.

(24) Haynes, B.F.; Warren, R.W.; Buckley, R.H.; McClure, J.E.; Goldstein, A.L.; Henderson, F.W.; Hensley, L.L.; and Eisenbarth, G.S. 1983. Demonstration of abnormalities in expression of thymic epithelial surface antigens in severe cellular immunodeficiency diseases. J. Immunnol. 130: 1182-1188.

(25) Hodes, R.J. 1982. Lyt antigens as markers for functional T-cell subpopulations. Immunol. Today 3: 235-236.

(26) Janossy, G.; Thomas, J.A.; Goldstein, G.; and Bollum, F.T. 1981. The human thymic microenvironment. In Microenvironments in Haemopoietic and Lymphoid Differentiation. Ciba Foundation Symposium 84, pp. 193-214. London: Pitman Medical.

(27) Jerne, N.K. 1971. The somatic generation of immune recognition. Eur. J. Immunol. 1: 1-9.

(28) Jordan, R.K. 1976. Development of sheep thymus in relation to in utero thymectomy experiments. Eur. J. Immunol. 6: 693-698.

(29) Kindred, B.; Corley, R.B.; and Schirrmacher, V. 1980. The relationship between alloantigen responses in nude mice injected with a low number of congenic thymus cells. Thymus 2: 83-92.

(30) Komuro, K.; Goldstein, G.; and Boyse, E.A. 1975. Thymus re-populating capacity of cells that can be induced to differ to T cells in vitro. J. Immunol. 115: 195-198.

(31) Kruisbeek, A.M.; Fultz, M.J.; Sharrow, S.D.; Singer, A.; and Mond, J.J. 1983. Early development of the T cell repertoire. In vivo treatment of neonatal mice with anti-Ia antibodies interferes with differentiation of I-restricted T cells but not K/D-restricted T cells. J. Exp. Med. 157: 1932-1946.

(32) Kruisbeek, A.M.; Hodes, R.J.; and Singer, A. 1981. Cytotoxic T lymphocyte responses by chimeric thymocytes, self-recognition is determined early in T cell development. J. Exp. Med. 153: 13-26.

(33) Kyewski, B.A., and Kaplan, H.S. 1982. Lymphoepithelial interactions in the mouse thymus: phenotypic and kinetic studies on thymic mouse cells. J. Immunol. 128: 2287-2294.

(34) Le Douarin, N.; Jotereau, F.; Houssaint, E.; Martin, C.; and Dieterlen-Lievre, F. 1982. Ontogeny of avian lymphocytes. In The Reticuloendothelial System: Phylogeny and Ontogeny, eds. N. Cohen and M.M. Sigel, vol. 3, pp. 589-616. New York: Plenum Press.

(35) Lepault, F.; Coffman, R.L.; and Weissman, I.L. 1983. Characteristics of thymus-homing bone marrow cells. J. Immunol. 131: 64-69.

(36) Longo, D.L., and Davis, M.L. 1983. Early appearance of donor-type antigen presenting cells in the thymuses of 1200R radiation-induced bone marrow chimeras correlates with self-recognition of donor I region gene products. J. Immunol. 130: 2525-2527.

(37) Loor, F.W., and Kindred, B. 1973. Differentiation of T-cell precursors in nude mice demonstrated by immunofluorescence of T-cell membrane markers. J. Exp. Med. 138: 1044-1055.

(38) Maryanski, J.L.; MacDonald, H.R.; Sordat, B.; and Cerottini, J.C.

1981. Cytolytic T lymphocyte precursor cells in congenitally athymic C57 BL/6 nu/nu mice: quantitation, enrichment, and specificity. J. Immunol. 126: 871-876.

(39) Mathieson, B.J.; Sharrow, S.O.; Rosenberg, Y.; and Hammerling, U. 1981. Lyt $1^{+}23^{-}$ cells appear in the thymus before Lyt 123^{+} cells. Nature 289: 179-181.

(40) Miller, J.F.A.P. 1979. Experimental thymology has come of age. Thymus 1: 3-25.

(41) Miller, J.F.A.P., and Osoba, D. 1967. Current concepts of the immunological function of the thymus. Physiol. Rev. 47: 437-487.

(42) Miller, R.G.; Derry, H.R.; and Garjeant, B.J. 1983. The extent of self MHC restriction of cytotoxic T cells in nude mice varies from mouse to mouse. J. Immunol. 130: 63-68.

(43) Mitchison, N.A., and Pettersson, G. 1983. Does clonal selection occur among T cells? Ann. Immunol. (Inst. Pasteur) 134D: 37-45.

(44) Morrissey, P.J.; Kruisbeek, A.M.; Sharrow, S.O.; and Singer, A. 1982. Tolerance of thymic cytotoxic T lymphocytes to allogeneic H-2 determinants encountered pre-thymically: evidence of expression of anti-H2 receptors prior to entry to the thymus. Proc. Natl. Acad. Sci. USA 79: 2003-2007.

(45) Muraoka, S., and Miller, R.S. 1983. Cells in immune fetal liver and in lymphoid colonies grown from fetal liver can suppress generation of cytotoxic T lymphocytes directed against their self antigens. J. Immunol. 131: 45-49.

(46) Owen, F.L. 1982. Products of the IgT-C region of chromosóme 12 are maturational markers for T cells. Sequence of appearance in immunocompetent T cells parallels ontogenetic appearance of T thy^{d}, T ind^{d}, and Tsu^{d}. J. Exp. Med. 156: 703-718.

(47) Owen, F.L. 1983. Tpre, a new alloantigen encoded in the IgT-C region of chromosome 12, is expressed on bone marrow of nude mice, fetal T cell hybrids and fetal thymus. J. Exp. Med. 157: 419-432.

(48) Owen, J.J.T., and Jenkinson, E.J. 1981. Embryology of the lymphoid system. Progr. Allergy 29: 1-34.

(49) Owen, J.J.T.; Jenkinson, E.J.; and Kingston, R. 1983. The ontogeny of T lymphocytes. Ann. Immunol. (Inst. Pasteur) 134D: 115-122.

(50) Piguet, P.F.; Irle, C.; Kollatte, E.; and Vassalli, P. 1981. Post-thymic T lymphocyte maturation during ontogenesis. J. Exp. Med. 154: 581-584.

(51) Ranges, S.E.; Goldstein, G.; Boyse, E.A.; and Schield, M.P. 1982. T cell development in normal and thymopentin-treated nude mice. J. Exp. Med. 156: 1057-1064.

(52) Rouse, R.V., and Weissman, I.L. 1981. Microanatomy of the thymus: its relationship to T cell differentiation. In Microenvironments in Haemopoietic and Lymphoid Differentiation. Ciba Foundation Symposium 84, pp. 161-177. London: Pitman Medical.

(53) Scollay, R. 1982. Thymus cell migration: cells migrating from thymus to peripheral lymphoid organs have a "mature" phenotype. J. Immunol. 128: 1566-1577.

(54) Sharrow, S.O.; Mathieson, B.J.; and Singer, A. 1981. Cell surface appearance of unexpected host MHC determinants on thymocytes from radiation bone marrow chimeras. J. Immunol. 126: 1327-1335.

(55) Shortman, K. 1977. The pathway of T-cell development within the thymus. In Progress in Immunology III, eds. T.E. Mandel, C. Cheers, C.S. Hosking, I.F.C. McKenzie, and G.J.V. Nossal, pp. 197-205. New York: Elsevier/North-Holland.

(56) Shortman, K.; Wilson, A.; Scollay, R.; and Chen, W-F. 1983. Development of large granular lymphocytes with anomalous non-specific cytotoxicity in clones derived from Ly-2^+ T cells. Proc. Natl. Acad. Sci. USA 80: 2728-2732.

(57) Stutman, O. 1978. Intrathymic and extrathymic T cell maturation. Immunol. Rev. 42: 138-184.

(58) Teh, H.S.; Bennink, J.; and von Boehmer, H.V. 1982. Selection of the T cell repertoire during ontogeny: limiting dilution analysis. Eur. J. Immunol. 12: 887-892.

(59) Van Ewijk, W.; Jenkinson, E.J.; and Owen, J.J.T. 1982. Detection of Thy-1, T-200, Lyt 1 and Lyt 2 bearing cells in the developing lymphoid organs of the mouse embryo in vivo and in vitro. Eur. J. Immunol. 12: 262-271.

(60) Van Ewijk, W.; Rouse, R.V.; and Weissman, I.L. 1980. Distribution of H-2 microenvironments in the mouse thymus. Immuno-electron microscopic identification of I-A and H-2K bearing cells. J. Histochem. Cytochem. 28: 1089-1099.

(61) Von Boehmer, H.; Bennink, J.; Teh, H.S.; and Haas, W. 1983. Selection of the T-cell repertoire during ontogeny. Ann. Immunol. (Inst. Pasteur) 134D: 17-24.

(62) Wallis, V.; Leuchars, E.; Chwalinski, S.; and Davies, A.J.S. 1975. On the sparse seeding of bone marrow and thymus in radiation chimaeras. Transplantation 19: 2-11.

(63) Wei-Feng, C.; Scollay, R.; and Shortman, K. 1982. The functional capacity of thymus subpopulations: limit-dilution analysis of all precursors of cytotoxic lymphocytes and of all T cells capable of proliferation in subpopulations separated by the use of peanut agglutinin. J. Immunol. 129: 18-24.

(64) Weissman, I.L. 1967. Thymus cell migration. J. Exp. Med. 126: 291-297.

(65) Zielinski, C.C.; Waksal, S.D.; and Datta, S.K. 1982. Thymic epithelium is programmed to induce preleukemic changes in retrovirus expression and thymocyte differentiation in leukemia susceptible mice: studies on bone marrow and thymic chimeras. J. Immunol. 129: 882-889.

(66) Zinkernagel, R.M. 1978. Thymus and lymphohaemopoietic cells: their role in T-cell maturation in selection of T cells' H-2 restriction specificity and in H-2 linked gene control. Immunol. Rev. 42: 224-270.

(67) Zinkernagel, R.M. 1982. Selection of restriction specificities of virus-specific cytolotoxic T cells in the thymus: no evidence for a crucial role of antigen-presenting cells. J. Exp. Med. 156: 1842-1847.

Leukemia, ed. I.L. Weissman, pp. 131-145. Dahlem Konferenzen 1985. Berlin, Heidelberg, New York, Tokyo: Springer-Verlag.

Effects of Acute Leukemia Viruses on the Differentiation of Hematopoietic Cells

T. Graf
European Molecular Biology Laboratory *
6900 Heidelberg, F.R. Germany

Abstract. The interaction of defective acute leukemia viruses (DLVs) with hematopoietic cells leading to cell transformation provides a useful model for studying various aspects of leukemogenesis. The major conclusions drawn in this review are: a) DLVs carry host-derived oncogenes which they can reintroduce into cells via infection. b) DLVs cause leukemias within a period of weeks to months in a non-clonal fashion. c) The majority of DLV target cells are committed to differentiation and are clearly past the level of pluripotent progenitors. d) Some DLV strains appear to be highly lineage-specific while others are not. e) DLV-transformed cells of different lineages retain specific factor/hormone requirements. f) In certain virus strains two oncogenes cooperate to induce an "advanced" type of leukemia. g) Some DLV strains stimulate the proliferation of infected hematopoietic cells without impairing their differentiation while others also block differentiation. h) No examples are known of DLV-transformed cells which express differentiation markers of more than one lineage, although DLV-transformed cells within a given lineage may express an aberrant phenotype.

INTRODUCTION

Leukemias are disorders of differentiation manifested by the abnormal proliferation of hematopoietic cells. While much has been learned about the classification and origin of human leukemias, a number of important issues still need to be resolved. First, it appears that most types of human

* On leave of absence from the German Cancer Center, 6900 Heidelberg, F.R. Germany.

leukemias can be assigned to one particular differentiation lineage, and yet some of the common forms of leukemia can be traced to an aberration in a single hematopoietic stem cell rather than in a committed progenitor (see Fialkow and Singer, this volume). It is not known how an aberrant stem cell gives rise to proliferating leukemic cells within one lineage and normally differentiating cells within other lineages. Second, human leukemic cells have often undergone changes which make them refractory to normal regulatory mechanisms (see Moore, this volume). It is not clear whether these regulatory defects are primary alterations which result from the initial transformation event itself or whether they reflect secondary changes which occur as a result of tumor progression. A third interesting question is whether human leukemia cells express a normal pattern of differentiation-specific phenotypes or whether they tend to express abnormal combinations of lineage-specific markers (i.e., lineage "infidelity"). While the first interpretation is favored by Greaves (this volume) and others, McCulloch and his school favor the latter (see, for example, (20)).

In this article I attempt to address some of the above questions by reviewing results obtained with acute leukemia viruses in animals. These viruses cause leukemias within short periods of time (weeks to months) following injection into susceptible animals. In addition, they are able to transform hematopoietic cells in vitro; the leukemic cells can thus be studied shortly after transformation (without the complicating process of tumor progression and diversification). The virus strains which will be discussed are all members of the defective leukemia virus (DLV) family, a group of retroviruses containing cell-derived sequences which encode the viral transforming capacity and which are known as oncogenes (for review, see (8, 24), and Hayman, this volume).

Aspects of Hematopoietic Differentiation That Can Be Affected by DLV Infection

First, I will consider some basic concepts of normal hematopoietic differentiation. It is assumed that hematopoietic cells of all lineages are derived from a small population of pluripotent stem cells. These stem cells are capable of self-renewal and of differentiation along several pathways, each of which is regulated by specific growth and/or differentiation factors. As they become committed to one lineage, their capacity for self-renewal gradually diminishes. As a rule, differentiation along a given pathway involves a fixed program of cell divisions. It is not clear whether growth and differentiation are coupled processes, that is, whether cell division is always a prerequisite for differentiation or whether the two processes can be separated.

In principle, DLVs might affect hematopoietic cells in a variety of ways. For example, virus infection could lead to an altered sensitivity to growth or differentiation factors. On the target cell level, DLVs might affect any of several cell populations: pluripotent stem cells, committed cells of one or more lineage(s), or possibly even all dividing hematopoietic cells (retroviruses require at least one cell division to establish an infection). Once infection is established, the differentiation program may become frozen, accelerated, reversed, or altered in other ways. As will be shown below, DLV infection of hematopoietic cells provide examples for most of these possibilities. The different DLV strains discussed, along with a summary of some of their properties, are listed in Table 1.

TABLE 1 - Differentiation phenotypes of DLV-transformed hematopoietic cells.

Virus strain	Oncogene	Tissue infected	Phenotype of transformed cell
1. Murine viruses			
AbMuLV	abl	bone marrow	immature B cells
		fetal liver	erythroid cells at different stages and immature B cells
2. Avian viruses			
AEV-H	erbB	bone marrow	erythroid cells at different stages
AEV-R[a]	erbA, erbB	bone marrow	immature erythroid cells
AMV	myb	bone marrow	immature myeloid cells
E26	myb, ets	bone marrow	erythroid and immature myeloid cells at different stages
		blastoderm	myeloid/erythroid cells
MC29	myc	bone marrow	macrophage-like cells

[a] or the ES4 strain

The factor/hormone requirements of hematopoietic cells are not always lost upon transformation with DLVs

Although neoplastic cells often show a lack of growth factor dependence, there are several examples of hematopoietic cells which have retained this requirement after DLV transformation. For example, most lymphoid cells freshly transformed by Abelson virus in vitro initially require a feeder layer that provides a growth factor. Only after prolonged time in culture do the cells become factor-independent ((22), and Witte et al., this volume). Whether or not in vivo transformed cells are factor-dependent is not clear from the literature. Other examples of factor-dependent leukemia cells are erythroid and myeloid cells transformed in vivo and in vitro by E26 virus. These two cell types require different culture conditions for growth (13, 15). The transformed erythroid cells grow only under conditions which will support the differentiation of normal erythroid cells, while the transformed myeloid cells require a growth factor which is characterized by its stimulatory effect on colony formation by normal myelomonocytic cells. In contrast, avian erythroblastosis virus (AEV ES4 strain)-transformed erythroblasts appear to have no factor requirement (such as chick erythropoietin) for growth (Beug and Graf, unpublished).

The majority of DLV target cells are recruited from committed hematopoietic precursors

To delineate the transforming specificity of DLVs, two approaches are possible. The first consists in determining which lineage(s) is transformed by a given DLV strain in vivo. The disadvantage of this approach is that the type of neoplasms obtained may depend on various factors such as the route of inoculation. As a consequence, only some of the cell types potentially susceptible to DLV transformation might actually be observed. For example, AEV induces exclusively erythroblastosis when injected i.v. but also causes sarcomas when injected i.m. The birds seem to die of the disease which is manifested more rapidly (7). A more direct and convenient approach consists of analyzing in vitro transformed cultures for their phenotype of differentiation, although this approach is limited by the state of art in tissue culture. Ideally, infection experiments should be performed under culture conditions which permit the growth and differentiation of all normal progenitor cells. Such conditions, including the necessary factors, have been worked out for a variety of avian and mammalian hematopoietic progenitor cells. Historically, as new culture conditions were developed and refined, and as a wider variety of tissues were examined, some DLV strains originally believed to be unilineage-specific were found to be capable of transforming cells from more than one lineage. For example, Abelson virus was initially found to transform B-cells only when bone marrow was infected but could be subsequently shown to transform erythroid cells as well when fetal liver was tested (for review, see (18), and Witte et al., this volume).

At this point it is useful to make a distinction between transformation specificity and target cell specificity. The first terms refers to the differentiation phenotype (with respect to both lineage and stage) of the transformed cells. The second term refers to the normal (untransformed) cells, that is, prior to infection. Although in practice the two cell populations are often quite similar, the distinction of these terms becomes important in cases where the transformed cells differ from the target cells. Such a difference could arise if pluripotent stem cells infected by a given DLV strain would be induced to differentiate along a given lineage, with a subsequent expression of the transformed phenotype expressed.

So far, target cell studies indicate that none of the known DLVs appears to affect exclusively multipotent stem cells. In contrast, all DLVs are capable of transforming committed cells. A few strains, like AEV and avian myeloblastosis virus (AMV), transform cells of a single lineage only (erythroid and myeloid, respectively; for review, see (12)), while others such as the Abelson virus (for review, see (18)) and the E26 virus (13) affect more than one lineage. In both of these cases, the transformed cells and the target cells have a similar phenotype. It is not entirely clear whether some DLVs are in addition capable of transforming uncommitted stem cells. A possible candidate is E26. Early chick embryo cells infected with this virus give rise to a variety of transformed colonies, including some which contain both myeloid-erythroid progeny, suggesting that in these colonies the originally transformed cell is bipotent ((13), and Graf and Kahn, unpublished).

How wide is the target cell "window" within a specific lineage for a given DLV strain? A well studied case is the Abelson virus. This virus can transform early B cells, pre-B cells, as well as virgin B cells ((23), and Witte et al., this volume), that is, essentially all dividing cells within the B cell lineage. In contrast, AEV transforms early, but not late, erythroid precursors (1, 19). Whether these late precursors can be infected by the virus is not clear.

However, the ability of DLVs to infect a given cell type does not ensure that the cell will become transformed. For example, AEV is capable of infecting macrophages but does not transform them (6). This observation suggests that expression of DLV-transforming proteins induces transformation only in those cells which belong to a particular hematopoietic lineage.

The question of whether DLV strains exist that can transform cells from a single lineage in a stage-specific manner is not clear at present. Transformation of bone marrow cells with myc- or myb-containing viruses gives rise to transformants which resemble somewhat immature or more immature myelomonocytic cells, respectively. In addition, myc-viruses efficiently transform macrophages (for review, see (12)).

Whether or not the myb-containing viruses AMV and E26 can also transform mature macrophages is a matter of controversy. Durban and Boettiger (3) and Gazzolo et al. (5) have reported that they can, while our own data suggest that these viruses are extremely inefficient at doing so ((9), and Kahn and Graf, unpublished). In order to explain this discrepancy, Durban and Boettiger (3) have argued that the macrophage cultures used in our studies may have lacked the capacity to divide (a prerequisite for a successful retrovirus infection). However, the same cultures which showed only a low susceptibility to AMV and E26 viruses were highly susceptible to transformation by MC29-type viruses ((9), and Kahn and Graf, unpublished). Possible explanations for this apparent discrepancy will be discussed later.

Effects of DLVs on Growth and Differentiation of Hematopoietic Cells

In the following sections, we have attempted to divide DLV-transformed cells into various categories, based on whether or not the cells have retained their capacity to differentiate. It should be noted that these categories are somewhat arbitrary, since each interaction of a DLV strain with cells from a given lineage may result in a unique phenotype. In addition, the boundaries between the different categories sometimes overlap, due to the clonal variability often observed in DLV-transformed cells.

Abelson virus can stimulate immature cells to grow and to differentiate

Abelson virus infection of fetal liver cells from 9-12 day gestation mouse embryos leads to the formation of large colonies of erythroid cells. Cells in these colonies differentiate terminally, apparently in the absence of erythropoietin ((21), and Rosenberg, personal communication). It is somewhat questionable whether or not these cells should be designated as "transformed," since they cannot be propagated in culture. The "transformed" cells, however, appear to arise from the direct action of the viral transforming protein on immature target cells. Viral infection in this instance, therefore, does not lead to the acquisition of an increased self-renewal capacity but somehow alters the program of growth and differentiation in erythroid target cells. Similar results (induction of colony formation without induction of self-renewal) have also been obtained with murine erythroid cells "transformed" by the Friend leukemia virus complex or the Harvey or Kirsten sarcoma viruses. It is possible that the inability of these cells to self-renew in vitro is peculiar to the mouse system, since virus-transformed chicken erythroid cells do not behave in this way.

MC29-type viruses can stimulate differentiated cells to proliferate

Macrophages are probably the only example of terminally differentiated hematopoietic cells (lymphocytes not included) which retained the potential for cell division. As mentioned earlier, mature macrophages can be transformed by MC29 virus as well as by other DLVs containing the myc gene (2, 5). Transformation in all instances is associated with a drastic growth stimulation of the target cells. It is doubtful whether MC29-transformed macrophages are truly neoplastic, since the virus itself does not induce monocytic leukemia (and only occasionally induces myelocytomatosis), and since transformed macrophages injected into birds do not form tumors.

Several DLV strains can stimulate cells to grow without eliminating their capacity to differentiate

The majority of DLV-transformed cell types belong in this category. A first example is lymphoid cells transformed by the Abelson virus (for review, see (16, 18, 24)). Some (but not all) freshly transformed clones show ongoing rearrangements of their immunoglobulin genes. Most clones show rearrangements only in their heavy chain genes and express cytoplasmic μ chains. These clones are often heterogeneous and lose μ chain expression as they are cultured, possibly because of the accumulation of deletions around their heavy chain genes. Very few clones have rearrangements in both heavy and light chain genes and even fewer express surface IgM.

Another example of this category is AEV (erbB)-transformed hematopoietic cells. AEV (erbB) is a deletion mutant of the ES4 strain of AEV which lacks a functional erbA gene (4). (Recently, another erythroblastosis-inducing strain (AEV-H) which naturally lacks the erbA gene has been described. The biological properties of this strain have not yet been fully characterized (see Hayman, this volume).) Cells transformed by AEV (erbB) in vitro or in vivo consist of erythroblast-like cells as well as of erythroid cells at various stages of differentiation, including mature erythrocytes (4). Erythroid cells transformed by E26 virus exhibit a similar phenotype (15). It is not yet clear whether the viral ets or the myb gene or both are responsible for erythroid transformation.

AEV and E26 viruses induce cells to proliferate and also block their ability to differentiate

It is interesting that the two best documented examples of DLVs which can block differentiation are strains carrying two oncogenes. Cells transformed in vitro or in vivo by the ES4 strain of AEV (containing the erbA and erbB genes) resemble rapidly growing erythroblasts which are completely blocked in differentiation. The phenotype of these cells thus differ significantly from the AEV (erbB)-transformed cells which, as discussed above, are still able to differentiate. However, studies using temperature-sensitive mutants of wild-type AEV (with lesions probably in erbB) have shown that tsAEV-transformed cells can differentiate into mature erythrocytes if the mutated viral oncogene product is inactivated by raising the temperature of cultivation (1, 19).

The second example in this category is E26. This virus is capable of transforming hematopoietic cells resembling myeloblasts or, perhaps more correctly, monoblasts. These cells weakly express some of the functional markers of mature macrophages and exhibit cell surface antigens characteristic of macrophage precursors. E26-transformed myeloid cells can be grown in culture for prolonged periods of time without showing a significant rate of spontaneous differentiation. In contrast, cultured AMV-transformed cells (despite having a phenotype which closely resembles that of E26-transformed cells) often show a sudden spontaneous differentiation into macrophage-like cells. Myeloblasts transformed by ts mutants of E26 virus can be induced to differentiate into macrophage-like cells if shifted from the permissive to the non-permissive temperature (Graf et al., in preparation). A similar but less well-defined ts mutant has also been described for AMV (14).

The mechanisms by which AEV and E26 arrest the differentiation of erythroid and myeloid cells, respectively, are not known. The primary effect of these viruses might consist in increasing the probability of self-renewal at each cell division and consequently decreasing the probability of differentiation. According to this view, self-renewal and differentiation might represent opposite sides of the same coin. Another possibility is that AEV and E26 induce both self-renewal and a block of differentiation as separate events and that each of the viral-encoded oncogenes is responsible for one of these functions.

Aberrant Versus Normal Differentiation Phenotypes of DLV-transformed Cells

This complex issue will be discussed in three parts: a) Are DLV-transformed cells capable of terminal differentiation into cells with a normal phenotype? b) Do DLV-transformed cells exhibit lineage infidelity? c) How do the phenotypes of DLV-transformed cells compare with those of their normal counterparts?

At least some DLV-transformed cells are capable of terminal differentiation

In the preceding sections we have discussed examples of DLV-transformed cells which have retained their capacity to differentiate. It has to be pointed out, however, that in most instances the criteria used to identify terminally differentiated cells have not included the study of functional markers. In the case of Abelson-transformed B cells, which show ongoing immunoglobulin gene rearrangements after cell transformation, mature plasma cells have not been described. It is unclear whether the Abelson-transformed cells do not reach the terminal stages of differentiation because of a direct effect of the Abelson-transforming protein, because of secondary changes that occur in the cells as they are kept in culture, or because the culture conditions are not suitable for terminal differentiation.

For those DLV strains which arrest hematopoietic cell differentiation, temperature-sensitive mutants provide a useful approach to the question of whether or not these "blocked" DLV-transformed cells have retained their capacity to differentiate. Such mutants have been extensively characterized for AEV in the erythroid lineage and for E26 virus in the myeloid lineage. As summarized in Table 2, transformed cells shifted from the permissive to the non-permissive temperature can be induced to differentiate terminally and to resume a near-normal phenotype (provided that they are grown in the presence of appropriate differentiation factors). It has to be emphasized, however, that these cells still exhibit morphological as well as quantitative differences in the expression of certain markers, relative to their normal counterparts. In addition, in both systems there is a considerable clonal heterogeneity with respect to the differentiation potential of individually transformed cells. These

TABLE 2 - Differentiation parameters of chick hematopoietic cells infected with temperature-sensitive DLV mutants.

	Differentiation phenotype of cells grown at		
	37°C	shifted to 42°C	-
	tsAEV cells		normal bone marrow cells
Morphology	erythroblast	erythrocyte-like	erythrocyte
Hemoglobin	+	+++	+++
Histone 5	++	+++	+++
Erythroblast antigen	+++	-	-
Erythrocyte antigen	-	+++	+++
Spectrin	+	+++	+++
	tsE26 cells		
Morphology	myeloblast	macrophage-like	macrophage
Motility in methylcellulose	-	+++	+++
Adherence capacity	-	+	+++
Phagocytic capacity	+	++	+++
Growth factor dependence	+++	+	+
Myeloblast antigen	+++	+	+
Macrophage antigens	-	++	+++

differences relative to normal terminal differentiation could be due to either a leakiness of the mutants used or to microenvironmental factors operating in vivo.

Do DLV-transformed cells exhibit lineage infidelity?

The question of whether or not transformed hematopoietic cells express markers of more than one lineage (interlineage infidelity, (20)) rests largely on the specificity of the differentiation markers used. This is a difficult problem and there have been several instances in which markers (e.g., spectrin) originally thought to be specific for one lineage were later detected in other lineages as well.

Even with this proviso, however, DLV-transformed cells have not been found to express markers of more than one lineage. In experiments carried out in our laboratory over the past eight years, testing hundreds of DLV-transformed cell clones for the expression of differentiation markers, we have not found a single instance of interlineage infidelity. Table

3 shows results obtained with AEV-transformed erythroblasts and E26-transformed myeloblasts.

The apparent discrepancy between these results and those obtained with human leukemia cells (which possibly express markers from more than one lineage) might be explained by the fact that the viral leukemias are non-clonal in origin while most human leukemias are clonal diseases. The constant generation of new leukemic cells by virus spread in the viral leukemias obviates the necessity for immortalization and progression of the leukemic cells, processes that are necessary in nonviral leukemias in order to maintain the disease. On the other hand, these latter processes may be associated with the extinction and/or aberrant expression of differentiation markers, a phenomenon which is occasionally also observed during the establishment of hematopoietic cell lines in vitro.

In the avian system a change of DLV-transformed cells from one lineage to another has never been reported. An interesting example for a possible lineage conversion has, however, recently been described: passage of Abelson-transformed B cells for several generations in vivo led to the recovery of cells which were derived from the original injected cells but which expressed more T cell markers than B cell markers (17). Since

TABLE 3 - Lineage-specific expression of differentiation markers in DLV-transformed chicken cells.

Markers tested	AEV-transformed erythroblasts	AMV- or E26-transformed myeloblasts
Hemoglobin	+ (500)	- (50)
Histone H5	+ (100)	- (50)
Erythroblast antigen(s)[a]	+ (100)	- (50)
MC 4.6.C.1[b]	+ (30)	- (20)
Myeloblast antigen(s)[a]	- (20)	+ (100)
MC 51/2[c]	- (10)	+ (20)
MC 61/8[c]	- (10)	+ (20)

In parenthesis: approximate number of transformed cell clones tested.
[a]Erythroblast and myeloblast antigens were detected with rabbit antisera (2).
[b]Monoclonal 4.6.C.1 (10).
[c]Monoclonals 51/2 and 61/8 (11).

a similar conversion was not observed in cultured cells, this phenomenon is likely to be related to events that occur during tumor progression.

Aberrant expression of stage-specific antigens within a given lineage in single DLV-transformed (intralineage infidelity (20)) cells has not yet been well documented, possibly due to the lack of appropriate markers. Suggestive evidence exists, however, that individual E26-transformed erythroid cells express both early and late erythroid-specific cell surface antigens (15).

Does the phenotype of DLV-transformed cells differ from that of their normal counterparts?

As discussed earlier, DLV-transformed cells are generally recruited from committed cells of the same lineage, that is, transformed and target cells both exhibit the same gross phenotype. The question remains, however, whether or not there is an aberrant, transformation-specific phenotype (such as seen in DLV-transformed fibroblasts) that is superimposed upon the differentiation phenotype.

The most direct experimental approach to this question would be to compare homogeneous populations of target cells with the corresponding transformed cells. This is, unfortunately, very difficult for both theoretical and practical reasons. First, unlike fibroblasts, most hematopoietic DLV target cells do not significantly self-renew but pass through transient stages along a fixed pathway which culminates in terminal differentiation. (It is probably also for this reason that the target cells for certain DLVs (e.g., AEV) are less mature than the transformed cells.) Second, DLV target cells are very difficult to purify from any of the hematopoietic organs or tissues. So far, only two cases exist where relatively homogeneous, growing target cell populations have been obtained: B cells, at various stages of differentiation, and macrophages. A comparison of murine B cells before and after infection with Abelson virus have not revealed any striking differences between the two (23), while macrophages transformed by MC29 virus (or any of the other myc-containing viruses) seem to be slightly less differentiated than normal macrophages with respect to phagocytic capacity, adherence, and levels of Fc and C3 receptors (2, 5).

How can these differences between MC29-transformed macrophages and normal mature macrophages be explained? One possibility is that the virus arrests macrophages at an early stage of maturation, either by inducing a partial dedifferentiation or by selectively transforming the more immature cells present in the cell population used for infection (MC29 virus transforms only up to 5% of the cells in a standard macrophage culture). An alternative interpretation is that MC29 induces the proliferation of resting macrophages and as a consequence the cells assume the slightly less differentiated phenotype described above.

As mentioned earlier, chicken macrophage cultures can also be transformed by AMV and E26 viruses. The transformed cells are even more immature (or aberrant?) by a number of criteria than the myc-virus transformed macrophage-derived cells (3). However, the transformation efficiencies with AMV and E26 are approximately 20-fold lower than those seen with MC29-type viruses. This originally suggested to us that with myc and myb viruses, each transforms a different target cell population. Recent experiments have revealed at least one instance in which E26 can transform the same population of cells as can MC29. We have found that individual macrophage clones transformed by MC29 can be "supertransformed" by E26 virus, resulting in the outgrowth of cells resembling myeloblasts (Graf and Beug, unpublished results). This observation may be interpreted as suggesting that MC29 stimulates resting macrophages into proliferation and that once they are cycling they can be transformed by E26. The observed reversal from the relatively mature MC29 phenotype to the immature E26 phenotype could again represent either a true virus (oncogene)-induced dedifferentiation or the expression of a dominant transformation-specific phenotype.

A change from a differentiated into an undifferentiated myelomonocytic cell has also been observed using ts mutants of E26 virus: macrophage-like cells obtained after temperature-induced differentiation of ts E26 myeloblasts can revert to a myeloblast-like phenotype upon shift back to the permissive temperature (Graf and Beug, unpublished results). However, this finding still does not resolve the issue of whether E26-transformed cells exhibit a normal or abnormal phenotype. Only careful comparisons of different combinations of differentiation markers on normal and transformed cells might provide a final answer.

Acknowledgements. I would like to thank H. Beug and P. Kahn for stimulating discussions.

REFERENCES

(1) Beug, H.; Palmieri, S.; Freudenstein, C.; Zentgraf, H.; and Graf, T. 1982. Hormone-dependent terminal differentiation in vitro of chicken erythroleukemia cells transformed by ts mutants of avian

erythroblastosis virus. Cell 28: 907-919.

(2) Beug, H.; von Kirchbach, A.; Doederlein, G.; Conscience, J.F.; and Graf, T. 1979. Chicken hematopoietic cells transformed by seven strains of defective leukemia viruses display three distinct phenotypes of differentiation. Cell 18: 375-390.

(3) Durban, E.M., and Boettiger, D. 1981. Replicating, differentiated macrophages can serve as in vitro targets for transformation by avian myeloblastosis virus. J. Virol. 37: 488-492.

(4) Frykberg, L.; Palmieri, S.; Beug, H.; Graf, T.; Hayman, M.J.; and Vennström, B. 1983. Transforming capacities of avian erythroblastosis virus mutants deleted in the erbA or erbB oncogenes. Cell 12: 227-238.

(5) Gazzolo, L.; Moscovici, C.; Moscovici, M.G.; and Samarut, J. 1979. Response of hemopoietic cells to avian acute leukemia viruses: Effects on the differentiation of the target cells. Cell 16: 627-638.

(6) Graf, T.; Beug, H.; and Hayman, M.J. 1980. Target cell specificity of defective avian leukemia viruses: hematopoietic target cells for a given virus type can be infected but not transformed by strains of a different type. Proc. Natl. Acad. Sci. USA 77: 389-393.

(7) Graf, T.; Fink, D.; Beug, H.; and Royer-Pokora, B. 1977. Oncornavirus-induced sarcoma formation obscured by rapid development of lethal leukemia. Cancer Res. 37: 59-63.

(8) Graf, T., and Stehelin, D. 1982. Avian leukemia viruses. Oncogenes and genome structure. Biochim. Biophys. Acta 651: 245-271.

(9) Graf, T.; von Kirchbach, A.; and Beug, H. 1981. Characterization of the hematopoietic target cells of AEV, MC29 and AMV avian leukemia viruses. Exp. Cell Res. 131: 331-343.

(10) Hayman, M.J.; Savin, K.; and Beug, H. 1982. Changes in the expression of membrane antigens during the differentiation of chicken erythroblasts. J. Cell Biochem. 18: 351-362.

(11) Kornfeld, S.; Beug, H.; Doederlein, G.; and Graf, T. 1983. Detection of avian hematopoietic cell surface antigens with monoclonal antibodies to myeloid cells: their distribution on normal and leukemic cells of various lineages. Exp. Cell Res. 143: 383-394.

(12) Moscovici, C., and Gazzolo, L. 1982. Tranformation of hemopoietic

cells with avian leukemia viruses. In Advances in Viral Oncology, ed. G. Klein, vol. 1, pp. 83-106. New York: Raven Press.

(13) Moscovici, M.G.; Jurdic, P.; Samarut, J.; Gazzolo, L.; Mura, C.V.; and Moscovici, C. 1983. Characterization of hemopoietic target cells for the avian leukemia virus E26. Virology 129: 65-78.

(14) Moscovici, M.G., and Moscovici, C. 1983. Isolation and characterization of a temperature-sensitive mutant of avian myeloblastosis virus. Proc. Natl. Acad. Sci. USA 80: 1421-1425.

(15) Radke, K.; Beug, H.; Kornfeld, S.; and Graf, T. 1982. Transformation of both erythroid and myeloid cells by E26, an avian leukemia virus that contains the myb gene. Cell 31: 643-653.

(16) Risser, R. 1982. The pathogenesis of Abelson virus lymphomas of the mouse. Biophys. Biochim. Acta 651: 213-244.

(17) Risser, R. 1983. In Mechanisms of B-cell Neoplasia, eds. F. Melchers, M. Potter, and M. Weigert. Basel, Switzerland: Editiones Roche.

(18) Rosenberg, N. 1982. Abelson leukemia virus. Curr. Top. Microbiol. Immunol. 101: 93-126.

(19) Samarut, J., and Gazzolo, L. 1982. Target cells infected by avian erythroblastosis virus differentiate and become transformed. Cell 28: 921-929.

(20) Smith, L.J.; Curtis, J.E.; Messner, H.A.; Senn, J.S.; Furthmayr, H.; and McCulloch, E.A. 1983. Lineage infidelity in acute leukemia. Blood 61: 1138-1145.

(21) Waneck, G.L., and Rosenberg, N. 1981. Abelson leukemia virus induces lymphoid and erythroid colonies in infected fetal cell cultures. Cell 26: 79-89.

(22) Whitlock, C.A., and Witte, O.N. 1981. Abelson virus-infected cells can exhibit restricted in vitro growth and low oncogenic potential. J. Virol. 40: 577-584.

(23) Whitlock, C.; Ziegler, S.F.; Treiman, L.J.; Stafford, J.I.; and Witte, O.N. 1983. Differentiation of cloned populations of immature B cells after transformation with Abelson murine leukemia virus. Cell 32: 903-911.

(24) Witte, O.N. 1983. Molecular and cellular biology of Abelson virus transformation. Curr. Top. Microbiol. Immunol. 103: 127-146.

Leukemia, ed. I.L. Weissman, pp. 147-162. Dahlem Konferenzen 1985. Berlin, Heidelberg, New York, Tokyo: Springer-Verlag.

Multiple Mechanisms of Oncogene Activation in Viral and Nonviral Neoplasia

W.S. Hayward
Sloan-Kettering Institute for Cancer Research
New York, NY 10021, USA

Abstract. The oncogenic potential of a proto-oncogene can be "activated" by many different types of mutational events, including insertion of proviral control sequences, gene amplification, translocation, and point mutations within regulatory or coding sequences. The mechanisms by which a specific proto-oncogene can most readily be activated probably reflects unique structural and biological characteristics of the gene involved. The c-myc gene can be activated by a variety of mechanisms, but each appears to induce changes in expression of the gene. By contrast, members of the c-ras gene family appear to be preferentially activated by point mutations within coding sequences. Induction of a fully malignant state may require activation of more than one proto-oncogene and/or multiple mutational events within a single gene.

INTRODUCTION

Recent studies have implicated a class of cellular genes (termed proto-oncogenes or c-onc genes) in neoplasms induced by both viral and nonviral agents. These genes, first identified as oncogenes (v-onc genes) in the genomes of acute retroviruses, have been highly conserved throughout evolution and are thought to play an essential role in normal cell growth control or development (2, 48). Mutational events that cause changes in the regulation of these genes, or in the properties of their gene products, can lead to abnormal cell growth patterns and neoplastic disease.

Studies of model systems, as well as naturally occurring tumors, have revealed quite diverse mechanisms for activating the oncogenic potential of a proto-oncogene (7, 9, 22, 49, 52). The general patterns that have emerged from these studies can be stated, with varying degrees of certainty, as follows: a) At least two dozen distinct proto-oncogenes are present in the DNA of normal vertebrate cells. Most, but not all, of those identified thus far are homologous to the known v-onc genes. (This bias, however, may reflect in part the ease with which v-onc gene homologs can be identified.) b) Proto-oncogenes can be "activated" by many different mechanisms. These include insertion of proviral regulatory sequences, chromosomal translocations, gene amplifications, and base substitutions within coding sequences. The mutational events fall into two classes: regulatory (altering the expression of the gene) and structural (altering the properties of the gene product). c) Oncogenes are not all alike. Likewise, the mechanisms by which specific proto-oncogenes are most efficiently activated probably differ, reflecting unique structural features of each gene, the different enzymatic properties of the gene products, and the characteristics of the target cells involved. d) The type of neoplasm induced by a specific agent would be determined to a certain extent by the type of mutational event induced by the agent. (This follows from point c) above and assumes that the phenotype associated with a specific neoplasm is determined, in part, by the characteristics of the oncogene(s) involved.) e) More than one mutational event may be required to activate the full oncogenic potential of a specific gene. f) More than one activated oncogene may be required to induce a fully malignant state. g) Certain oncogenes, specifically the c-myc gene and members of the ras gene family, have been implicated in a surprisingly high number of neoplasms. These genes may be more susceptible to activation by simple mutational events. h) Although much has been learned about the molecular basis for activation of proto-oncogenes, little is known about the functions of their gene products in either the normal or the malignant cell. (This subject, therefore, will not be discussed here.)

In the present paper I will use the ALV-induced B cell lymphoma system as a basis for discussion of many of the points listed above. Other systems will also be mentioned in order to draw parallels or contrasts with the ALV system.

ACTIVATION OF c-myc BY AVIAN LEUKOSIS VIRUS

By far the most abundant retroviruses in nature - and probably most important in naturally occurring viral cancers - are the "slowly transforming" retroviruses. Although they lack oncogenes, retroviruses of this type induce neoplasms in infected animals after long latent periods

(9, 22, 48, 49). The avian leukosis viruses (ALVs), which belong to this class, induce B cell lymphomas, fibrosarcomas, erythroleukemias, and nephroblastomas. Analyses of ALV-induced B cell lymphomas have provided strong evidence that induction of these tumors results from insertion of proviral sequences adjacent to, and transcriptional activation of, the host c-myc gene (21). This conclusion is based on the following lines of evidence: a) In more than 80% of ALV-induced lymphomas a provirus was found to be integrated adjacent to the c-myc gene. b) Levels of c-myc mRNA were elevated 30-100-fold in the lymphomas, compared to equivalent normal tissues. c) In most tumors, the myc-specific mRNA contained viral sequences derived from the long terminal repeat (LTR) of the integrated provirus. This indicated that transcription initiates within the viral LTR and reads into the adjacent c-myc gene, causing transcriptional activation of the gene.

The coding sequences of the avian c-myc gene are located within two exons, interrupted by an intron of about 1 kb (30, 40, 50). Two potential promoters, mapping approximately 1 and 1 kb upstream of the coding sequences, have been identified by cell-free transcription of cloned c-myc DNA (Neel, unpublished). However, it is not yet known which of these functions in vivo in the avian system. In the vast majority of ALV-induced B cell lymphomas, the provirus is integrated upstream of the c-myc coding sequences, but downstream from both potential c-myc promoters ((22), Goodenow and Hayward, unpublished). Thus, insertion of the provirus presumably results in displacement of the cellular promoter and regulatory sequences, and placement of the c-myc gene under the transcriptional control of viral regulatory sequences. Integration at these sites results in synthesis of a truncated message, lacking sequences derived from the first exon (non-coding) of c-myc. A model has been proposed in which loss of these sequences would result in enhanced translational efficiency of the mRNA (43, 45). If this model is correct, a single integration event might alter c-myc expression at both the transcription and translation levels.

Payne et al. (37) have identified one tumor in which integration was downstream from c-myc and several tumors in which integration was upstream, but in the opposite transcriptional orientation. Since the viral promoter could not be utilized directly for transcription of c-myc in these tumors, it seems likely that c-myc transcription is augmented by viral enhancer sequences which act on a cellular promoter. These orientations have been observed in only a small minority of cases (5-10%) (9, 22, 49), suggesting that integration in the same transcriptional orientation, with the viral promoter and enhancer in their proper juxtaposition, is a more efficient mechanism for activating the c-myc gene. (This orientation, however, is the exception in the MMTV system (see below).)

Point mutations have been detected within the c-myc coding sequences of one ALV-induced lymphoma (Westaway and Varmus, personal communication). Although the functional significance of these mutations is unknown, this finding raises the interesting possibility that changes in the structure of the gene product may contribute to the oncogenic properties of an activated c-myc gene. Changes within the coding region are not, however, an essential feature of c-myc activation, at least in human neoplasia. In two independent cases, the rearranged c-myc genes in Burkitt lymphomas have been sequenced and shown not to carry a single point mutation within the coding sequences (P. Leder, personal communication, and Wiman and Hayward, unpublished).

Interestingly, most, and perhaps all, of the proviruses integrated next to c-myc are defective (16, 31, 37). In most cases, the 5'-proximal sequences of the provirus, including the 5' LTR, are deleted. This observation suggests that defectiveness plays an essential role in c-myc activation. One explanation is that transcription from the 3' LTR is enhanced by removal of 5' transcriptional signals. (Normal transcription of viral RNA, from the 5' LTR, proceeds into, and beyond, the initiation site within the 3' LTR; this might partially inhibit the efficient utilization of the 3' promoter.) Loss of 5' sequences might also allow the cell to escape detection by the host immune system, because viral antigens would no longer be synthesized.

The insertional activation mechanism is not unique to ALV, nor is it restricted to the c-myc gene. Activation of c-myc by the same mechanism has been observed in B cell lymphomas induced by reticuloendotheliosis virus (a retrovirus that has no apparent sequence homology with ALV) (34) and in a minority of cases of T cell lymphoma induced by MuLV in rats (Steffan, personal communication). Fung et al. (17) have demonstrated that the c-erb gene is activated by the same mechanism in ALV-induced erythroleukemias. Common sites of integration were found in a high proportion of fibrosarcomas induced by ring-necked pheasant virus, but the putative oncogene involved has not yet been identified (Simon and Hayward, unpublished). Activation of c-mos, apparently resulting from insertion of A-type particle sequences, has been reported in one human tumor line (38). However, efforts to demonstrate an insertional activation mechanism have been unsuccessful thus far in many systems (e.g., bovine leukemia virus)(24).

A high percentage of carcinomas induced by murine mammary tumor viruses (MMTV) contain proviruses integrated within a single 20 kb domain (49). A candidate oncogene (termed int-1) located within this domain was found to be transcriptionally activated. Proviruses were integrated on either side of int-1 - often at a considerable distance - and oriented such that viral transcription reads away from int-1. Presumably, activation of int-1 results from insertion of enhancer sequences located within the LTR of the integrated provirus. Regional integration of this type, which is very difficult to identify by restriction analysis, may account for some of the negative results obtained in certain other retroviral systems. However, the possibility that completely novel mechanisms are responsible for some retroviral neoplasms must also be considered (24).

ACTIVATION OF ONCOGENES IN NONVIRAL NEOPLASMS

Many types of neoplasms are characterized by specific, nonrandom, chromosomal translocations (25, 35, 41). These observations, together with the demonstration of c-myc activation by ALV integration, have led to the suggestion that proto-oncogenes might be activated by translocations that join the coding sequences of a proto-oncogene to a positive control element from another gene (21, 25, 42). In support of this notion, recent studies have demonstrated that the c-myc gene is translocated to another chromosomal location in murine plasmacytomas (4, 44, 47) and in human Burkitt lymphomas (10, 47). In both types of neoplasms, the c-myc gene is joined to one of the immunoglobulin (Ig) genes.

Efforts to deduce the mechanism by which translocation causes activation of c-myc have been complicated by the fact that the sequence arrangement of the two loci is variable from one tumor to another ((4, 19, 20, 33); Wiman et al., in preparation). In a high proportion of Burkitt lymphomas and plasmacytomas the breakpoint in c-myc is located within the first intron, but breakpoints within, or considerably upstream of, the first exon are also common. Breakpoints in the Ig locus often occur within the switch region, but sites have also been observed both upstream and downstream of this region. A number of models have been presented to explain one or more of the observed rearrangements. a) Transcriptional control may be altered by removal of c-myc regulatory sequences, and/or placement of Ig enhancer sequences adjacent to the rearranged c-myc gene (20, 27). b) Loss of non-coding sequences in the 5' exon may result in synthesis of a truncated mRNA with enhanced translational efficiency (33, 43). c) Placement of c-myc adjacent to the Ig locus (a genetically "unstable" region) might result in an enhanced mutational frequency within the gene, thus increasing the probability of mutational events that might alter regulatory or coding sequences of the gene in a way that favors neoplastic growth (Wiman et al., in preparation). Experimental support for each of these models has been presented in specific cases, but no single model has emerged to explain all of the observed rearrangements.

In some tumors, activation of proto-oncogenes may result from gene amplification. The c-myc gene, for example, is amplified some 20-30-fold in two cell lines, a promyelocytic leukemia cell line (HL-60) (6, 11) and a human colon carcinoma line (1). Gene amplification is accompanied by a corresponding increase in c-myc mRNA. Several other cases of gene amplification involving other proto-oncogenes have also been demonstrated (Bishop, personal communication).

Point mutations play a central role in activation of proto-oncogenes belonging to the ras gene family. The ras genes have been implicated in a wide variety of neoplasms (13, 18, 36), including bladder, colon, and lung carcinomas (Ki-ras and Ha-ras), neuroblastomas and T cell leukemias (N-ras), one cell line derived from a promyelocytic leukemia (N-ras), and one Burkitt lymphoma cell line (N-ras). These genes were first identified by transfection of tumor cell DNA onto NIH3T3 cells (7, 52). Analyses of various constructs between the cloned oncogenes and their normal counterparts have provided compelling evidence that the ability to transform NIH3T3 cells can be attributed to a single base substitution within one of two domains in the coding sequences of the ras gene (39, 46, 53). The ras oncogenes are the only examples in which activation by a single point mutation has been documented. It is interesting to note that transformation of NIH3T3 cells can also apparently result from over-expression of the normal c-ras gene (5, 12).

REGULATORY VS. STRUCTURAL CHANGES

The mechanisms that activate proto-oncogenes can be classified into two groups: those that alter the expression of the gene ("regulatory") and those that alter the structure of the gene product ("structural"). Examples of the first group include provirus insertion, translocation, and gene amplification. This mechanism has been demonstrated experimentally by constructing recombinant molecules in which proto-oncogene sequences are linked to a viral LTR (3, 5, 12). The best documented examples of changes in protein structure are the point mutations in the coding sequences of activated c-ras genes.

Although it has been argued that only structural changes are important in oncogene activation (15), it is more likely that both regulatory and structural changes play important roles in different cancers. The mechanism that most efficiently activates a specific gene would depend on the sequence organization of that gene, enzymatic properties of the gene product, and the presence of sites that can be easily altered by mutation to generate a malignant phenotype.

What role(s) might regulatory changes play in induction of neoplastic disease? a) Clearly, an oncogene must be expressed if it is to exert any influence on the cell. Although many normal c-onc genes (e.g., c-src, c-ras) are expressed in a wide variety of tissues, others (e.g., c-fps, c-myc) are expressed differentially in different tissues, and at least one (c-mos) has not been found to be expressed in any tissue (2, 19, 23, 28). b) Constitutive expression of the gene may be required to maintain the transformed state. If the expression of a particular proto-oncogene normally fluctuates in response to cellular regulatory signals, replacement or alteration of control sequences may be necessary to allow uninterrupted expression of the gene. A hypothetical example would be a gene required for proliferation. This gene would presumably be turned on at appropriate times to allow cell division (e.g., during embryogenesis), but turned off when the tissue has reached maturity. c) Over-expression of a proto-oncogene may induce altered phenotypes. Increasing the concentration of the gene product might result in interactions with low affinity substrates that do not interact significantly when the proto-oncogene product is present at normal physiologic concentrations.

Mutations affecting protein structure can be envisioned as causing two types of changes: a) altered substrate affinity or specificity, or b) a change in the intracellular localization of the protein (e.g., by loss or gain of a hydrophobic signal sequence).

Both regulatory and structural changes may be involved in some systems. For example, it is likely that the highly oncogenic properties of the v-onc genes of many acute retroviruses can be attributed both to the fact that these genes are placed under the control of retroviral regulatory sequences (and hence are expressed constitutively, and at high levels in the infected cell), and to mutational events that alter the properties of the oncogene products.

MULTISTAGE PROGRESSION OF NEOPLASIA

Pathologists have long recognized that the development of cancer is a multi-step process (32), but it is only recently that experimental evidence has provided a molecular basis for this phenomenon. Recent studies indicate that a) more than one mutational event may be required to activate the full oncogenic potential of a single proto-oncogene, and b) more than one oncogene may be required to induce a fully malignant state. There are many examples of multiple mutations in the v-onc genes of acute viruses, but the functional significance of each mutation has not been fully evaluated in any viral system. As many as three independent mutational events may be involved in activation of c-myc by ALV (see below), but the evidence that all three events are required for activation is, at the moment, only circumstantial.

The first evidence implicating more than one oncogene in a single neoplasm was obtained in the ALV-induced lymphoma system. Two different approaches were used to identify candidate oncogenes. The c-myc gene, identified by screening with a series of v-onc probes, is activated by insertion of proviral sequences. A second oncogene (termed Blym), which is unrelated to c-myc, was identified by transfection of NIH3T3 cells with lymphoma DNA (8). Activation of this gene apparently results from some mechanism that does not involve direct interaction with proviral DNA.

The same two experimental approaches have also yielded evidence for participation of multiple oncogenes in a number of human tumor cell lines, including a promyelocytic leukemia line (myc plus N-ras), neuroblastoma (N-myc plus N-ras), and one Burkitt lymphoma cell line (myc plus N-ras) (1, 18, 29, 51). Diamond et al. (14) have presented evidence that Blym is activated in Burkitt lymphoma (presumably in addition to c-myc), and that another gene participates along with c-myc in murine plasmacytomas.

More recently, several groups have presented evidence that primary tissue culture cells must be supplied with at least two activated oncogenes in order to induce complete transformation (26, 42). This is in contrast to the NIH3T3 cells (and several other established cell lines) which can often be transformed by transfection with a single oncogene (3, 7, 12, 52). Certain oncogenes (e.g., myc) do not score well on NIH3T3 cells. Presumably, a gene equivalent to c-myc, representing one stage in transformation, has already become activated in NIH3T3 cells during establishment of the cell line. Land et al. (26) have tentatively placed oncogenes into two complementary groups: a) myc, polyoma large T, adenovirus E1A, and the postulated gene that is activated in NIH3T3 cells, and b) polyoma middle T, ras, and Blym.

SOMATIC SELECTION

Cancer can be viewed as the result of two processes: a continuing exposure of cell DNA to environmental mutagens (e.g., viruses, irradiation, chemical carcinogens) and a selection for mutations that confer a selective advantage to the cell. (Although we have discussed here only mutational events, such quasi-stable changes as altered methylation patterns might also play an important role.) Selection would occur at two levels - with entirely different consequences. At the germ line level, selection would be directed against any mutation that was deleterious to the whole organism. In somatic cells, however, the fate of the whole organism would be of little consequence. Selective pressure would favor any cell that had acquired a growth advantage over other cells in the population, regardless of the effect on the whole organism.

In the ALV-induced lymphoma system we can envision as many as four distinct mutational events (see below). If each event occurs with a frequency of 10^{-8} per cell per generation, the probability that all four events would occur in the same cell would be 10^{-32}, a frequency too low to occur within the lifetime of the animal. However, if we assume that each event confers a selective advantage to the cell, then the population carrying this mutation would expand, providing a vastly increased number of target cells in which a second rare event might occur. This would result in the expansion of a subpopulation carrying two mutational events, providing, therefore, an expanded target population for a third event, etc. The long latent period characteristic of B cell lymphoma would result from the time required to sequentially expand the clonal population or subpopulation after each mutational event. (If we assume that cells divided every 24 h, it would take approximately one month to expand from a single cell to a population of 10^9 cells at each step.)

The following scenario can be proposed for ALV-induced B cell lymphoma. Each stage is assumed to confer a growth advantage that would result in clonal expansion of a single cell from within the population. a) The ALV provirus becomes integrated adjacent to the c-myc gene. This is a rare event (perhaps at a frequency of 10^{-6} to 10^{-7}), since integration is thought to be random. Integration may induce two important changes. First, the regulatory sequences of the c-myc gene are displaced by the inserted provirus. The gene is now placed under control of viral control sequences and is expressed constitutively. (We must assume here that some transcription from the 3' LTR can occur, even in the presence of normal transcription from the 5' LTR.) Second, as mentioned above, the translational efficiency of the resultant truncated c-myc mRNA may be enhanced because of the loss of sequences from the first exon. b) Most of the 5' portion of the integrated provirus is deleted, resulting in enhanced transcription from the 3' LTR into c-myc and termination of synthesis of viral gene products that might be recognized by the host immune system. c) Random mutations within the coding sequences of c-myc may result occasionally in the synthesis of a protein with enhanced transforming activity, thus conferring an additional growth advantage on a single cell within the clonal subpopulation. d) The Blym gene is activated by an as yet unknown mechanism. (Presumably, a mutation within the coding sequences is involved, since no change in expression has been detected.)

Although it may not be essential that the events described above occur in the order shown, it is likely that certain events (for example, activation of Blym) would provide a selective advantage only at a specific stage in tumor development.

CONCLUSIONS

More than twenty different oncogenes are now known. Each of these is in some way unique. Thus, it is not surprising that different proto-oncogenes are activated by different mechanisms, and, conversely, that similar mechanisms appear to be responsible for activation of the same oncogene in different biological systems. The c-myc gene has been implicated in a wide range of neoplasms. Although activation of c-myc can occur by such diverse mechanisms as insertion of retroviral regulatory sequences, translocation, and gene amplification, it is perhaps significant that in each case the mutational event induces a change in gene expression. In contrast, all of the naturally occurring examples of ras gene activation appear to involve point mutations within the coding sequences of the gene.

The myc gene and members of the ras gene family have been implicated in an unusually high proportion of tumors. Although the statistics now available are subject to certain technical biases (for example, the NIH3T3 transfection assay is particularly efficient for scoring members of the ras gene family), the preponderance of cases involving these two groups of genes is quite striking. A possible explanation for this higher than expected frequency is that these genes are more readily activated by single mutational events, or by multiple mutations, each of which confers a selective advantage on the cell. The latter requirement may be partially circumvented in the conversion of a c-onc gene to a v-onc gene in an acute retrovirus, because of the huge number of copies of the gene generated during virus replication and the enhanced rate of mutations inherent in the replication process. (The viral reverse transcriptase apparently introduces an unusually high frequency of transcriptional errors.) Thus genes that have been detected as v-onc genes in one or more retroviruses may be activated only rarely in nonviral neoplasms.

The molecular basis for neoplastic disease is in some ways more simple, and in some ways more complex than originally believed. On the one hand, we have a proto-oncogene that can apparently be activated by a single point mutation, and on the other hand, we find that multiple mutations, in one or more genes, may be required for induction of a fully malignant state. Undoubtedly more complexities will be encountered, new oncogenes will be discovered, and new mechanisms of activation will be found. Each proto-oncogene will have to be studied independently to determine the unique features of the gene that allow it to be mutationally altered in a way that leads to abnormal cell growth.

Acknowledgments. The author would like to thank L. O'Connor for help in preparation of this manuscript. Work in the author's laboratory was supported by grant CA34502 from the National Institutes of Health, and by grants from Bristol Meyers, The Flora E. Griffin Fund, and The Kleberg Foundation.

REFERENCES

(1) Alitalo, L.; Schwab, M.; Lin, C.C.; Varmus, H.E.; and Bishop, J.M. 1983. Homogeneously staining chromosomal regions contain amplified copies of an abundantly expressed cellular oncogene (c-myc) in malignant neuroendocrine cells from a human colon carcinoma. Proc. Natl. Acad. Sci. USA 80: 1707-1711.

(2) Bishop, J.M. 1981. Enemies within: The genesis of retrovirus oncogenes. Cell 23: 5-6.

(3) Blair, D.G.; Oskarsson, M.; Wood, T.G.; McClements, W.L.; Fischinger, P.J.; and Vande Woude, G.F. 1981. Activation of the transforming potential of a normal cell sequence: A molecular model for oncogenesis. Science 212: 941-943.

(4) Calame, K.; Kim, S.; Lalley, P.; Hill, R.; Davis, M.; and Hood, L.

1982. Molecular cloning of translocations involving chromosome 15 and the immunoglobulin C gene from chromosome 12 in two murine plasmacytomas. Proc. Natl. Acad. Sci. USA 79: 6994-6998.

(5) Chang, E.H.; Furth, M.E.; Scolnick, E.M.; and Lowy, D.R. 1982. Tumorigenic transformation of mammalian cells induced by a normal human gene homologous to the oncogene of Harvey murine sarcoma virus. Nature 297: 479-483.

(6) Collins, S., and Groudine, M. 1982. Amplification of endogenous myc-related DNA sequences in a human myeloid leukemia cell line. Nature 298: 679-681.

(7) Cooper, G.M. 1982. Cellular transforming genes. Science 217: 801-806.

(8) Cooper, G.M., and Neiman, P.E. 1981. Two distinct candidate transforming genes of lymphoid leukosis virus induced neoplasms. Nature 292: 857-858.

(9) Crittenden, L.B., and Kung, H.J. 1984. Mechanisms of induction of lymphoid leukosis and related neoplasms by avian leukosis viruses. In Mechanisms of Viral Leukemogenesis, eds. J.M. Goldman and J.W. Jarret, pp. 64-88. Edinburgh, Scotland: Churchill Livingston Books.

(10) Dalla-Favera, R.; Bregni, M.; Erikson, J.; Patterson, D.; Gallo, R.C.; and Croce, C.M. 1982. Human c-myc onc gene is located on the region of chromosome 8 that is translocated in Burkitt lymphoma cells. Proc. Natl. Acad. Sci. USA 79: 7824-7827.

(11) Dalla-Favera, R.; Wong-Staal, F.; and Gallo, R.C. 1982. Onc gene amplification in promyelocytic leukemia cell line HL-60 and primary leukaemic cells of the same patient. Nature 299: 61-63.

(12) DeFeo, D.; Gonda, M.A.; Young, H.A.; Chang, E.H.; Lowy, D.R.; Scolnick, E.M.; and Ellis, R.W. 1981. Analysis of two divergent rat genomic clones homologous to the transforming gene of Harvey murine sarcoma virus. Proc. Natl. Acad. Sci. USA 78: 3328-3332.

(13) Der, C.J.; Krontiris, T.G.; and Cooper, G.M. 1982. Transforming genes of human bladder and lung carcinoma cell lines are homologous to the ras genes of Harvey and Kirsten sarcoma viruses. Proc. Natl. Acad. Sci. USA 79: 3637.

(14) Diamond, A.; Cooper, G.M.; Ritz, J.; and Lane, M.-A. 1983. Identification and molecular cloning of the human Blym transforming gene

activated in Burkitt's lymphomas. Nature 305: 112-116.

(15) Duesberg, P.H. 1983. Retroviral transforming genes in normal cells? Nature 304: 219-226.

(16) Fung, Y.-K.; Fadly, A.M.; Crittenden, L.B.; and Kung, H.-J. 1981. On the mechanism of retrovirus-induced avian lymphoid leukosis: Deletion and integration of the proviruses. Proc. Natl. Acad. Sci. USA 78: 3418-3422.

(17) Fung, Y.-K.; Lewis, W.G.; Kung, H.-J.; and Crittenden, L.B. 1983. Activation of the cellular oncogene c-erb B by LTR insertion: Molecular basis for induction of erythroblastosis by avian leukosis virus. Cell 33: 357-368.

(18) Goldfarb, M.; Shimizu, K.; Perucho, M.; and Wigler, M. 1982. Isolation and preliminary characterization of a human transforming gene from T24 bladder carcinoma cells. Nature 296: 404-409.

(19) Gonda, T.J.; Sheiness, D.K.; and Bishop, J.M. 1982. Transcripts from the cellular homologs of retroviral oncogenes: distribution among chicken tissues. Mol. Cell Biol. 2: 617-624.

(20) Hayday, A.C.; Gillies, S.D.; Saito, H.; Wood, C.; Wiman, K.; Hayward, W.S.; and Tonegawa, S. 1984. Activation of translocated human c-myc gene transcription in a non-Hodgkin's lymphoma by an immunoglobulin gene-associated transcriptional enhancer element. Nature 307: 334-340.

(21) Hayward, W.S.; Neel, B.G.; and Astrin, S.M. 1981. Activation of a cellular onc gene by promoter insertion in ALV-induced lymphoid leukosis. Nature 290: 475-480.

(22) Hayward, W.S.; Neel, B.G.; and Astrin, S.M. 1982. Avian leukosis viruses: Activation of cellular oncogenes. In Advances in Viral Oncology, ed. G. Klein, vol. 1, pp. 207-233. New York: Raven Press.

(23) Hayward, W.S.; Shih, C.-K.; and Moscovici, C. 1983. Induction of bursal lymphoma by myelocytomatosis virus-29 (MC29). In Cetus-UCLA Symposium on Tumor Viruses and Differentiation, pp. 279-287. New York: Liss.

(24) Kettman, R.; Deschamps, J.; Couez, D.; Claustriaux, J.J.; Palm, R.; and Burny, A. 1983. Chromosome integration domain for bovine leukemia provirus in tumors. J. Virol. 47: 146-150.

(25) Klein, G. 1981. Changes in gene dosage and gene expression: a

common denominator in the tumorigenic action of viral oncogenes and non-random chromosomal changes. Nature 294: 313-318.

(26) Land, H.; Parada, L.F.; and Weinberg, R.A. 1983. Tumorigenic conversion of primary embryo fibroblasts requires at least two cooperating oncogenes. Nature 304: 596-602.

(27) Marcu, K.H.; Harris, L.J.; Stanton, L.W.; Erikson, J.; Watt, R.; and Croce, C.M. 1983. Transcriptionally active c-*myc* oncogene is contained within NIARD, a DNA sequence associated with chromosome translocations in B-cell neoplasia. Proc. Natl. Acad. Sci. USA 80: 519-523.

(28) Muller, R.; Tremblay, J.M.; Adamson, E.D.; and Verma, I.M. 1983. Tissue and cell-type specific expression of two human c-*onc* genes. Nature 304: 454-456.

(29) Murray, M.J.; Cunningham, J.M.; Parada, L.F.; Dautry, F.; Lebowitz, P.; and Weinberg, R.A. 1983. The HL60 transforming sequence: a *ras* oncogene coexisting with altered *myc* genes in hematopoietic tumors. Cell 33: 749-757.

(30) Neel, B.G.; Gasic, G.P.; Rogler, C.E.; Skalka, A.M.; Papas, T.; Astrin, S.M.; and Hayward, W.S. 1982. Molecular cloning of virus-cell junctions from ALV-induced lymphomas: Comparison with the normal c-*myc* gene. J. Virol. 44: 158-166.

(31) Neel, B.G.; Hayward, W.S.; Robinson, H.L.; Fang, J.; and Astrin, S.M. 1981. Avian leukosis virus-induced tumors have common proviral integration sites and synthesize discrete new RNAs: Oncogenesis by promoter insertion. Cell 23: 323-334.

(32) Neiman, P.E.; Jordon, L.; Weiss, R.A.; and Payne, L.N. 1980. *In* Viruses in Naturally Occurring Cancers, eds. M. Essex, G. Todaro, and H. zer Hausen, pp 519-528. Cold Spring Harbor Laboratories.

(33) Nishikura, K.; ar-Rushdi, A.; Erikson, J.; Watt, R.; Rovera, G.; and Croce, C.M. 1983. Differential expression of the normal and of the translocated human c-*myc* oncogenes in B cells. Proc. Natl. Acad. Sci. USA 80: 4822-4862.

(34) Noori-Daloii, M.R.; Swift, R.A.; Kung, H.-J.; Crittenden, L.B.; and Witter, R.L. 1981. Specific integration of REV proviruses in avian bursal lymphomas. Nature 294: 574-575.

(35) Nowell, P.C., and Hungerford, D.A. 1960. A minute chromosome in human chronic granulocytic leukemia. Science 132: 1497-1499.

(36) Parada, L.F.; Tabin, C.J.; Shih, C.; and Weinberg, R.A. 1982. Human EJ bladder carcinoma oncogene is homologue of Harvey sarcoma virus ras gene. Nature 297: 474-478.

(37) Payne, G.S.; Bishop, J.M.; and Varmus, H.E. 1982. Multiple arrangements of viral DNA and an activated host oncogene (c-myc) in bursal lymphomas. Nature 295: 209-213.

(38) Rechavi, G.; Givol, D.; and Canaani, E. 1982. Activation of a cellular oncogene by DNA rearrangement: possible involvement of an IS-like element. Nature 300: 607-611.

(39) Reddy, E.P.; Reynolds, R.K.; Santos, E.; and Barbacid, M. 1982. A point mutation is responsible for the acquisition of transforming properties by the T24 human bladder carcinoma oncogene. Nature 300: 149-152.

(40) Robins, T.; Bister, K.; Garon, C.; Papas, T.; and Duesberg, P. 1982. Structural relationship between a normal chicken DNA locus and the transforming gene of the avian acute leukemia virus MC29. J. Virol. 41: 635-642.

(41) Rowley, J.D. 1982. Identification of the constant chromosome regions involved in human hematologic malignant disease. Science 216: 749-751.

(42) Ruley, H.E. 1983. Adenovirus early region 1A enables viral and cellular transforming genes to transform primary cells in culture. Nature 304: 602-606.

(43) Saito, H.; Hayday, A.C.; Wiman, K.; Hayward, W.S.; and Tonegawa, S. 1983. Activation of c-myc gene by translocation: a model for translational control. Proc. Natl. Acad. Sci. USA 80: 7476-7480.

(44) Shen-Ong, G.L.C.; Keath, E.J.; Piccoli, S.P.; and Cole, M.D. 1982. Novel myc oncogene RNA from abortive immunoglobulin gene recombination in mouse plasmacytomas. Cell 31: 443-452.

(45) Shih, C.-K.; Linial, M.; and Hayward, W.S. 1984. Nucleotide sequence of the 5' flanking region of avian c-myc coding region: localization of a noncoding exon that is absent from myc transcripts in most ALV induced lymphomas. Proc. Natl. Acad. Sci. USA 81: 4697-4701.

(46) Tabin, C.J.; Bradley, S.M.; Bargmann, C.I.; Weinberg, R.A.; Papageorge, A.G.; Scolnick, E.M.; Dhar, R.; Lowy, D.R.; and Change, E.H. 1982. Mechanism of activation of a human oncogene. Nature

300: 143.

(47) Taub, R.; Kirsch, I.; Morton, C.; Lenoir, G.; Swan, D.; Tronick, S.; Aaronson, S.; and Leder, P. 1982. Translocation of the c-myc gene into the immunoglobulin heavy chain locus in human Burkitt lymphoma and murine plasmacytoma cells. Proc. Natl. Acad. Sci. USA 79: 7837-7841.

(48) Teich, N.; Wyke, J.; Mak, T.; Bernstein, A.; and Hardy, W. 1982. Molecular Biology of Tumor Viruses: Part III. RNA Tumor Viruses, eds. R. Weiss, N. Teich, H.E. Varmus, and J. Coffin. Cold Spring Harbor Laboratory.

(49) Varmus, H.E. 1982. Form and function of retroviral proviruses. Science 216: 812-820.

(50) Vennstrom, B.; Sheiness, D.; Zabielski, J.; and Bishop, J.M. 1982. Isolation and characterization of c-myc, a cellular homolog of the oncogene (v-myc) of avian myelocytomatosis virus strain 29. J. Virol. 42: 773-779.

(51) Watt, R.; Stanton, L.W.; Marcu, K.B.; Gallo, R.C.; Croce, C.M.; and Rovera, G. 1983. Nucleotide sequence of cloned cDNA of human c-myc oncogene. Nature 303: 725-728.

(52) Weinberg, R.A. 1982. Transforming genes of nonvirus-induced tumors. In Advances in Viral Oncology, ed. G. Klein, vol. I, pp. 235-241. New York: Raven Press.

(53) Yasuhito, Y.; Srivastava, S.K.; Dunn, C.Y.; Rhim, J.S.; Reddy, E.P.; and Aaronson, S.A. 1983. Acquisition of transforming properties by alternative point mutations within c-bas/has human proto-oncogene. Nature 303: 775-779.

Leukemia, ed. I.L. Weissman, pp. 163-178. Dahlem Konferenzen 1985. Berlin, Heidelberg, New York, Tokyo: Springer-Verlag.

Oncogenes of Avian Leukemia Viruses

M.J. Hayman
Imperial Cancer Research Fund Laboratories
St. Bartholomew's Hospital
London EC1A 7BE, England

Abstract. Avian acute leukemia viruses can be divided into three main classes based on the oncogene contained within their genomes. These three oncogenes, erb, myc, and myb, are responsible for the neoplastic diseases observed in chickens infected by acute leukemia viruses. The purpose of this paper is to summarize what is known about the gene products of these oncogenes with an emphasis on the possible functions of these proteins.

INTRODUCTION

Acute leukemia viruses are so called because upon injection into young chickens they cause rapidly progressing neoplasms of hematopoietic cells resulting in the death of the animal. It should be stressed, however, that while the viruses are associated mainly with hematological neoplasms, neoplastic diseases of other tissues are also observed. Indeed, certain laboratory strains of virus are no longer able to transform hematopoietic cells but are still able to transform other tissue types. This aspect of the biology of acute leukemia viruses will be taken into account when mechanisms of transformation are discussed.

The acute leukemia viruses to be discussed here fall into three groups on the basis of the oncogenes that are contained in their genomes. The oncogenes are erb, which is found in viruses which cause erythroid leukemias and sarcomas; myc which is associated with a wide variety of neoplasms including myelocytoma, sarcoma, and carcinoma; and myb which is primarily associated with myeloblastic leukemia. The viruses which contain these oncogenes are listed in Table 1, as are the most common diseases associated with these viruses.

There are two other classes of avian acute leukemia viruses, the reticuloendotheliosis viruses which contain the oncogene known as rel, and the erythroblastosis virus S13. However, this review is concerned mainly with the gene products of the oncogenes, and as little is known about the rel gene product and since the oncogene of S13 has yet to be identified, they will not be included here. We are only going to consider three oncogenes out of almost twenty identified; therefore, certain very interesting features of other oncogenes will naturally be excluded from this review. However, these three oncogenes will allow us to consider most of the central features of the research that is under way to understand the function of oncogene products.

In considering how oncogene proteins transform cells, one question that has to be addressed by any proposed mechanism of action is the target cell specificity observed amongst acute leukemia viruses. For example, AMV only causes myeloblastic leukemia and not erythroblastosis or sarcomas. In order to try and gain insight into the function of these proteins and their specificity of action, the approaches taken have been the following: first, identification of the viral oncogene product, its sequence, and its cellular location. Second, mutants which are altered in their ability to transform have been analyzed to see if the mutations alter

TABLE 1 – Three classes of avian acute leukemia viruses.

Oncogene	Virus	Disease
erb	AEV-ES4	Erythroblastosis, sarcoma
	AEV-H	Erythroblastosis, sarcoma
myc	MC29	Myelocytoma, carcinoma, endothelioma
	CM11	Myelocytoma
	OK10	Endothelioma
	MH2	Endothelioma
myb	AMV	Myeloblastosis
	E26	Myeloblastosis, Erythroblastosis

the expression of the oncogene protein and provide clues to the function. Finally, the product of the viral gene is compared to its cellular counterpart to see if there are differences between the products. Although the cellular sequences are referred to as cellular oncogenes, c-onc, they do not usually exhibit the same ability to bring about malignant transformation as their viral counterparts. Hence, there must be crucial differences between the v-onc and its cellular counterpart. The oncogene products under discussion here will be reviewed individually and then their general features will be considered.

THE erb ONCOGENE

There have been two independent isolates of viruses containing erb sequences, AEV-ES4 and AEV-H (18, 21). Both cause erythroblastosis and fibrosarcoma in vivo. The best understood of these two viruses is AEV-ES4, and consequently the gene products of this virus will be considered in most detail. Figure 1 shows the genome structure and products of both AEV-ES4 and AEV-H.

Both viruses contain a gene referred to as erb B, whereas AEV-ES4 contains an additional gene termed erb A. Deletion of the erb A sequences from AEV-ES4 generates a virus which can still transform both fibroblasts and erythroblasts (14). These data, together with the isolation of AEV-H, demonstrated that erb B is the gene responsible for malignant transformation. However, in the case of AEV-ES4 the presence of the erb A gene renders the virus more tumorigenic, and therefore it must play some role in the development of the malignant phenotype.

Characterization of the erb B gene products of AEV-H and AEV-ES4 has shown them to be membrane glycoproteins, see Fig. 1 ((20, 33) and Kawai, personal communication). In the case of AEV-ES4, mutants that are temperature-sensitive for transformation have been analyzed, and it has been possible to correlate the synthesis of the plasma membrane gp74 protein with transformation. At the non-permissive temperature gp68 is not processed into gp74 and no cell surface immunofluorescence with erb B-specific antiserum is seen (Hayman and Beug, unpublished observations). Interestingly, nucleic acid sequence analysis of molecularly cloned erb B genes from both AEV-ES4 and AEV-H have revealed that they contain a region of homology with the sequence associated with the tyrosine-specific protein kinase activity found in the sarcoma-inducing viruses, i.e., Rous sarcoma virus src gene and Y73 yes gene (Privalsky and Bishop, and Kawai, both personal communications). Various growth factor receptors are associated with a similar protein kinase activity

(7, 11, 25), therefore it is intriguing to speculate that the erb B protein could itself be a growth factor receptor. The specific growth factor for the erb B glycoprotein would have to be either a serum protein or a protein secreted by the transformed cell in an autocrine fashion if it is responding to growth factor.

Alternatively, the erb B protein may be mutated in such a way that it can function as a receptor in the absence of its normal signal. These are all intriguing possibilities that undoubtedly deserve and will get further attention.

The role of erb A in the transformation process is unclear, although it undoubtedly enhances the effect of erb B alone. It is found mainly in the cytoplasm (8, 20), and therefore any direct interaction with erb B may be considered unlikely. However, this cannot be ruled out since

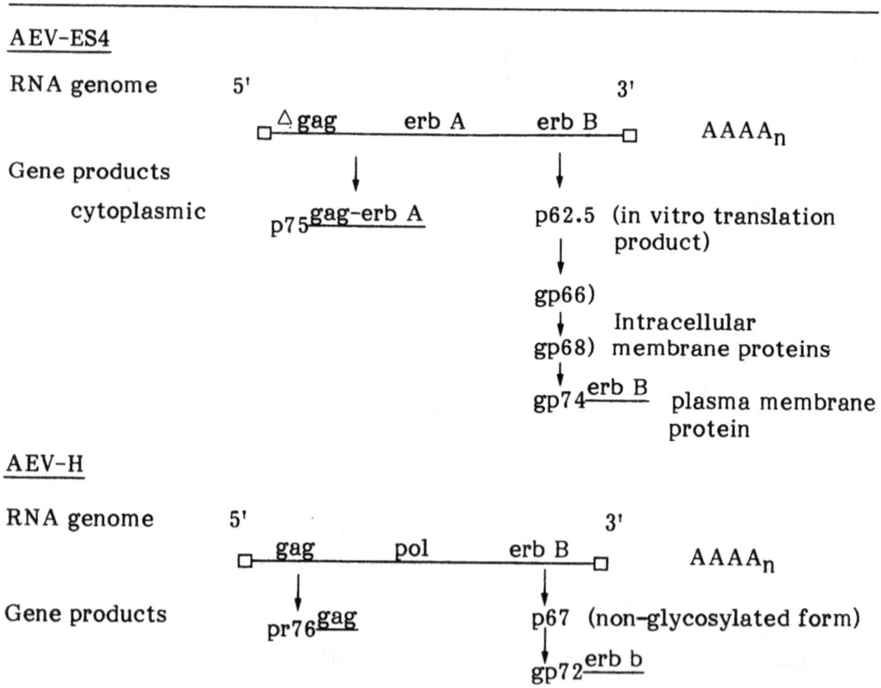

FIG. 1 - Genome structure and products of avian erythroblastosis virus.

a small fraction of erb A is found in membrane fractions (20) where it could be exerting an effect on the erb B protein found there.

Attempts to identify the normal cellular counterparts of either erb A or erb B have so far been unsuccessful. This has been due to the inability to find a tissue in which these erb genes are expressed in any appreciable amount (16). However, in avian leukemia virus-induced erythroblastosis which is associated with an insertional mutation of the cellular erb B locus, c-erb B, very high expression of c-erb B is observed (15). Analysis of these leukemic cells has shown that c-erb B products can be found that range in size from 60,000-90,000 daltons, and they all appear to be plasma membrane glycoproteins (Hayman et al., in preparation). It is not known whether the c-erb B gene is mutated in any way in these leukemic cells, but given the size range, it is likely that these products represent truncated versions of the normal protein. Therefore, as yet there is no direct evidence that the normal c-erb B gene is transforming.

Both the c-erb A and c-erb B genes have been molecularly cloned from both chicken and human genomic DNA (24, 44). Attempts to show that these two genes are linked in the chicken genome were unsuccessful, the genes being at least 15 kb apart. In addition, they give rise to specific distinct mRNA species (44). Chromosomal mapping of the human loci has placed c-erb A on chromosome 17 and c-erb B on chromosome 7 (Spurr and Vennström, personal communication). These data are consistent with recent observations on the recovery of erb sequences by avian leukosis viruses in which the viruses appear to pick up erb B first and then occasionally erb A sequences also.

THE myb ONCOGENE

There are two isolates of viruses containing the myb gene, AMV and E26. Interestingly, these viruses have significantly differing pathogenic properties: AMV causes only myeloblastic leukemia, whereas E26 causes both myeloblastic and erythroblastic leukemia (30, 35, 41). Examination of the genome structure of these viruses shows that whereas AMV has only the myb gene (10), E26 contains an additional cellular sequence termed ets (see Fig. 2).

The myb gene product in AMV has been identified as a protein of 45-48,000 molecular weight (5, 26), preliminary observations indicate that it is phosphorylated and is a nuclear protein (Bishop, personal communication). Although a conditional mutant of AMV does exist (31), there is no published information about the myb gene product in this mutant.

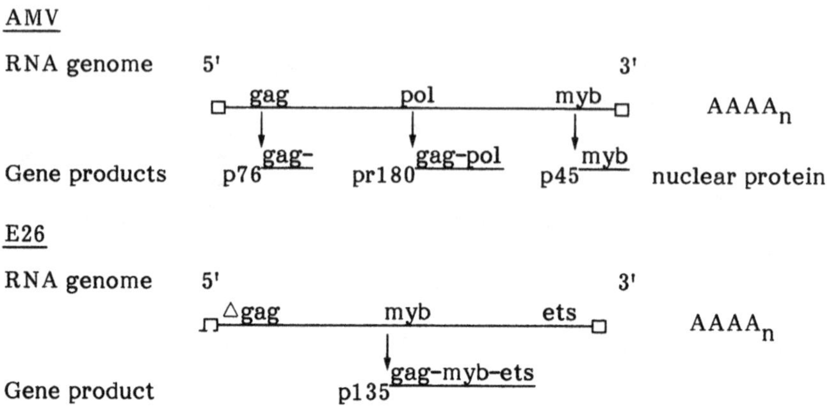

FIG. 2 - Genome structure and products of the *myb*-containing viruses AMV and E26.

Using the available antisera, two proteins here have been identified as products of the *c-myb* gene. A 75,000 molecular weight protein has been identified in chicken erythroleukemia cells (26), whereas a 105,000 molecular weight protein was identified in normal thymus cells using a different anti-*myb* serum (5). These differences may reflect differences in the antisera used (i.e., cross-reacting proteins are occasionally precipitated by antisera raised against peptides), or they may be pointing to a mechanism by which expression of the *c-myb* gene is controlled in different tissues (i.e., differential splicing). Nevertheless, it is clear that the *v-myb* gene, present in AMV, represents a truncated version of the *c-myb* gene, suggesting that the *v-myb* protein is a mutated version of the cellular gene. This difference may alter its function sufficiently to make it a transforming protein.

The *myb* gene in E26 is expressed as a large fusion protein of 135,000 molecular weight (3, 4); the remaining information includes the 5' remnant of the *gag* gene and the *ets* gene (see Fig. 2). It appears that even less of the *c-myb* gene is found in E26 (28, 32). It is presumed that it is this *myb* gene information that is responsible for the myeloblastosis associated with E26. The additional cellular sequence *ets* is thought to enable E26 to cause erythroblastosis. Whether it does this in its own right or by acting in concert with myb is not known. No data is available on the cellular location of this protein. Obviously this protein is very interesting as it apparently has two transforming activities. If, as appears likely, the myb gene and the ets gene act independently, then the characterization of this protein will be extremely interesting. Already it has been shown that the synthesis of this protein in myeloblasts is affected by myeloid growth factors (3); it is not yet known at what level the growth factor acts or, indeed, if it is acting on the myb or ets sequence. The recent isolation of temperature-sensitive mutants of E26 (Graf, personal communication) will undoubtedly help resolve these questions. More information is obviously needed on this virus.

THE myc ONCOGENE

Four avian viruses have been isolated which contain the myc gene, and these viruses are capable of transforming a relatively large variety of cell types (Table 1). As with the myb gene, the myc gene is expressed in one of two different ways, either as a gag fusion protein or as an entity in its own right (Fig. 3).

Whether this difference in mode of expression has any effect on the disease spectrum is unknown. However, both the gag-myc fusion proteins and the myc proteins are found in the nucleus of transformed cells (1, 2, 9, 19). Their function in the nucleus is unknown, but the gag-myc fusion proteins have been shown to bind DNA in vitro, including chromatin (6, 9). Preliminary evidence suggests that they are components of the nuclear matrix (Hann and Eisenman, personal communication).

Nonconditional mutants of MC29 have been isolated that are essentially nonpathogenic in vivo and have lost the ability to transform macrophage-like cells efficiently (36, 37). They do, however, morphologically transform fibroblasts, but apparently these fibroblasts are not malignantly transformed since no sarcomas are seen in vivo (12). All three of these mutants were shown to have deletions in the 3' half of the myc gene (37), and although they encode smaller proteins than wt that locate to the nucleus (8), these mutant proteins were no longer phosphorylated on the amino acid threonine (38).

No mutants of OK10 or CM11 have been reported, however, mutants of MH-2 have been isolated. These mutants are still transforming but are no longer able to synthesize the p100 protein (Fig. 3) (29). MH-2 is unusual among the other myc viruses in that it contains an additional cellular sequence termed mil (23, 39), which is contained in the cytoplasmic

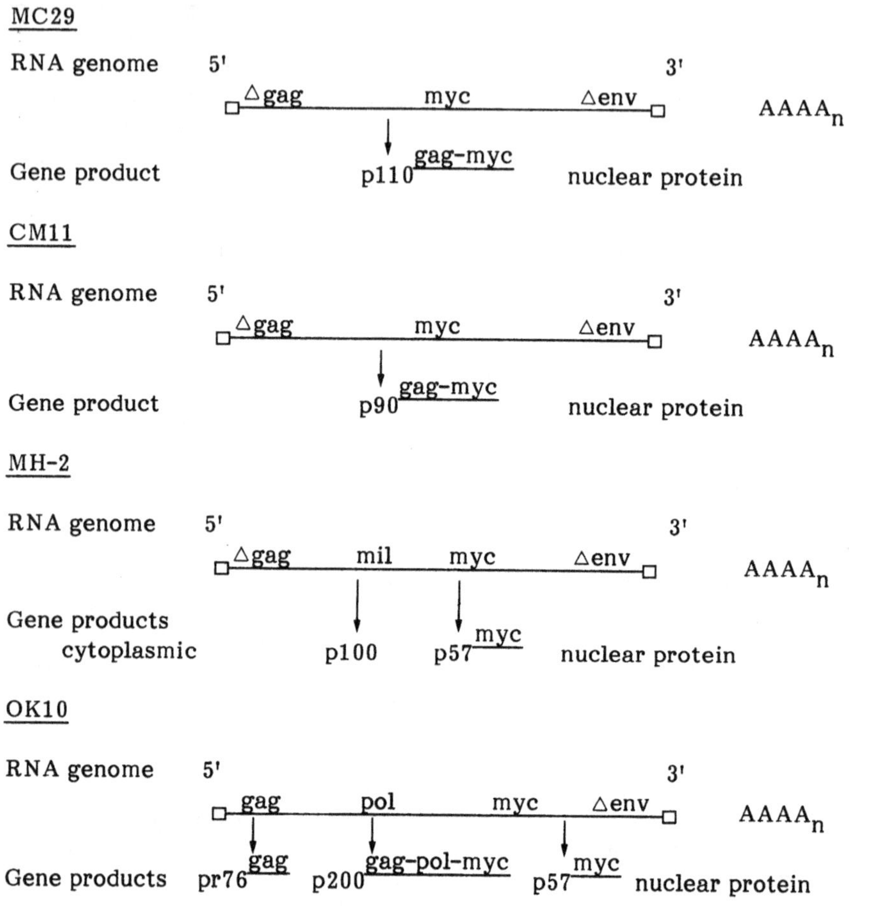

FIG. 3 - Genome structure and products of the myc-containing viruses.

p100 protein. These data imply that the p100 is not essential for transformation by MH-2 and that it is the myc gene which is responsible for transformation by MH-2. However, the recent finding that v-mil is homologous to the murine oncogene v-raf (22) indicates that mil probably can play a role in oncogenesis.

The c-myc gene has recently been identified in normal fibroblasts and erythroid leukemic cells (2, 19) and appears to be very similar to the v-myc product found in OK10. The c-myc product found in avian leukosis virus-induced B cell lymphoma has also been identified and again is very similar to the OK10 v-myc product ((2, 19) and Hayman, unpublished observation). However, all these comparisons are based on size and cellular localization, and there may well be subtle changes in the v-myc gene which affect its function. It is known from sequencing data that there are seven amino acid changes between the v-myc and c-myc gene (43), and there are possibly extra 5' exons in the c-myc gene. Also, recent data on a recovered MC29 virus termed HB1, which is suspected of having a hybrid, v-myc-c-myc, gene transforms lymphoid cells in vivo rather than the endothelial cells transformed by wt MC29 (13). Therefore, small changes in the myc gene may have profound effects on its function.

DNA transfection experiments have also been used to analyze the myc gene. Cellular DNA from B cell lymphomas which have a transcriptionally activated c-myc gene will transform NIH-3T3 cells, but it is a "gene" termed B-lym which is responsible for the transformation and not c-myc (17). Also, if primary rat embryo cells are used as recipients, myc will only transform them if co-transfected with the ras oncogene (27). These data have been interpreted as implying that activation of c-myc is a necessary but insufficient stage in a multistage progression to tumorigenicity. From a functional standpoint they imply that myc exerts its effect by immortalizing cells and activating other genes which in turn are responsible for malignant transformation. It is not clear in this case why the myc gene in a retroviral genome is sufficient to elicit malignant transformation in vivo, in a relatively short period of time. However, it should be remembered that fibroblasts tranformed by wt MC29 are not tumorigenic, and nonpathogenic deletion mutants of MC29 are still capable of transforming fibroblasts morphologically. Therefore, the myc protein may be a multi-functional protein, and care should be taken about which function is being scored in the different systems.

In considering possible functions for the myc gene, its conservation throughout evolution has to be accounted for. Finding myc-related genes in Drosophila and yeast as well as mammalian species (40) implies that the myc gene may have a rather general function as opposed to one associated with the differentiation of a specialized cell type. If it is a nuclear matrix protein that can apparently affect other genes and immortalize cells, then a possible role in control of cell division is suggested. If myc does have a function such as this, then the cell-type specificity of transformation seen in vivo would have to be explained by secondary factors that do not bear directly on the primary function of the myc gene. It is known that the genetic makeup of the host affects the pathology of myc-containing viruses (13, 29), and it is possible that these effects are not acting on the myc gene but on other genetic elements.

CONCLUSION

From the data reviewed here, it is obvious that there is no single mechanism by which the oncogenes function, although there may only be a limited number of strategies that can be employed to bring about malignant transformation. This can be implied from the large number of oncogenes which encode tyrosine-specific protein kinases. There is also no obvious key compartment within the cell in which oncogenes exert their action - oncogene products being found in the plasma membrane, under the plasma membrane, in the cytoplasm, and within the nucleus. The most reasonable hypothesis is that they represent various kinds of effector molecules which are normally engaged in regulatory functions. In the transformed cell these molecules would then have to be considered as functioning in an uncontrolled way such that the cell can no longer control its own growth. The oncogenes could then represent all kinds of molecules from growth factors, for example, sis (42); growth factor receptors - perhaps erb B; intracellular regulatory molecules such as protein kinase - src, etc.; and nuclear proteins that can directly influence transcription and division - possible myb and myc.

If in the transformed state these proteins are acting in an uncontrolled manner due to mutation, how can we envisage that this might take place? It seems probable that in the cases of myb and myc the transforming domain of the protein may normally be accompanied by regulatory domains (i.e., c-myb and c-myc genes have more information than their viral counterparts). V-myb represents a truncated version of the cellular protein, whereas v-myc may not contain information from a 5' exon found in c-myc. The v-myc protein itself appears to have two domains - a 5' domain sufficient to locate the molecule in the nucleus and transform fibroblasts and a 3' domain required for malignancy in vivo. It is likely that functional domains will also be identified on the fusion, p135, encoded by E26. In this case, myb sequences make up only 25-30% of the protein, a small portion, but sufficient for cellular transformation. The recent finding of a domain for cell adhesion on fibronectin of only a few amino acids in length (34) suggests that oncogene proteins will have to be studied in great detail to understand the subtleties of their activities. One of the major problems to be overcome in understanding how these molecules work is to identify exactly the functional region(s) on the v-onc and c-onc proteins and how these regions control the activity of the molecule. In other words, the normal function of the molecule has to be identified and compared with the function carried out by its oncogenic counterpart.

The possibility also exists that the oncogenic protein is not mutated and that it is the inappropriate expression that is the problem. For example, if the oncogene were a growth factor or growth factor receptor, inappropriate expression could result in an autocrine-like situation where a cell was now expressing both the growth factor and its receptor and as a result was stimulating itself to divide. This mechanism would predict that the target cell for transformation would not normally express the oncogene in question, but would express the molecule it interacts with.

A third mechanism hypothesized is over-expression of the oncogene product. Although this was a popular hypothesis, it has lost favor to the mutation hypothesis in recent years as more examples of mutation have been discovered. However, it is still a viable hypothesis and may be the mechanism used by some oncogenes.

The oncogenes represent a diverse group of genes whose only common feature is their ability to induce malignant transformation. Since this can undoubtedly be achieved by a wide variety of means, we should beware seeking one overriding mechanism of action. Consequently, these three different mechanisms are not meant to be mutually exclusive. Indeed, it is quite likely that an example will be found for all three mechanisms. In every case the mechanism will have to address three aspects of malignant transformation: what is the function of the oncogene product? How does this function affect the cell? And why does it only affect certain cell types? Only when all three questions can be answered will the model for the mode of action be truly viable.

Acknowledgements. I would like to thank P.J. Enrietto for her help with the manuscript and my many colleagues who provided information prior to publication. I would also like to thank J. Newton for typing the manuscript.

REFERENCES

(1) Abrams, H.D.; Rohrschneider, L.R.; and Eisenman, R.N. 1982. Nuclear localization of the putative protein of avian myelocytomas virus. Cell 29: 427-439.

(2) Alitalo, K.; Ramsay, G.; Bishop, J.M.; Pfeifer, S.O.; Colby, W.W.; and Levinson, A.D. 1983. Identification of nuclear proteins encoded by viral and cellular myc oncogenes. Nature 306: 274-277.

(3) Beug, H.; Hayman, M.J.; and Graf, T. 1982. Myeloblasts transformed by the avian acute leukemia virus E26 are hormone-dependent for growth and for the expression of a putative gag-myb containing protein, p135 E26. EMBO J. 9: 1069-1073.

(4) Bister, K.; Nunn, M.; Moscovici, C.; Perbal, B.; Baluda, M.; and Duesberg, P. 1982. Acute leukemia viruses E26 and avian myeloblastosis viruses have related transformation-specific RNA sequences but different genetic structures, gene products and oncogenic properties. Proc. Natl. Acad. Sci. USA 79: 3677-3681.

(5) Boyle, W.J.; Lipsick, J.S.; Reddy, E.P.; and Baluda, M.A. 1983. Identification of the leukemogenic protein of avian myeloblastosis virus and of its normal cellular homologue. Proc. Natl. Acad. Sci. USA 80: 2834-2838.

(6) Bunte, T.; Greiser-Wilke, I.; Donner, P.; and Moelling, K. 1982. Association of gag-myc proteins from avian myelocytomatosis virus wild-type and mutants with chromatin. EMBO J. 1: 919-927.

(7) Cohen, S.; Carpenter, G.; and King, L.E. 1980. Epidermal growth factor-receptor protein kinase interactions. J. Biol. Chem. 255: 4834-4842.

(8) Donner, P.; Bunte, T.; Greiser-Wilke, I.; and Moelling, K. 1983. Decreased DNA binding ability of purified transformation-specific proteins from deletion mutants of the acute avian leukemia virus MC29. Proc. Natl. Acad. Sci. USA 80: 2861-2865.

(9) Donner, P.; Greiser-Wilke, I.; and Moelling, K. 1982. Nuclear localization and DNA binding of the transforming gene product of avian myelocytomatosis virus. Nature 296: 262-266.

(10) Duesberg, P.H.; Bister, K.; and Moscovici, C. 1980. Genetic structure of avian myeloblastosis virus, released from transformed myeloblasts as a defective virus particle. Proc. Natl. Acad. Sci. USA 77: 5120-5124.

(11) Ek, B.; Westermark, B.; Wasteson, A.; and Heldin, C.H. 1982. Stimulation of tyrosine-specific phosphorylation by platelet-derived growth factor. Nature 295: 419-420.

(12) Enrietto, P.J.; Hayman, M.J.; Ramsay, G.M.; Wyke, J.A.; and Payne,

L.N. 1982. Altered pathogenicity of avian myelocytomatosis (MC29) viruses with mutations in the v-myc gene. Virol. 124: 164-172.

(13) Enrietto, P.J.; Payne, L.N.; and Hayman, M.J. 1984. A recovered Avian myelocytomatosis virus which induces lymphomas in chickens: Pathogenic properties and their molecular basis. Cell 35: 369-379.

(14) Frykberg, L.; Palmieri, S.; Beug, H.; Graf, T.; Hayman, M.J.; and Vennström, B. 1983. Transforming capacities of avian erythroblastosis virus mutants deleted in the erb A or erb B oncogenes. Cell 32: 227-238.

(15) Fung, Y.K.T.; Lewis, W.G.; Kung, H.-J.; and Crittenden, L.B. 1983. Activation of the cellular oncogene c-erb B by LTR insertion: Molecular basis for induction of erythroblastosis by avian leukosis virus. Cell 33: 357-368.

(16) Gonda, T.J.; Sheiness, D.K.; and Bishop, J.M. 1982. Transcripts from the cellular homology of retroviral oncogene: Distribution among chicken tissues. Mol. Cell. Biol. 2: 617-624.

(17) Goubin, G.; Foldman, D.S.; Luce, J.; Neiman, P.E.; and Cooper, G.M. 1983. Molecular cloning and nucleotide sequence of a transforming gene detected by transfection of chicken B-cell lymphoma DNA. Nature 302: 114-119.

(18) Graf, T., and Beug, H. 1978. Avian leukemia viruses: Interaction with their target cells in vivo and in vitro. Biochim. Biophys. Acta 516: 269-299.

(19) Hann, S.R.; Abrams, H.D.; Rohrschneider, L.R.; and Eisenman, R.N. 1984. Proteins encoded by the v-myc and c-myc oncogenes: identification and localization in acute leukemia virus transformants and bursal lymphoma cell lines. Cell 34: 789-798.

(20) Hayman, M.J.; Ramsay, G.; Savin, K.; Kitchener, G.; Graf, T.; and Beug, H. 1983. Identification and characterization of the avian erythroblastosis virus erb B gene product as a membrane glycoprotein. Cell 32: 579-588.

(21) Hihara, H.; Yamamoto, H.; Shimohira, H.; Arai, K.; and Shimizu, T. 1983. Avian erythroblastosis virus isolated from chicken erythroblastosis induced by lymphatic leukemia virus subgroup A. J. Natl. Canc. Inst. 70: 891-898.

(22) Jansen, H.W.; Lurz, R.; Bister, K.; Bonner, T.I.; Mark, G.E.; and

Rapp, U.R. 1984. Homologous cell-derived oncogenes in avian carcinoma virus MH2 and murine sarcoma virus 3611-MSV. Nature 307: 281-284.

(23) Jansen, H.W.; Patschinsky, T.; and Bister, K. 1983. Avian oncovirus MH2: Molecular cloning of proviral DNA and structural analysis of viral RNA and protein. J. Virol. 48: 61-73.

(24) Jansson, M.; Philipson, L.; and Vennström, B. 1983. Isolation and characterization of multiple human genes homologous to the oncogenes of avian erythroblastosis virus. EMBO J. 2: 561-565.

(25) Kasuga, M.; Fujita-Yamaguchi, Y.; Blithe, D.L.; and Kahn, C.R. 1983. Tyrosine-specific protein kinase activity is associated with the purified insulin receptor. Proc. Natl. Acad. Sci. USA 80: 2137-2141.

(26) Klempnauer, K.-H.; Ramsay, G.; Bishop, J.M.; Moscovici, M.G.; Moscovici, C.; McGrath, J.P.; and Levinson, A.D. 1983. The product of the retroviral transforming gene v-myb is a truncated version of the protein encoded by the cellular oncogene c-myb. Cell 33: 345-355.

(27) Land, H.; Parade, L.F.; and Weinberg, R.A. 1983. Tumorigenic conversion of primary embryo fibroblasts requires at least two cooperating oncogenes. Nature 304: 596-601.

(28) Leprince, D.; Gegonne, A.; Cell, J.; de Taisne, C.; Schneeberger, A.; Lagrou, C.; and Stehelin, D. 1983. A putative second cell-derived oncogene of the avian leukaemia retrovirus E26. Nature 306: 395-397.

(29) Linial, M. 1982. Two retroviruses with similar transforming genes exhibit differences in transforming potential. Virology 119: 382-391.

(30) Moscovici, C. 1975. Leukemic transformation with avian myeloblastosis virus: Present status. Curr. Top. Microbiol. Immunol. 71: 79-101.

(31) Moscovici, G.M., and Moscovici, C. 1983. Isolation and characterization of a temperature-sensitive mutant of avian myeloblastosis virus. Proc. Natl. Acad. Sci. USA 80: 1421-1425.

(32) Nunn, M.F.; Seeburg, P.; Moscovia, C.; and Duesberg, P.H. 1983. Tripartite structure of the avian erythroblastous virus E 26 transforming gene. Nature 306: 391-395.

(33) Pierschbacher, M.; Hayman, E.G.; and Ruoslahti, E. 1983. Synthetic peptide with cell attachment activity of fibronectin. Proc. Natl. Acad. Sci. USA 80: 1224-1227.

(34) Privalsky, M.L.; Sealy, L.; Bishop, J.M.; McGrath, J.P.; and Levinson, A.D. 1983. The product of the avian erythroblastosis virus erb B locus is a glycoprotein. Cell 32: 1257-1267.

(35) Radke, K.E.; Beug, H.; and Graf, T. 1982. Transformation of both erythroid and myeloid cells by E26, and avian erythroleukemic virus which contains the myb gene. Cell 31: 643-653.

(36) Ramsay, G.M.; Graf, T.; and Hayman, M.J. 1980. Mutants of avian myelocytomatosis virus MC29 with smaller gag gene related protein have an altered transforming ability. Nature 288: 170-172.

(37) Ramsay, G.M., and Hayman, M.J. 1982. Isolation and biochemical characterization of partially transformation-defective mutants of avian myelocytomatosis virus MC29. J. Virol. 41: 745-753.

(38) Ramsay, G.M.; Hayman, M.J.; and Bister, K. 1982. Phosphorylation of specific sites in the gag-myc polyproteins encoded by MC29 type viruses correlates with their transforming ability. EMBO J. 9: 1111-1116.

(39) Saule, S.; Coll, J.; Righi, M.; Lagrou, C.; Raes, M.B.; and Stehelin, D. 1983. Two different types of transcription for the myelocytomatosis viruses MH2 and CM11. EMBO J. 2: 805-809.

(40) Shilo, B.Z., and Weinberg, R.A. 1981. DNA sequences homologous to vertebrate oncogenes are conserved in Drosophila melanogaster. Proc. Natl. Acad. Sci. USA 78: 6789-6792.

(41) Sotirov, N. 1981. Histone H5 in the immature blood cells of chickens with leukosis induced by avian leukosis virus strain E26. J. Natl. Canc. Inst. 66: 1143-1147.

(42) Waterfield, M.D.; Scrace, G.T.; Whittle, N.; Stroobant, P.; Johnsson, A.; Wasteson, A.; Westermark, B.; Heldin, C.H.; Huang, J.S.; and Deuel, T.F. 1983. Platelet-derived growth factor is structurally related to the putative transforming protein $p28^{sis}$ of simian sarcoma virus. Nature 304: 35-39.

(43) Watson, D.K.; Reddy, E.P.; Duesberg, P.H.; and Papas, T.S. 1983. Nucleotide sequence analysis of the chicken c-myc gene reveals homologous and unique coding regions by comparison with the transforming gene of avian myelocytomatosis virus MC29. Proc. Natl.

Acad. Sci. USA 80: 2146-2150.

(44) Vennström, B., and Bishop, J.M. 1982. Isolation and characterization of chicken DNA homologous to the two putative oncogenes of avian erythroblastosis virus. Cell 28: 135-143.

Leukemia, ed. I.L. Weissman, pp. 179-202. Dahlem Konferenzen 1985. Berlin, Heidelberg, New York, Tokyo: Springer-Verlag.

Significance of Chromosome Rearrangements in Leukemia and Lymphoma

J.D. Rowley
Dept. of Medicine, University of Chicago
Chicago, IL 60637, USA

Abstract. Nonrandom chromosome changes have been identified in a number of malignant tumors, of which the leukemias are the best studied. In chronic myeloid leukemia, a reasonably consistent translocation [t(9;22) (q34;q11)] is observed in 93% of all Ph^1-positive patients. In acute nonlymphocytic leukemia, two translocations are each specifically associated with leukemic cells arrested at two different stages of maturation. One of these, t(8;21) (q22;q22), is found almost exclusively in patients with acute myeloblastic leukemia with maturation (AML-M2). The other, t(15;17) (q22;q21), is seen only in patients with acute promyelocytic leukemia (APL-M3). An inversion of chromosome 16(p13q22) has recently been described in patients with AMMoL and abnormal marrow eosinophils; other patients with marrow eosinophilia have had a deletion of 16 at q22. Translocations or deletions involving 11q23 have recently been described in patients with AMoL, particularly of the monoblastic type. Various translocations have been observed in B cell acute lymphoblastic leukemia or in Burkitt lymphoma. The most common is t(8;14) (q24;q32), but varients of this, namely, t(2;8) (p13?;q24) and t(8;22) (q24;q11), have also been observed; in all of these, the consistent change involved 8q24. The various immunoglobulin loci are located on chromosomes 2, 14, and 22 in the same chromosome band affected by the translocations in B cell leukemia. More recently it has been shown that the myc gene is located at 8q24 and that the translocation results in the movement of the myc gene adjacent to the Ig locus on No. 14. These translocations may occur randomly. If a specific translocation provides a particular cell type with a growth advantage, then selection could act to cause the proliferation of this aneuploid cell line vis-a-vis cells with a normal karyotype. The chromosome change could then be the initial event leading to the leukemic transformation of an otherwise normal cell. The challenge for the future is to define the genes located at the sites of consistent translocations in myeloid leukemias and to determine the alterations in gene function that are associated with the translocation.

INTRODUCTION

The study of the chromosome pattern in the affected cells of a number of human tumors has been one of the most rapidly advancing areas in cancer research over the last twenty years. Major advances in our understanding of the specificity of some of the abnormalities have occurred in the last ten years with the application of new chromosome banding techniques. These techniques allow the identification of each human chromosome and of parts of chromosomes as well. Thus, the hypothesis put forward by Boveri at the turn of the century, namely, that an abnormal chromosome pattern was intimately associated with the malignant phenotype of the tumor cell, can now be tested with substantial hope of obtaining a valid answer (7).

Except for the detection of the Philadelphia (Ph^1) chromosome in chronic myeloid leukemia (27), no specific chromosome abnormalities were observed prior to the application of the new banding techniques. With the use of banding techniques, other specific abnormalities were found to be associated with certain leukemias and lymphomas. Moreover, banding techniques revealed that the gains and losses of chromosomes were distinctly nonrandom. The specific abnormalities that have been identified in human leukemia during the last ten years will be described in this review. The data obtained prior to 1970 have been reviewed in a number of reports and they will not be considered here (25, 37, 38). The data presented here have been gathered primarily during the period 1974-1982. The observations and conclusions are based on our increased ability to identify abnormal chromosomes with banding. However, most of the studies, especially those before 1980, used chromosomes that were relatively contracted, and the banding pattern often was fuzzy and poorly defined. For this reason, subtle abnormalities such as a deletion or a duplication of one third of a chromosome band, involving about $3x10^6$ nucleotide pairs, would be undetectable. Substantial improvements have occurred in the quality of the chromosome preparations used for analysis. Yunis et al. (43) have reported that with the use of elongated (prophase) chromosomes from patients with acute non-lymphocytic leukemia (ANLL), everyone of twenty-four patients had an abnormal karyotype. Thus, the future emphasis will be to identify the abnormalities we have all overlooked in the past.

Several major types of chromosome abnormalities have been identified in human leukemias and in other malignant diseases as well. These include gain of a whole chromosome or a portion thereof, loss of part or all of a chromosome, consistent translocations, and other structural rearrangements. This diversity of abnormalities implies an equal diversity in the mechanisms of genetic changes that can be associated with malignant transformation. Thus, a gain of all or part of a chromosome implies amplification of a gene, suggesting that an increase in a gene product is an important factor in the malignant process. Deletion of part or all of a chromosome suggests that loss of certain elements regulating cell growth may be significant. Consistent translocations, on the other hand, imply that a more complex process is involved because two chromosomes are affected by this rearrangement. It should be emphasized that for each type of aberration certain chromosomes are preferentially affected. Thus, a gain of No. 8 is the most frequent aberration in a variety of myeloid disorders (25, 37, 38). When a chromosome is lost, No. 7 is most commonly affected. The consistent translocations in myeloid disorders are t(9;22) in CML, t(8;21) in AML-M2, and t(15;17) in APL-M3; more recently translocations or deletions involving chromosome No. 11 have been observed primarily in AMoL (5), and an inversion of No. 16 has been described in AMMoL (21). Different chromosomes are involved in lymphoid disorders, for example, t(8;14), t(2;8), t(8;22), and t(14;18) (37). These various aberrations will be discussed in detail in subsequent sections.

METHODS

An analysis of chromosome patterns, to be relevant to a malignant disease, must be based on a study of the karyotype of the tumor cells themselves. In the case of leukemia, the specimen is usually a bone marrow aspirate that is processed immediately or is cultured for 24 to 48 hours (40). In patients with a white blood cell count higher than 15.500, with about 10% immature myeloid cells, a sample of peripheral blood can be cultured for 24 to 48 hours without adding phytohemagglutinin (PHA). The karyotype of the dividing cells will be similar to that obtained from the bone marrow. The use of amethopterin to synchronize dividing cells provides cells with elongated chromosomes that have a larger number of bands (43).

The observation of at least two "pseudodiploid" or hyperdiploid cells or three hypodiploid cells, each showing the same abnormality, is considered evidence for the presence of an abnormal clone; patients with such clones are classified as abnormal. However, in some tumors with a low mitotic index, a single abnormal cell may be the only malignant cell dividing in the particular sample examined. In the following discussion, the chromosomes are identified according to the ISCN (15), and the karyotypes are expressed as recommended under this system. The total chromosome number is indicated first, followed by the sex chromosomes, and then by the gains, losses, or rearrangements of the autosomes. A "+" sign or "-" sign before a number indicates a gain or loss, respectively, of a whole chromosome; a "+" or "-" after a number indicates a gain or loss of part of a chromosome. The letters "p" and "q" refer to the short and long arms of the chromosome, respectively. Translocations are identified by "t" followed by the chromosomes involved in the first set of brackets; the chromosome bands in which the breaks occurred are indicated in the second brackets. Uncertainty about the chromosome or band involved is signified by "?".

CHRONIC MYELOGENOUS LEUKEMIA (CML)

Chronic Phase of CML

Chromosome banding techniques were first used in the cytogenetic study of leukemia for identification of the Ph^1 chromosome as a No. 22q-. The nature of the Ph^1 (22q-) chromosome was revealed in 1973, when Rowley (29) reported that the Ph^1 chromosome resulted from an apparently balanced reciprocal translocation t(9;22) (q34;q11). Subsequent measurements of the DNA content of the affected chromosomes have shown that the amount of DNA added to No. 9 is equal to that missing from the Ph^1. The reciprocal nature of the translocation was only established recently when the gene, <u>c-abl</u>, normally on No. 9, was identified on the Ph^1 chromosome (8). Other studies with fluorescent markers or chromosome polymorphisms have shown that, in a particular patient, the same No. 9 or No. 22 is involved in each cell. These observations confirm earlier work, based on enzyme markers, indicating that CML cells originated from a single cell and are therefore clonal in origin. The original report on the translocation, and a number of reports confirming it, noted that the translocation occurred only between No. 9 and No. 22. The karyotypes of 1129 Ph^1+ patients with CML have been examined with banding techniques and have been reported by a number of investigators, and the 9;22 translocation has been identified in 1036 (92%) (for review, see (37)).

Variant translocations occur in addition to the typical t(9;22). For 10 years, we thought that about 4% of all translocations were simple two-way translocations that involved some chromosome other than No. 9. Mitelman and Levan (25) noted that the breakpoints in the simple translocations were, with rare exceptions, located at the ends of the chromosome. On the other hand, in the complex translocations involving at least three chromosomes including No. 9, the breakpoints in the third chromosome (other than Nos. 9 and 22) were in the middle of the arm of the affected chromosome; these complex translocations also occurred in about 4% of patients. As will be discussed in detail in a later section, we now have clear genetic evidence that the simple translocations are also three-way translocations that involve No. 9. These translocations were not detected previously because the size and staining characteristics of the other chromosome involved were similar to No. 9 and the involvement of No. 9 was overlooked. The great specificity of the translocation involving Nos. 9 and 22 remains an enigma. The consistency of the breakpoints in chromosomes 9 and 22 is a matter of considerable biologic importance, but these breakpoints appear to be the same in all patients. A more precise answer will be obtained when the breakpoint in the Ph^1 translocation has been isolated.

Acute Phase of CML

When patients with CML enter the terminal acute phase, some appear to retain the 46, Ph^1+ cell line unchanged, whereas the majority of patients show additional chromosome abnormalities. Bone marrow chromosomes from 392 patients with Ph^1+ CML, who were in the acute phase, have been analyzed with banding techniques (for summary, see (37)). Eighty-nine (22%) showed no change in their karyotype, whereas 303 patients had additional chromosome abnormalities. The most common changes frequently occur in combination to produce modal numbers of 47 to 50. Different abnormal chromosomes occur singly or in combinations in a distinctly nonrandom pattern during the acute phase of CML. The significance of these patterns will be understood only when we have more information about the genes carried on these chromosomes. When patients had only a single new chromosome change, this most commonly involved a second Ph^1, an i(17q), or a +8, in descending order of frequency. An extra No. 8 and i(17q) occurred together as the only changes in twenty-eight patients; a +8 and +17 were never seen as the only changes. On the other hand, if the patient's cells also had a second Ph^1, then +8, i(17q) and +8, +17, +Ph^1 were seen with equal frequency. Chromosome loss is very low; that most often seen is minus 7 which occurred in only eight of 297 patients (37). The relatively restricted nature of the common chromosome abnormalities in the acute phase implies that these chromosomes carry genes that provide a proliferative advantage to the Ph^1+

myeloid cell that has an extra copy of one or a combination of these chromosomes.

The Ph^1 Chromosome As a Biological Marker

Our interpretation of the biologic implications of the Philadelphia chromosome has been modified as our clinical experience with this marker has widened. Earlier cases of acute leukemia in which the Ph^1 chromosome was present were classified as chronic myeloid leukemia presenting in blast transformation. More recently, however, the tendency has been to refer to patients who have no prior history suggestive of CML as having Ph^1+ acute leukemia (31). It is becoming increasingly evident that the observed interrelations of Ph^1+ leukemia are complex, indeed, and that the distinctions between some categories, which are difficult to make, will be determined by the arbitrary judgment of the investigator.

The question as to which cells in CML contain a Philadelphia chromosome is not completely resolved. It was shown relatively early that the Ph^1 chromosome was present in granulocytic, erythroid, and megakaryocytic cells (38). It was assumed that the Ph^1 chromosome was not present in lymphoid cells because most PHA-stimulated peripheral blood cells lacked a Ph^1 chromosome. As techniques in cell separation improved and immunologic markers were developed, it could be established that some B cells were also Ph^1+. In blast crisis, some blasts had intracytoplasmic IgM which is characteristic of pre-B cells. The fact that B cells from patients in the chronic phase were also Ph^1+ was shown by Martin et al. (23) who established Epstein-Barr virus (EBV) transformed B lymphoblastoid cell lines from a patient with Ph^1+ CML who was also heterozygous for glucose-6-phosphate dehydrogenase (G6PD) isoenzymes. Nine of the 74 cell lines were Ph^1+ and G6PD type B which was the isoenzyme type of the myeloid leukemia clone. Moreover, each cell line expressed a single immunoglobulin class providing further evidence for their monoclonal nature. Bernheim et al. (6) also showed more directly that some B cells have a Ph^1 chromosome. Seven of eight patients had a Ph^1 chromosome in SIgM+ cells that were stimulated with pokeweed mitogen or nocardia opaca antigen. In unstimulated cultures, all cells were Ph^1+ and they lacked SIgM; they were considered to be granulocytes or monocytes.

The final question concerns the relationship of the Ph^1 translocation and malignant transformation; in an individual patient, does the Ph^1 occur in a single normal cell which becomes the progenitor of the leukemic clone, or is there expansion of a clone, possibly leukemic, in which a translocation occurs in one of these already abnormal cells? This question is not easily resolved because of the lack of independent markers for the leukemic cell; it is considered by Fialkow (this volume). Rare patients with CML have been reported whose marrow cells appeared to be Ph^1- at presentation which later became Ph^1+. On the other hand, atomic bomb survivors who were followed regularly had virtually 100% Ph^1+ cells prior to the development of clinically evident CML, which indicates that the Ph^1 aberration can be a very early event in the disease process. What is required to resolve this issue is a reliable marker for leukemic cells independent of the karyotype; one could then correlate the presence of the Ph^1 with this marker and determine how many Ph^1- cells were positive for the leukemia marker.

ACUTE NON-LYMPHOCYTIC LEUKEMIA (ANLL)

There have now been numerous reports on cytogenetic analyses, with banding techniques, of relatively large series of unselected patients with ANLL as well as of single cases or selected patients. Abnormal karyotypes have been reported in approximately 50% of all patients with ANLL de novo whose bone marrow cells were examined with banding techniques (25, 37, 38). However, the incidence of cytogenetic abnormalities will be significantly greater when techniques for culturing leukemic cells and for obtaining prophase chromosomes are generally applied (43). This discussion will focus on certain specific aberrations that appear to be of exceptional biologic interest. These include two translocations that are each specifically associated with a particular type of leukemia and two related abnormalities that are especially common in other types of acute leukemia. The two translocations are the t(8;21), seen with rare exceptions only in acute myeloblastic leukemia with maturation (AML, M2), and t(15;17), seen only in acute promyelocytic leukemia (APL, M3). Myeloblasts and promyelocytes are two sequential stages in normal granulocyte differentiation. The rearrangements of 11q are more variable and can be translocations, deletions, or duplication involving 11q23-24 preferentially (5). They are most commonly seen in acute monocytic leukemia (AMoL, M5) but have been reported in acute myelomonocytic leukemia (AMMoL, M4) and in AML (M2). Most recently, an association between increased bone marrow eosinophils and a deleted No. 16 (1) or abnormal marrow eosinophils and an inverted No. 16 (21) has been identified.

It should be pointed out that these associations have only become apparent as investigators have examined the relationship of particular chromosome changes to a well-defined type of leukemia. The special significance of these specific translocations was not apparent when chromosome changes were related to ANLL in general. Whereas this point seems obvious now, it merits emphasis because of the apparently confusing array of karyotypic patterns seen in acute lymphocytic leukemia and in other lymphoproliferative disorders. In those lymphoid neoplasms that appear to be well-defined entities, clear karyotypic patterns have emerged. In other lymphoid disorders the karyotypic findings are chaotic; the T cell disorders, except for ataxia-telangiectasia, are good examples. As more sophisticated monoclonal antibodies and other reagents are developed, these disorders will be divided into more homogeneous groups, and it will almost certainly be possible to show the same types of chromosome-morphology correlations that have been established in the myeloid leukemias. As will be mentioned in the discussion of APL, the karyotypic pattern can provide clues as to the correct cytologic classification of cells with atypical morphology. Thus a close interaction between cytogenetics, cytology, and immunology will be required for future progress in establishing a rational classification of the various malignant diseases affecting hematopoietic cells.

The 8;21 Translocation in Acute Myeloblastic Leukemia (AML, M2)

A translocation between chromosomes 8 and 21 [t(8;21) (q22;q22)] was first identified in 1973 (30). The frequency with which this translocation occurs seems to vary from one laboratory to another, but it accounted for 10% (25/249) of the abnormal cases recently reviewed by Rowley and Testa (37). A similar but somewhat lower incidence of the t(8;21) was reported in patients reviewed at both the First and Fourth International Workshops on Chromosomes in Leukemia (10, 11); 11 of 139 (7.9%) and 44 of 353 (12.5%), respectively, de novo ANLL patients who had abnormal karyotypes had a t(8;21). In the review by Rowley and Testa (37), the t(8;21) was found to be the most frequent abnormality in children with ANLL, being reported in 17% (10 of 60) of karyotypically abnormal cases.

The abnormality initially appeared to be restricted to patients with a diagnosis of M2 (acute myeloblastic leukemia with maturation), according to the FAB classification. However, 7% (3 of 44) of patients analyzed at the Fourth Workshop (11) whose cells had a t(8;21) and adequate bone marrow material available for cytological review had a diagnosis of M4.

The 8;21 translocation is also of interest for three other reasons. First, chromosomes 8 and 21 can participate in three-way rearrangements similar to those involving chromosomes 9 and 22 in CML. Second, the t(8;21) is often accompanied by the loss of a sex chromosome; of the cases reviewed at the Second International Workshop on Chromosomes in Leukemia (39), 32% of the males with the t(8;21) were -Y, and 36% of the females were missing one X; these figures are higher for the Fourth Workshop (11) with 28 of 33 (85%) males -Y and 8/12 (67%) females -X. This association is particularly noteworthy because sex chromosome abnormalities are otherwise rarely observed in ANLL. Third, this translocation has never been reported as a constitutional abnormality or in other malignant diseases (Rowley, unpublished observations). Thus, it may be lethal in all cells except granulocytes.

The 15;17 Translocation and Acute Promyelocytic Leukemia (APL)
A structural rearrangement involving chromosomes 15 and 17 in APL was first recognized by Rowley et al. (36). Of the eighty patients with APL who were reviewed at the Second Workshop (39), thirty-three (41%) had a t(15;17) alone (23 cases) or with other abnormalities, seven had other types of chromosome changes, and forty had a normal karyotype. With improved techniques including widespread use of marrow culture, only 15 of 61 (25%) patients analyzed at the Fourth Workshop (11) had a normal karyotype. Forty-three patients (70%) had a t(15;17) and three had other abnormalities. The rearrangement was not found in patients with any other type of leukemia or other solid tumor. Two cases with complex translocations involving Nos. 15 and 17 and either No. 2 or No. 3 were reported. Thus, the same pattern of variation of a specific translocation can involve the t(15;17) as well as the t(9;22) and the t(8;21). The usefulness of these variant translocations will be illustrated in a later section.

In some cases, the granules typically seen in the leukemic promyelocytes may be too small to be seen by light microscopy, although they are present when the cells are examined ultrastructurally. The FAB Co-operative Group recently recognized that not all APL patients have coarse granules and has thus added a category called the M3 variant. The variant category was identified largely on the basis of the clinical features and the presence of the t(15;17).

The t(15;17) is of special interest for several reasons. The first relates to the controversy over the exact breakpoints in both chromosome No. 15 and No. 17. The problem arises because the critical regions of both 15 and 17 have relatively similar banding patterns so the breakpoints are ambiguous. Moreover, the chromosomes from these patients frequently have unusually poor morphology with contracted chromosomes and fuzzy banding. We have recently been successful in obtaining longer chromosomes and have identified the breakpoints as 15q22 and 17q21.1 (20); these are both closer to the centromere than those proposed earlier (39).

The second interesting feature of APL relates to the difficulty in demonstrating the t(15;17). In our experience, all twenty-five patients with APL whom we have studied have had a t(15;17) (20). However, in three patients, no abnormal metaphase cells were observed when BM cells were studied directly; 9-64% of marrow cells had a t(15;17) when the cells were cultured for 24 hours. Similar observations have been reported by others. The reason for this difficulty in obtaining mitoses in cells with the translocation is not known. However, Berger et al. (2) have presented evidence that the translocation is present only in myeloblasts and promyelocytes, whereas the erythroid cells are normal. The erythroblasts apparently stop dividing in culture, leaving only dividing granulocytic cells. Thus, it is entirely possible that the difference in frequency is related more to technical factors such as culture methods than to actual differences in the frequency of the translocation.

Structural Alterations of 11q in Acute Monocytic Leukemia (M5)

In addition to the consistent translocations just discussed, a new chromosome-morphology relationship has recently been described. Berger et al. (5) presented ten cases of acute monocytic leukemia (AMoL, M5) that had an unexpectedly high incidence of rearrangements of the long arm of chromosome 11. They recently reported on thirty-four patients, twenty-four of whom had type a or monoblastic and ten of whom had type b or well differentiated monocytic leukemia (3). Thirteen of the thirty-four appeared to have a normal karyotype, nine had various abnormalities, and twelve had aberrations involving 11q. Abnormalities of 11q occurred most frequently in children with monoblastic leukemia (type a), 6 of 8; adults with monoblastic leukemia had the next highest incidence, 5 of 16; the incidence in monocytic (type b) leukemia was low, namely, 1 of 3 children and 0 of 7 adults.

In the Fourth Workshop (11), thirty-three patients had some structural rearrangement involving 11q, and the slides of these patients were reviewed for FAB classification. Twenty-one of the thirty-three (63.6%) were M5, five were M4, and three were M2; single cases fell into other FAB types. Of the twenty-one patients with M5, fifteen were of monoblastic type, three were monocytic, and slides from three could not be subclassified. Five of the patients were under 1 year of age and seven others were under 20 years. When all patients with M5 leukemia were considered, about 22% had an aberration involving 11q.

Aberrations of 11q differ from the t(8;21) and t(15;17) in three ways. First, the breakpoint in 11q usually involves band 11q23-24 but can also occur in 11q13-14; in Berger's series (3,5), 11q23-24 was affected in nine patients and 11q13-14 in three others. In the Fourth Workshop, twenty-four of the thirty-three breaks occurred in 11q23-24; the others usually involved 11q13-14. Second, the other chromosome involved in the translocation is variable, although 9p and 19 appear to be affected more often than others. Finally, 11q aberrations have been reported in patients with acute leukemia other than AMoL M5. In a series of children reported by Kaneko et al. (19) a translocation involving 11q was seen in a patient with AML-A2, although the cytochemical reaction of the leukemic cells was of the monocytic type. It may be that the chromosome analyses have revealed a spectrum of morphologic features in AMoL not heretofore suspected, noting that in APL, the M3 variant or microgranular type was identified in large measure because of the consistent t(15;17) seen in the leukemic cells.

The most recent clinical-cytogenetic association to be identified involves myelomonocytic (M4) leukemia with unusual eosinophils. Arthur and Bloomfield (1) described five cases (three with M2 and two with M4 leukemia) whose bone marrow contained an excess of eosinophils; four of the cases were said to have a deleted No. 16 [del(16)(q22)]. Le Beau et al. (21) have reported on a related entity in eighteen patients, all of whom had M4 leukemia, with eosinophils that showed unique morphologic changes including large and irregular basophilic granules. Many of these patients did not have an increased frequency of marrow eosinophils. All patients had an inv(16) (p13q22). Based on our data, 23% of our patients with M4 have an inv(16). The breakpoint in the long arm of the del(16) and the inv(16) is the same.

Unique Biologic Features of Consistent Aberrations

It seems reasonable from a biologic point of view to consider 11q aberrations, despite the "irregularities," along with t(8;21) and t(15;17) for several reasons. In addition to the close association with a particular type of leukemia, they all show a relatively similar age distribution which differs from other ANLL patients. All three abnormalities are more common in children and young adults. In the collaborative study of 503 patients with ANLL published recently by Rowley et al. (34), the age distribution for APL and AMoL was relatively similar and the median age was much younger than for the other types of leukemia. This suggests that the factors that are important in the etiology of these types of leukemia differ from those that are associated with leukemia in older adults. One factor associated with leukemia is the occupation of the leukemic patient. In the initial study by Mitelman in 1978 that was recently confirmed by a larger series (26), patients who were occupationally exposed to some potentially mutagenic agent (petroleum products, chemical solvents, pesticides) were more likely to have chromosomally abnormal leukemic cells than were non-exposed patients (children, students, housewives, and white-collar workers). This study has also been confirmed by Golomb et al. (14). Occupational data were available for patients included in the Fourth Workshop (11); an analysis of 361 patients over 16 years of age with adequate chromosomes revealed that of patients 30 years and older, 67% of occupationally exposed compared with 49% of non-exposed patients and an abnormal karyotype ($p < 0.005$). In all series the incidence of certain chromosome changes such as -5, -7, or +8 was much higher in the exposed than in the non-exposed population. In general, other aberrations, particularly the consistent translocations, were less common in the exposed group, suggesting that mutagenic exposure was a less important factor in their production.

These data suggest that some other mechanism is associated with the high frequency of consistent aberrations in the younger age group. The young age is particularly prominent in Berger's thirty-four patients with AMoL; of eight children under 9 years of age, 5 of 6 with an 11q rearrangement were under 2 years of age (3). This same distribution was noted in the Fourth Workshop with eight patients with 11q aberrations being under 2 years of age. This change in age distribution is reminiscent of that seen in retinoblastoma due to autosomal dominant inheritance compared with those that are sporadic. In this instance, the inherited genetic change is a mutation present in all cells, including the retina; in the two-step theory of carcinogenesis, only one more mutation is required to produce a malignant cell. By analogy, in applying this model to the t(8;21) and t(15;17) and the aberration of 11q, one could postulate that there is a genetic polymorphism or a mutation in the gene(s) located at the site of one or both breakpoints such that a translocation in a granulocytic precursor involving these specific breakpoints would result in a leukemic transformation. As the population at risk decreases with age, because those who are "susceptible" have already developed leukemia, the incidence of t(8;21), t(15;17), and 11q aberrations would decline, which it does. Those adult patients whose leukemic cells show these aberrations may represent individuals who were genetically normal and whose cells have acquired mutations/translocations due to other causes.

Another area in which these three rearrangements share a common feature is in the nature of the cell carrying the rearrangement. The work of Berger and his colleagues has provided evidence that in the t(8;21), t(15;17), and 11q rearrangements, the chromosome aberration occurs only in the granulocytic or monocytic cell and that the erythroid cells are chromosomally normal (2, 3). In one patient, direct marrow preparations revealed seven cells with t(8;21) and thirteen cells with a normal karyotype; determination of the cytology of the dividing blast cells from the same sample showed that twenty-three were myeloblasts and twenty-eight were erythroblasts. In a sample cultured for 48 hours, all mitoses were t(8;21) and all dividing blasts were myeloblasts. Studies of the other 9 patients provided similar results. The results for the t(15;17) are similar, the translocation occurs in myeloblasts and promyelocytes and not in erythroid cells. In the monocytic leukemias, the evidence suggests the aberration occurs in monocytes and not in granulocytes (except for possibly one patient) or in erythroblasts.

These data are in agreement with a recent report by Fialkow et al. showing that in some patients the red cells do not share the same G6PD isoenzyme as the leukemic granulocytes (9). These observations have significant biologic and therapeutic implications. One possibility is that all of the cells are leukemic, and the chromosome change has occurred secondarily only in the granulocytic or monocytic cells. The other possibility is that the leukemic transformation is restricted to the granulocytes or monocytes. The data of Fialkow et al. would support the latter interpretation since in some patients only the granulocytes were monoclonal. The clinical implications are clear; if the red cells are normal, then therapy should be directed toward sparing the red cells while destroying the leukemic granulocytes.

MALIGNANT DISEASES AFFECTING LYMPHOCYTES

The evidence presented in this section represents a small fraction of all that has been collected over the past ten years regarding the chromosome abnormalities seen in acute and chronic lymphocytic leukemia, multiple myeloma, and the various lymphomas. Recent reviews by Mitelman (24), Rowley and Fukuhara (35), Rowley and Testa (37), and Sandberg (38) cover all aspects of lymphoid disorders in considerable detail. The data that will be presented are selected because they provide the background for illustrating the next step in our understanding of the role of consistent chromosome changes in malignant transformation. This section will review the chromosome pattern in acute lymphocytic leukemia (ALL) and the consistent translocations seen in Burkitt's lymphoma and in some patients with B cell ALL. As noted earlier, there are fewer specific clinical-chromosome associations for lymphoid compared with myeloid diseases.

Acute Lymphocytic Leukemia (ALL)
Based on earlier studies, it appeared that chromosome abnormalities occurred in about one half of the patients with ALL, and hyperdiploidy was predominant among aneuploid karyotypes. The recent study of 330 ALL patients (adults, 173; children, 157) at the Third International Workshop on Chromosomes in Leukemia (41) revealed that 65% of the patients had clonal abnormalities. Of the 213 aneuploid patients, 34.8% had pseudodiploidy, 24.5%, hyperdiploidy, and 6.7%, hypodiploidy. Our study of thirty-three ALL patients (19) also showed a high incidence of aneuploidy (70%); pseudodiploidy was predominant (13 of the 23 aneuploid patients). Although the karyotype in many of these patients may be very complex, certain patterns recur. It is now possible to analyze the clinical features of these patients, together with the morphology of the leukemic cells and the results of cell surface marker studies; this provides additional insight into the derivation of these malignant lymphoid cells.

The 8;14 translocation. A translocation involving the long arms of #8 and #14 has been detected in a large number of Burkitt's tumors of both African and non-African origin, independent of whether they are EBV-positive or -negative (16, 44). An apparently identical translocation has been observed in ALL patients with B cell markers and in patients with L3-type leukemia cells (24), indicating that Burkitt's lymphoma and most B cell ALL of the L3 type are probably different manifestations of the same disease. Sixteen patients with this rearrangement were reported at the Third Workshop. These patients had a poorer prognosis (a median survival of 5 months) than any other group of patients classified according to chromosome patterns. With one exception, all patients in whom the immunologic markers of leukemic cells were identified had B cell markers, and all but one had L3-type cells. In the exceptional patient, the leukemic cells had a pre-B cell phenotype and were of the L1 type (19); the morphology of the leukemic cells, however, changed to L3-type at relapse.

Recently, variant translocations have been reported in Burkitt's lymphoma; these variants include a t(2;8) (p12-13;q24) (42) and a t(8;22) (q24;q11) (4). Both variant translocations, t(2;8) and t(8;22), have also been found in ALL patients with the L3 type (19). Moreover, complex three-way translocations have also been observed affecting the t(8;14). We recently studied a patient with B cell ALL who had a complex translocation (19). In the leukemic cells, most of the long arm of No. 5 was translocated to No. 8, and the end of No. 8 was translocated to No. 14 producing the typical 14q+ marker chromosome; presumably the end of No. 14 was translocated to No. 5. Chromosome #8 is always involved in these translocations, with the breakpoint in band 8q24. Thus the consistent chromosome abnormality in some B-ALL and in Burkitt's lymphoma is a rearrangement of 8q rather than that of 14q.

A 14q+ chromosome not involving number 8. A 14q+ chromosome is frequently observed in malignant lymphomas, particularly, although not exclusively, in those of B cell origin (35). Fifteen ALL patients at the Third Workshop were reported to have a 14q+ chromosome (breakpoint in 14q32) that was not involved in a translocation with the terminal segment of chromosome #8. The leukemic cells in about one half of the patients had non-T, non-B immunologic markers, and the other one half had B cell markers. The 14q+ chromosome was due to a balanced translocation in six patients, in four of whom the donor chromosome was identified as #11. The t(11;14) is one of the common abnormalities seen in malignant lymphoma, poorly differentiated lymphocyte type (35), suggesting that there is a relationship between it and ALL with the 14q+ chromosome. The complete remission rate in the patients with a 14q+ chromosome was 53%, with a median survival of nine months.

The 4;11 translocation. A translocation involving the long arms of No. 4 and No. 11 [t(4;11) (q21;q23)] was observed in eighteen patients at the Third Workshop. These patients had very high leukocyte counts (median WBC, 183,000/mm^3) and a very poor prognosis; the complete remission rate was 67%, and the median survival was seven months. One half of the patients were adults; the other one half were children most of whom were less than 1 year of age. The association of the 4;11 translocation with neonatal or early-childhood ALL is particularly interesting in view of the low incidence of ALL in this age group.

Hyperdiploidy with 50 to 60 chromosomes. The karyotype of some patients is characterized by many extra chromosomes and few structural abnormalities, with chromosome numbers in the 50 to 60 range. Although identical karyotypes are rarely found, certain additional chromosomes are commonly seen. Among thirty patients with high hyperdiploidy, including twenty-two children and eight adults evaluated at the Third Workshop, +21 was seen in twenty-two, +6 in fifteen, +18 in fourteen, +14 in eleven, +4 or +10 each in ten patients. If the additional chromosomes that were common in this group are compared with the additional chromosomes in patients who have a near-haploid complement, the similarities are remarkable, because the most consistent changes in the latter group are +10, +18, and +21.

The median age of the twenty-two children with this abnormality was 3 years, and that of all thirty patients was 5 years, which was less than that of patients with other abnormalities. The WBC count in patients with hyperdiploidy was low, with a median of 6,000/mm^3; it was below 10,000/mm^3 in more than half of the patients. All patients had non-T, non-B ALL. The complete remission rate and the median survival of the thirty patients evaluated at the Third Workshop were 86% and thirty-four months, respectively. Thus, in patients who have hyperdiploidy with more than 49 chromosomes, all of the previously recognized factors that indicate a good prognosis, including age between 3 and 7 years, low WBC count, and non-T, non-B markers, were present. It should be emphasized that the median survival of the hyperdiploid patients, including both children and adults, was longer than that of patients with a normal karyotype.

The Ph^1 chromosome in ALL. A Ph^1 chromosome, which is formed by a reciprocal translocation between No. 22 and No. 9 or various other chromosomes, is seen in patients with ALL, as well as in patients with CML. Of the thirty-nine patients evaluated at the Third Workshop, thirty were adults and nine were children. The incidence of Ph^1+ patients with ALL was 5.7% for children and 17.3% for adults. Thus, the Ph^1 chromosome is the most frequent rearrangement in adult ALL. Thirty-six patients at the Workshop had the typical t(9q+;22q-), and the remaining three had variant translocations; the incidence of the variant form was 8%, which is similar to that observed in CML patients. The patients had a high leukocyte count, and all had non-T, non-B ALL. The complete remission rate was 55%. The median survival was 9 months, reflecting the poor prognosis for these patients. By identifying this chromosome abnormality, one can detect individuals in the non-T, non-B category who have a poor prognosis.

Based on the evidence gathered at the Third Workshop, plus that of individual reports, the cytogenetic study of leukemic cells from patients with ALL clearly can provide important information. At present, these data are clinically useful, providing another independent variable that has prognostic significance. Of more importance, however, is the ability to define subsets of patients with ALL on the basis of certain genetic (chromosome) changes and then to relate these changes to various functional and immunologic studies. In this way, we will gain a much more sophisticated and accurate understanding of the interrelationship of the various subsets of lymphoid cells.

Other Lymphoid Diseases

Overall, when the karyotypic aberrations seen in lymphoid diseases are considered, a break in No. 14 at q32 with translocation of material to the end of No. 14 is the single most common change (24, 35). The only other translocation that occurs in the majority of patients with a particular type of lymphoid malignant disease is a t(14;18) (q32;q21) which we have identified in the majority of our patients with poorly differentiated lymphocytic lymphoma, now called malignant lymphoma, follicular, predominantly small cleaved cell (FSC) in the International Classification System (12, 35). An extra chromosome No. 12 is the most common change in chronic lymphocytic leukemia of the B cell type (13). This observation has recently been confirmed by others. In addition, translocations involving both No. 14 chromosomes are seen in some patients with ataxia-telangiectasia (17).

BIOLOGIC USEFULNESS OF CONSISTENT CHROMOSOME ABNORMALITIES, PARTICULARLY TRANSLOCATIONS

Defining the Critical Recombinant Chromosome

It is now apparent that the sites of consistent translocations pinpoint chromosome segments that contain genes critically involved in malignant transformation. Isolation and analysis of these segments of DNA have high scientific priority. The evidence for Burkitt's lymphoma is exciting and clearly points the way to future research in this area. The loci for the immunoglobulin genes are on the three chromosomes other than No. 8, involved in translocations in Burkitt's lymphoma. Thus, the locus for the heavy chain complex is on No. 14, that for kappa is on No. 2, and that for lambda is on No. 22. Moreover, with the use of chromosome hybridization in situ, the kappa light chain genes have been mapped to the short arm of No. 2 (band 2p12-13), the heavy chain gene has been mapped to 14q32, and the lambda light chain gene has been mapped to 22q11 (reviewed in (32)).

An even more direct association between translocation types and gene function has been reported by Lenoir et al. (22). They analyzed the type of immunoglobulin produced in either Burkitt's tumor cell lines or in fresh tumor cells and correlated this information with the karyotype of the tumors. All three lines with a t(2;8) expressed kappa light chains and all five cell lines with a t(8;22) expressed lambda light chains. For seventeen cell lines with t(8;14), nine were kappa and eight were lambda producers.

There are two recombinant chromosomes in each translocation, and it would appear useful to determine which is the critical recombinant (32). As has been indicated earlier, each of the three common translocations in myeloid leukemia 9;22, 8;21, and 15;17 also occurs in a variant form in a limited number of patients, and one can use these to determine whether one recombinant chromosome is constant in these variant forms. The observations are illustrated in Fig. 1. The constant recombinant is enclosed in a box in the figure. For CML, we now recognize that the 4% of patients thought to have a simple two-way translocation also, in fact, have complex three-way translocations. Thus, in every patient with CML, the constant feature is the apposition of the end of 9q to the remainder of 22q. Based on these data the critical event leading to malignant transformation in these types of myeloid leukemia is related to the juxtaposition of 9q to 22q in CML, that of 21q to 8q in AML, and that of the end of 17q to 15q in APL.

Chromosome Location of Oncogenes

One of the most exciting revelations in the past year has involved the cellular oncogenes and their chromosome location. Much of the excitement derives from the observation that many oncogenes are located in the bands that are involved in consistent translocations (33) (Fig. 2). The specific rearrangement of the c-myc gene and the immunoglobulin loci is discussed by Vogt et al. (this volume) and will not be covered in this paper. The c-mos gene is located on band 8q22; what its relationship is to the t(8;21) in AML is currently unknown. The Abelson oncogene has been shown to translocate to the Ph^1 chromosome in the t(9;22) in CML (8). This is an important observation from the genetic viewpoint, because this is the first gene known to be on No. 9 that has been shown to translocate to No. 22. This establishes the fact that the translocation is reciprocal.

Some known oncogenes have not been implicated in structural rearrangements. Thus, it was assumed for some time that c-fes, known to be on No. 15, would be involved in the t(15;17) in APL. Such is not the case; first, we know that c-fes is not on the 15q+ chromosome. Moreover, c-fes has been localized to the end of No. 15 and thus is some distance from the breakpoint.

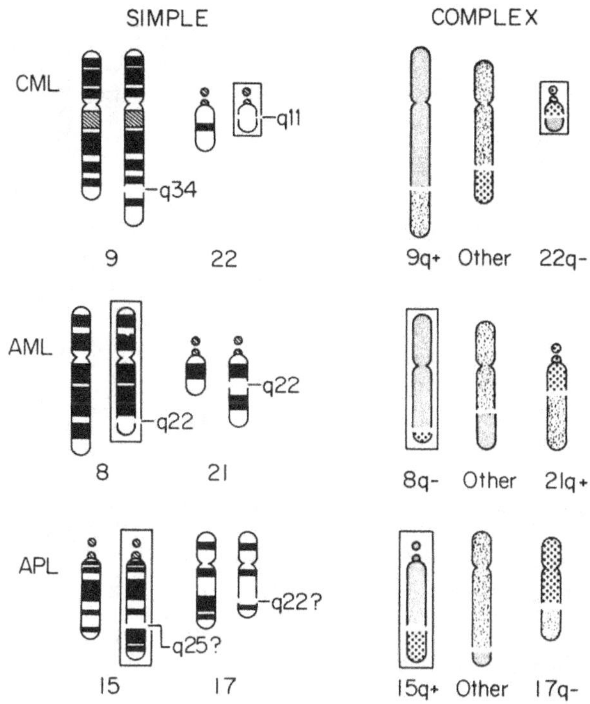

FIG. 1 - (Left) Diagrammatic representation of the breakpoints and the chromosome exchange in the simple consistent translocations in CML, AML, and APL. (Right) Schematic drawing of the breakpoints and the typical pattern of chromosome exchange observed in the complex variants affecting each of these translocations. The other chromosome involved in these complex rearrangements is variable. For each type of leukemia, the rearranged chromosome that is constant in both the simple and complex translocations is enclosed in a box. Reprinted with permission from Science (32).

Of particular interest is c-ras which is on 11p14; a deletion proximal to this band as a constitutional abnormality is associated with aniridia and a predisposition to Wilms' tumor (28). Moreover, we have described a patient with a normal karyotype whose Wilms' tumor cells had a deletion of 11p13 (18). Thus the c-ras is near the critical deletion, but the oncogene is outside of the deletion. Therefore, in a number of leukemias, lymphomas, or cancers, chromosome regions previously defined by cytogeneticists as sites of consistent rearrangements are found to be at or near the sites of oncogenes.

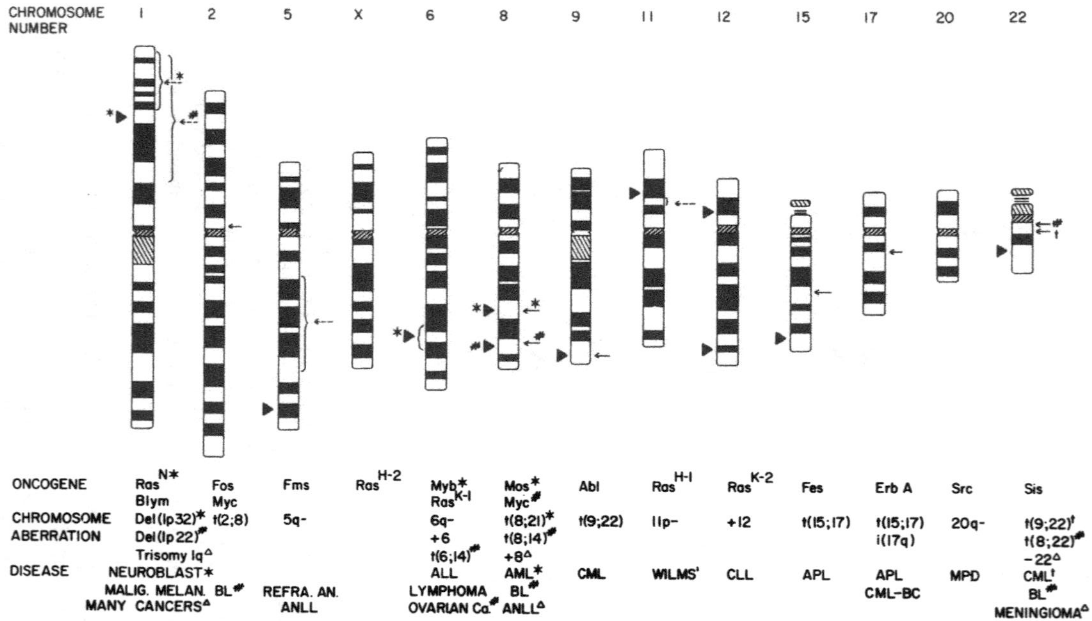

FIG. 2 - Diagram of chromosomes containing known cellular oncogenes; the number is above each chromosome, and the oncogenes, karyotypic aberrations, and neoplastic diseases associated with these aberrations are indicated below the chromosomes. The arrowhead (▶) to the left of each chromosome indicates the band carrying the cellular oncogene; the arrow to the right of a chromosome identifies specific bands involved in consistent translocations (←) or deletions (← -) observed in patients having the disorders listed. Under No. 1, B-lym has been localized to 1p32 (▶*); the deletions distal to 1p32 and 1p22 are associated with neuroblastoma or malignant melanoma, respectively. For chromosome No. 6, c-myb has been localized to 6q22-24 (▶*). The t(6;14) is found in ovarian cancer. Under No. 8, * indicates the c-mos and the t(8;21) in AML-M2 and # indicates c-myc and t(2;8), t(8;14), or t(8;22) in Burkitt's lymphoma (BL). In chromosome 12, the c-ras^{K-2} shows two regions of homology with in situ hybridization. REFRA. AN., refractory anemia; CLL, chronic lymphocytic leukemia; MPD, myeloproliferative disorders. p indicates the short arm and q the long arm of the chromosome.

The challenge for the future in the myeloid leukemias is first to find a way to isolate the DNA from the breakpoints, then to identify the genes involved, and finally to determine the alterations in gene function that are related to the translocations or deletions. Unless we are very lucky, this task will be more difficult in the myeloid leukemias than in Burkitt's lymphoma for two reasons. We do not have suitable cell lines available to provide a continuing source of cells for DNA analysis. There are, for example, no cell lines with a t(15;17) or a t(8;21). Those from patients with CML generally have a very rearranged karyotype. The second problem is the lack of information regarding which genes in myeloid cells will be analogous to the immunoglobulin genes in B cell tumors. It may be that the c-onc, such as c-mos or c-abl will be at the breakpoint, and cloned DNA from these genes can be used to isolate the breakpoint. If this is not the case, then the search for the DNA from each breakpoint may be a very tedious one. As is clear from the harvest of information regarding c-myc in B cell tumors, the reward is worth the search.

REFERENCES

(1) Arthur, D.C., and Bloomfield, C.D. 1983. Partial deletion of the long arm of chromosome 16 and bone marrow eosinophilia in acute nonlymphocytic leukemia: A new association. Blood 61: 944-998.

(2) Berger, R.; Bernheim, A.; and Flandrin, G. 1980. Absence d'anormalie chromosomique et leucemie aigue. CR Acad. Sci. Paris 290: 1557-1559.

(3) Berger, R.; Bernheim, A.; Francois, S.; et al. 1982. Acute monocytic leukemia chromosome studies. Leukemia Res. 6: 17-26.

(4) Berger, R.; Bernheim, A.; Weh, H.J.; et al. 1979. A new translocation in Burkitt tumor cells. Hum. Genet. 53: 111-112.

(5) Berger, R.; Bernheim, A.; Weh, H.J.; et al. 1980. Cytogenetic studies on acute monocytic leukemia. Leukemia Res. 4: 119-127.

(6) Bernheim, A.; Berger, R.; Preud'homme, J.L.; et al. 1981. Philadelphia chromosome positive blood B lymphocytes in chronic myelocytic leukemia. Leukemia Res. 5: 331-339.

(7) Boveri, T. 1914. Zur Frage der Entstehung maligner Tumoren. Jena: Gustav Fischer.

(8) De Klein, A.; van Kessel, A.G.; Grosveld, G.; et al. 1982. A cellular

oncogene is translocated to the Philadelphia chromosome in chronic myelocytic leukemia. Nature 300: 765-767.

(9) Fialkow, P.J.; Singer, J.W.; Adamson, J.W.; et al. 1981. Acute nonlymphocytic leukemia: Heterogeneity of stem cell origin. Blood 57: 1068-1073.

(10) First International Workshop on Chromosomes in Leukemia. 1978. Chromosomes in acute non-lymphocytic leukemia. Brit. J. Haem. 39: 311-316.

(11) Fourth International Workshop on Chromosomes in Leukemia. 1984. Cancer Genet. Cytogenet. 11: 249-360.

(12) Fukuhara, S.; Rowley, J.D.; Variakojis, D.; et al. 1979. Chromosome abnormalities in poorly differentiated lymphocytic lymphoma. Cancer Res. 39: 3119-3128.

(13) Gahrton, G.; Robert, K.-H.; Friberg, K.; et al. 1980. Nonrandom chromosomal aberrations in chronic lymphocytic leukemia revealed by polyclonal B-cell mitogen stimulation. Blood 56: 640-647.

(14) Golomb, H.M.; Alimena, G.; Rowley, J.D.; et al. 1982. Correlation of occupation and karyotype in adults with acute nonlymphocytic leukemia. Blood 60: 404-411.

(15) International System for Human Cytogenetic Nomenclature. 1978. Cytogenet. Cell Genet. 21: 309-404.

(16) Kaiser-McCaw, B.; Epstein, A.L.; Kaplan, H.S.; et al. 1977. Chromosome 14 translocation in African and North American Burkitt's lymphoma. Int. J. Cancer 19: 482-486.

(17) Kaiser-McCaw, B.; Hecht, F.; Harnden, D.G.; et al. 1975. Somatic rearrangement of chromosome 14 in human lymphocytes. Proc. Natl. Acad. Sci. USA 72: 2071-2075.

(18) Kaneko, Y.; Eques, M.C.; and Rowley, J.D. 1981. Interstitial deletion of 11p limited to Wilms' tumor cells in a patient without aniridia. Cancer Res. 41: 4577-4578.

(19) Kaneko, Y.; Rowley, J.D.; Variakojis, D.; et al. 1982. Correlation of karyotype with clinical features in acute lymphoblastic leukemia (ALL). Cancer Res. 42: 2918-2929.

(20) Kondo, K.; Larson, R.A.; Vardiman, J.W.; et al. 1982. Further evidence for the specificity of t(15;17) in acute promyelocytic leukemia.

Am. Soc. Hum. Genet. Abstract.

(21) Le Beau, M.M.; Larson, R.A.; Bitter, M.A.; et al. 1983. Association of inv(16)(p13q22) with abnormal marrow eosinophils in acute myelomonocytic leukemia: A unique cytogenetic-clinicopathologic association. New Engl. J. Med. 309: 630-636.

(22) Lenoir, G.M.; Preud'homme, J.L.; Bernheim, A.; et al. 1982. Correlation between immunoglobulin light chain expression and variant translocation in Burkitt's lymphoma. Nature 298: 474-476.

(23) Martin, P.J.; Najfeld, V.; Hansen, J.A.; et al. 1980. Involvement of the B-lymphoid system in chronic myelogenous leukaemia. Nature 287: 49-50.

(24) Mitelman, F. 1981. Marker chromosome 14q+ in human cancer and leukemia. Adv. Cancer Res. 34: 141-170.

(25) Mitelman, F., and Levan, G. 1981. Clustering of aberrations to specific chromosomes in human neoplasms. IV. A survey of 1,871 cases. Hereditas 95: 79-139.

(26) Mitelman, F.; Nilsson, P.G.; Brandt, L.; et al. 1981. Chromosome pattern, occupation, and clinical features in patients with acute nonlymphocytic leukemia. Cancer Genet. Cytogenet. 4: 197-214.

(27) Nowell, P.C., and Hungerford, D.A. 1960. A minute chromosome in human granulocytic leukemia. Science 132: 1497.

(28) Riccardi, V.M.; Sujansky, E.; Smith, A.C.; et al. 1978. Chromosomal imbalance in the aniridia-Wilms' tumor association: 11p interstitial deletion. Pediatrics 61: 604-610.

(29) Rowley, J.D. 1973. A new consistent chromosomal abnormality in chronic myelogenous leukemia. Nature 243: 290-293.

(30) Rowley, J.D. 1973. Identification of a translocation with quinacrine fluorescence in a patient with acute leukemia. Ann. Genet. 16: 109-112.

(31) Rowley, J.D. 1980. Ph^1 positive leukemia, including chronic myelogenous leukemia. Clinics Haem. 9: 55-86.

(32) Rowley, J.D. 1982. Identification of the chromosome region involved in human hematologic malignant disease. Science 216: 749-751.

(33) Rowley, J.D. 1983. Human oncogene locations and chromosome

aberrations. Nature 301: 290-291.

(34) Rowley, J.D.; Alimena, G.; Garson, O.M.; et al. 1982. A collaborative study of the relationship of the morphologic type of acute nonlymphocytic leukemia with patient age and karyotype. Blood 59: 1013-1022.

(35) Rowley, J.D., and Fukuhara, S. 1980. Chromosome studies in non-Hodgkin lymphomas. Sem. Onc. 7: 255-256.

(36) Rowley, J.D.; Golomb, H.M.; Vardiman, J.; et al. 1977. Further evidence for a non-random chromosomal abnormality in acute promyelocytic leukemia. Int. J. Cancer 20: 869-872.

(37) Rowley, J.D., and Testa, J.R. 1982. Chromosome abnormalities in malignant hematologic diseases. In Advances in Cancer Research, pp. 103-148. New York: Academic Press Inc.

(38) Sandberg, A.A. 1980. The Chromosomes in Human Cancer and Leukemia. New York: Elsevier North-Holland.

(39) Second International Workshop on Chromosomes in Leukemia. 1980. Cancer Genet. Cytogenet. 2: 89-113.

(40) Testa, J.R., and Rowley, J.D. 1981. Chromosomes in leukemia and lymphoma with special emphasis on methodology. In The Leukemic Cell, ed. D. Catovsky, pp. 184-202. Edinburgh: Churchill-Livingston.

(41) Third International Workshop on Chromosomes in Leukemia. 1981. Cancer Genet. Cytogenet. 4: 95-142.

(42) Van den Berghe, H.; Parloir, C.; Gosseye, S.; et al. 1979. Variant translocation in Burkitt lymphoma. Cancer Genet. Cytogenet. 1: 9-14.

(43) Yunis, J.J.; Bloomfield, C.D.; Ensrud, B.S. 1981. All patients with acute nonlymphocytic leukemia may have a chromosomal defect. N. Engl. J. Med. 305: 135-139.

(44) Zech, L.; Haglund, U.; Nilsson, K.; et al. 1976. Characteristic chromosomal abnormalities in biopsies and lymphoid-cell lines from patients with Burkitt and non-Burkitt lymphomas. Int. J. Cancer 17: 47-56.

Leukemia, ed. I.L. Weissman, pp. 203-222. Dahlem Konferenzen 1985. Berlin, Heidelberg, New York, Tokyo: Springer-Verlag.

Tracing Development and Cell Lineages in Human Hemopoietic Neoplasia

P.J. Fialkow* and J.W. Singer**
*Dept. of Medicine RG-20, University of Washington
Seattle, WA 98195
**Veterans Administration Medical Center
Seattle, WA 98108, USA

Abstract. Cellular mosaicism based on X-chromosome inactivation with glucose-6-phosphate dehydrogenase (G6PD) as a marker was used to investigate human hemopoietic neoplasms. The data indicate that chronic myelocytic leukemia (CML) is a clonal disease that involves a stem cell pluripotent for B lymphoid as well as myeloid cells. Although T cells may also arise from this stem cell, this question has not been definitively resolved. Elements that make up the in vitro hemopoietic microenvironment may be derived from the same stem cell in CML that gives rise to the clonal blood cells. By inference, there may be a pluripotent stem cell in normal people that is common to marrow stromal and hemopoietic cells. Acute myeloid leukemia is heterogeneous with respect to the pattern of stem cell involvement and the nature of remission. In some patients the disease involves stem cells with multipotent differentiative expression, whereas in others it involves progenitors with differentiative expression restricted to the granulocytic pathway. In some patients in remission the marrow is repopulated by normal stem cells, whereas in others, clonally derived stem cells persist. The two types of remission may not be distinguishable by morphologic or cytogenetic criteria. Lastly, data are presented that suggest that myeloid leukemias have a multistep pathogenesis with clonal proliferation of marrow stem cells preceding acquisition of distinctive chromosomal, morphologic, and clinical abnormalities.

INTRODUCTION

A convenient cell marker to use for tracing the development and cell lineages of human hemopoietic neoplasms is the X-chromosome-linked glucose-6-phosphate dehydrogenase (G6PD). Because the locus for this enzyme undergoes X-chromosome inactivation, only one of the two G6PD genes is active in each XX somatic cell. Therefore, women who are heterozygous for the usual B gene ($\underline{Gd}^B$) and a variant such as $\underline{Gd}^A$ have cellular mosaicism with two identifiable populations of cells: one with $\underline{Gd}^B$ active and synthesis of B-type enzyme and the other with $\underline{Gd}^A$ active and production of A-type G6PD. The B and A enzymes can easily be distinguished from one another after electrophoresis. Normal tissues are a mixture of the two cell types and show both B and A enzymes (double-enzyme phenotype), whereas proliferations that develop clonally show only one type of G6PD (single-enzyme phenotype).

This system has been used extensively to investigate hemopoietic and other neoplasms (reviewed in (6,7)). In this paper studies on myeloid leukemias are discussed with emphasis on five areas: a) lymphocyte origin from the pluripotent stem cells involved by many of these neoplasms, b) heterogeneity in the cells of origin of the acute myeloid leukemias, c) evidence for a stem cell common to marrow hemopoietic and microenvironmental cells, d) the heterogeneous nature of therapeutically induced clinical remission, and e) evidence for a multi-step pathogenesis of myeloid leukemias.

CELL LINEAGES IN MYELOID LEUKEMIAS

Chronic Myelocytic Leukemia (CML)

Early studies with the Philadelphia chromosome (Ph) as a marker suggested clonal development of CML. When present in a patient with CML, Ph is generally found in 90-100% of dividing marrow cells; it therefore seemed likely that the disease arose from a single cell in which Ph had occurred. Nonetheless, it was possible that Ph was induced simultaneously in several cells, as might have occurred if the involved regions on chromosomes 22 and 9 were particularly unstable or sensitive to a causative agent. Studies with G6PD provide strong evidence that the leukemic cells are members of a single clone, and the data suggest that clonal proliferation may even precede acquisition of Ph (see below).

Thus far, we studied twenty-six women with Ph-positive CML and heterozygous for G6PD ((7, 9), and Fialkow et al., unpublished). As anticipated, double-enzyme phenotypes were found in normal tissues, such as skin and cultured skin fibroblasts, but in each case a single-enzyme type was observed in the CML granulocytes (fifteen patients had type B and eleven had type A). These data indicate that CML develops clonally, a conclusion confirmed by other studies in which different enzymes or chromosomes were used as markers (reviewed in (7)). As with the granulocytes, single-enzyme G6PD types were found in red cells and platelets, confirming the suggestion based on studies with Ph that CML involves a stem cell multipotent for myelocytic cells, erythrocytes, and platelets. Similarly, single-enzyme types were found in cultured monocytes/macrophages and eosinophils. However, double-enzyme phenotypes were observed in cultured marrow fibroblasts, indicating that they did not arise from the multipotent stem cell involved by the myeloproliferative disorders, even in the presence of myelofibrosis (9, 19).

Several types of investigations indicate that lymphocytes also arise from the CML stem cell. For example, the finding of single-enzyme G6PD types in non-E-rosetting lymphocytes from two G6PD heterozygous women with CML and the observation that immunoglobulin (Ig) was detected in up to 46% of these non-T cells, suggested that cells from the abnormal clone differentiated along the B lymphoid pathway (8). This postulate was confirmed directly by G6PD typing of Epstein-Barr virus (EBV)-transformed B lymphoid cell lines (24) and by the demonstration of Ph in Ig-synthesizing cells (2, 24). However, these same studies also indicated that not all B lymphocytes in patients with CML arise from the abnormal stem cells.

The conclusion that B lymphoid cells are involved by CML receives support from studies in patients with blastic crisis of the disease. In one third of these cases the blast cells have characteristics which resemble those found in cells from patients with common-type acute lymphoblastic leukemia (reviewed in (16)). Less frequently the blast cells express cytoplasmic Ig (i.e., they have a "pre-B cell" phenotype).

The question of whether T cells emanate from CML stem cells has not been definitively resolved. Phytohemagglutinin (PHA)-stimulated blood lymphocytes from patients with CML are generally reported as Ph-negative (refs. in (16)). G6PD studies showed that at least the great majority of circulating T lymphocytes present during conventionally induced clinical remission or cultured in T cell colonies grown from patients at differing stages of their disease did not arise from the CML stem cell ((8), and Fialkow et al., unpublished). However, these findings do not necessarily indicate that the stem cell involved by CML does not have differentiative potential for the T cell lineage. One possibility is that most lymphocytes which are circulating during remission in vivo or are responsive to PHA in vitro are long-lived and antedated the development of leukemia. T cells derived from a neoplastic progenitor may be less responsive to mitogens and therefore more difficult to detect in vitro. Moreover, even if some mature T lymphoid cells did emanate from the CML stem cell, it would be difficult to detect them because they would be outnumbered by the long-lived T lymphocytes. Clonally derived T lymphoid cells might only be seen in vivo under circumstances that amplify the abnormal clonal population.

For example, E-rosette-positive lymphocytes from two G6PD heterozygotes with CML studied when the leukemia was under poor control had the same single-enzyme G6PD type as the CML granulocytes (8). Perhaps when the disease was under poor control, expansion of the CML clone, chemotherapy, or both, decreased proliferation of the antecedent normal T cells so that the ability to detect clonally derived T cells was enhanced. Another possibility is that these cells were not T lymphocytes but were other members of the abnormal clone that had acquired the attribute of forming E-rosettes during evolution of the leukemia. One case of blastic crisis with T cell characteristics has been reported recently (17). It is possible that the T cell phenotype in this patient's blast cells reflected the differentiative potential of the original CML clone, but the possibility cannot be excluded that its expression by the highly malignant blast phase cells resulted from alterations that occurred as a secondary consequence of malignancy.

In summary, the data indicate that B lymphocytes emanate from the pluripotent stem cell involved by CML; although the data suggest that T cells arise from this stem cell, the question has not been definitively resolved. Other evidence suggesting the existence of a hemopoietic stem cell common to the myeloid and T lymphoid lineages is provided by data from patients with the Tn syndrome (4), by G6PD studies of mixed-cell colonies (25), and by data from one patient with idiopathic sideroblastic anemia (28).

Acute Non-lymphocytic Leukemia (ANLL)

ANLL resembles the chronic form of myeloid leukemia in that it develops clonally (of the fourteen patients tested, eight had type B G6PD in their blast cells and six had type A) ((11,12) and Fialkow et al., unpublished). Cell lineage data are available for twelve patients. In four elderly women (ages 67, 69, 70, and 77 years), single-enzyme G6PD types were found in erythroid cells and platelets as well as in myeloblasts, indicating that the leukemias involved multipotent stem cells. A similar conclusion was reached earlier on the basis of chromosome studies (3, 21).

In contrast to the data for these elderly patients, in the four younger women (ages 18, 18, 34, and 38 years) and four children studied, double-enzyme phenotypes were found in erythroid cells or platelets, or both, despite the fact that the blast cells showed only a single G6PD. These erythroid cells and platelets arose from presumably normal stem cells. Thus, in these patients ANLL was expressed in cells with restricted differentiative ability. Two mechanisms could have been responsible for this restriction: the progenitors for the leukemia were cells analogous to granulocyte colony-forming units (e.g., progenitors restricted to granulocytic/monocytic differentiation), or they were multipotent stem cells incapable of erythroid and megakaryocytic differentiation. In any event, the data indicate that ANLL is heterogeneous with respect to the pattern of stem cell expression. The leukemias associated with the two patterns of stem cell expression were morphologically indistinguishable from each other, using criteria of the FAB classification.

The heterogeneity in differentiative expression of the stem cell involved in patients with ANLL may reflect causative differences and may have prognostic and other clinical implications. Thus far, all of the patients in whom multipotent stem cell differentiative expression has been demonstrated were elderly and may have had clinically undetected preleukemic syndromes. Patients with preleukemic syndromes or exposure as adults to an oncogen may develop ANLL different from that generally seen in most children and most younger adults. More G6PD heterozygotes with ANLL must be studied to determine the relative frequency of origin and expression in progenitors with restricted, as compared to multipotent differentiative expression, and to determine the relationship of pattern of cell involvement to other findings such as cell type, cytogenetics, and prognosis.

Myelodysplasia

Cell lineages have also been investigated with G6PD in a 61-year-old woman with a myelodysplastic refractory anemia (Jacobson et al., unpublished). Equal amounts of A- and B-type G6PD activities were found in skin and cultured skin fibroblasts, but erythrocytes, platelets, granulocytes, and marrow-nucleated cells expressed virtually exclusively type B enzyme. EBV-transformed Ig-synthesizing B lymphoid cell lines were established and tested for G6PD (29). Of twenty-four lines recovered, twenty-one showed G6PD type B and three manifested G6PD type A, markedly different from the 50:50 ratio predicted (X^2, $p < 0.01$). These results indicate that the stem cell involved by this disease can differentiate to mature granulocytes, erythrocytes, platelets, and B lymphocytes. Although a double-enzyme phenotype was found in pooled T lymphocyte colonies, the ratio was skewed towards type B G6PD, suggesting origin of some T lymphocytes from the pluripotent stem cells involved by the disease.

Marrow Microenvironment

More recently, we used G6PD and chromosomes as markers to study cells which grew in "long-term" cultures of human marrow. The technique for long-term culture of marrow cells in vitro was initially described by Dexter (5) and has been applied to human marrow (13). A feature necessary for the growth of hemopoietic stem cells in this system is the presence of an adherent "stromal layer" (5). The exact nature of these stromal cells is not known, but they may be an in vitro representation of the in vivo microenvironment required to sustain hematopoiesis. In previous studies, we demonstrated with the Y chromosome as a marker that the cell populations forming the adherent stromal layer in long-term human marrow cultures become increasingly donor-derived following marrow transplantation (23). This finding that some progenitors for the in vitro stromal layer are transplantable is consistent with the hypothesis that marrow hemopoietic and microenvironmental cells have a common progenitor stem cell.

To test this postulate, we studied four patients with clonal hemopoietic malignancies involving multipotent stem cells (31). At the time of study, Patient 1, a 31-year-old woman who had had CML for six years and had been treated with busulfan, was in an accelerated phase of the disease. All examined marrow metaphases were Ph-positive. Patient 2, a 74-year-old woman with newly diagnosed Ph-negative CML, had received no chemotherapy (22). Patient 3 was a 67-year-old untreated woman with newly diagnosed ANLL (20). Patient 4, a 7-year-old girl with newly diagnosed Ph-positive CML, had received no therapy. G6PD assays of cells from these patients documented multipotent hemopoietic stem cell involvement in each case (Table 1).

Long-term marrow cultures were established as described (23). After 3 to 4 weeks of culture, when stromal layers achieved confluence, nonadherent cells were harvested. Some stromal cells were recultured on glass slides for immunofluorescence tests; the remainder were assayed for G6PD. Collagen synthesis patterns were obtained from the media

TABLE 1 - G6PD analyses of uncultured tissues and blood cell colonies from four patients with clonal proliferations of multipotent hemopoietic stem cells.

			Uncultured tissues (%A/%B G6PD activity)			
Pt No.	Age (yrs)	Diagnosis	RBC	Platelets	Granulocytes	Skin
1	31	Ph+CML	0/100	0/100	0/100	50/50
2	74	Ph-CML	90/10*	100/0	100/0	60/40
3	67	ANLL	0/100	0/100	0/100	60/40
4	7	Ph+CML	100/0	100/0	100/0	60/40**

	Colonies	
Pt No.	Granulocytic (CFU-C) (#type A/# type B G6PD activity)	Pooled T cell (%A/%B G6PD activity)
1	0/55	50/50
2	42/3	60/40
3	3/25	40/60
4	27/1	NT

Ph - Philadelphia chromosome; CML - chronic myelocytic leukemia; ANLL - acute non-lymphocytic leukemia; NT - not tested.

* RBC studied two weeks after RBC transfusion. A pre-RBC transfusion specimen was not studied. Two days after transfusion, 70% of the G6PD activity was type A.

** Cultured marrow fibroblasts.

of companion cultures for Patients 1 and 2.

Non-involved tissues such as skin, cultured skin or marrow fibroblasts, and cultured, pooled T cell colonies showed approximately equal amounts of A and B G6PD activities (Table 1), but supernatant cells in the long-term cultures from the four patients showed only the single G6PD type found in the circulating blood cells. Similarly, washed stromal cells manifested the same single G6PD type as the neoplastic clone. In contrast, stromal layers grown from normal women and from a G6PD heterozygote whose ANLL involved progenitors with differentiative expression restricted to the granulocytic pathway showed double-enzyme phenotypes (data not given).

These results suggested that the multipotent stem cells involved by the leukemias in these four patients differentiated not only to hemopoietic elements, but also to cells with non-hemopoietic characteristics forming the in vitro microenvironment. However, before this suggestion could be accepted, it was necessary to exclude the possibility that the stromal cells themselves had a double-enzyme G6PD phenotype but were heavily "contaminated" with clonal hemopoietic cells (e.g., maturing granulocytes and macrophages) which masked their enzyme and resulted in the finding of single-enzyme G6PD types in the adherent layers.

Several techniques were used to study this possibility. Unfortunately, not all tests could be done for each patient. Synthesis by stromal cells of types I, III, and IV collagen was demonstrated for Patients 1 and 2, and up to 25% of the washed stromal cells from these patients reacted with an affinity-purified antibody to Factor VIII-associated antigen (kindly donated by G. Schmeer). These features are not characteristic of hemopoietic cells, but the assays are insufficiently quantitative. For example, it is possible that a minor population of cells was responsible for the collagen synthesis.

To refine the quantitative estimate of hemopoietic cells within the stromal layer, adherent cells from Patients 2, 3, and 4 were examined with monoclonals. The 9.4 antibody recognizes the T 200 cell surface glycoprotein, a determinant which has been found on almost all nucleated hemopoietic cells tested to date (27), but not on stromal cells or fibroblasts. Only 29%, 14%, and 20%, respectively, of the adherent cells from Patients 2, 3, and 4 were positive. And finally, 40% of the stromal cells from Patient 2 reacted with the CGA7 monoclonal, an antibody that appears to be specific for the alpha-actin determinant present on smooth muscle cells ((15), and A. Gown, unpublished) (the 9.4 and CGA7 were kindly donated by P. Martin and A. Gown, respectively). Approximately the same proportion of stromal cells cultured from normal marrows react with this antibody. Hemopoietic cells, fibroblasts, and endothelial cells do not express this antigen. With a rhodamine-conjugated second antibody, a dual labeling assay showed that Factor VIII-associated antigen-positive cells did not react with the CGA7 monoclonal. Thus, it seems very likely that less than 50% of the cells in the stromal layers shown to be clonal by G6PD analyses were "contaminating" hemopoietic cells.

Additional evidence that the G6PD activity in the stromal cells was not masked by hemopoietic cells was provided by mixture experiments. Stromal cells of G6PD type A (less than 10% positive with the 9.4

monoclonal) were mixed in varying proportions with nonadherent hemopoietic cells (99% positive with the 9.4 monoclonal) from long-term cultures of type B G6PD. The data indicate that the amount of G6PD activity in stromal cells is similar to what it is in granulocytes or macrophages derived from long-term cultures. Thus, if even 20% of the stromal cells were not derived from the abnormal clone, they would have been detected by G6PD analysis.

Although it is unlikely that the adherent layer contains a large proportion of hemopoietic cells, the characteristics of its major cell populations have not been defined. Stromal layers do not contain substantial numbers of fibroblasts since cultured, serially passaged marrow fibroblasts are not derived from the multipotent stem cells involved by the myeloproliferative disorders (9, 19), and since a 5% mixture of type B fibroblasts was detected in the presence of 95% type A stromal cells. The data suggest that the cells making up the major population of the adherent cell layer described by Dexter as "endothelial-like" (5) are an unusual population derived from a stem cell which also gives rise to hemopoietic elements and possessing biosynthetic and antigenic features of both endothelial and smooth muscle cells.

In summary, the G6PD data suggest that in certain myeloproliferative disorders involving multipotent hemopoietic stem cells, elements which make up the in vitro microenvironment are derived from the same clone that gives rise to the neoplastic hemopoietic cells. By inference, the results suggest that in normal people there is a pluripotent stem cell common to marrow stromal and hemopoietic cells.

Since it is presumed that the microenvironment plays a major role in hemopoietic cell regulation, clonal and thus "abnormal" stromal cells may be partly responsible for the disordered regulation of stem cells seen in patients with myeloproliferative diseases. For example, abnormal stromal cells could be causally related to the myelofibrosis commonly found in patients with CML and related conditions. The altered microenvironment might allow overgrowth of fibroblasts, either by failure to normally inhibit their growth or by abnormally stimulating their proliferation. This suggestion is compatible with observations that myelofibrosis in CML and agnogenic myeloid metaplasia is not part of the clonal proliferation of blood cells and, therefore, may represent a reaction secondary to the neoplastic process (9, 19). In addition, the abnormal microenvironment might play a role in the selective growth advantage enjoyed by the neoplastic hemopoietic stem cells, either by providing a poor environment for normal cell proliferation, or by selectively stimulating neoplastic cells. Studies of the interaction of clonally derived stromal cells and their synthetic products with normal and neoplastic hemopoietic stem cells are needed to elucidate further the role of stromal cells in blood cell regulation.

REMISSIONS IN CHRONIC MYELOCYTIC LEUKEMIA AND ACUTE NON-LYMPHOCYTIC LEUKEMIA

Chronic Myelocytic Leukemia

In most patients with CML whose clinical "remissions" are induced by conventional chemotherapy, the single-enzyme G6PD phenotypes in myeloid cells persist and the percentage of Ph-positive marrow metaphases does not decline. Thus, although the therapy is associated with decreased proliferation of leukemic cells, it does not lead to repopulation of the marrow by normal stem cells. However, large populations of Ph-negative marrow cells do reappear transiently in about 30 to 50% of patients treated with intensive combination chemotherapy (14). Nonetheless, it is possible that these Ph-negative cells were still members of the abnormal clone (see below). G6PD studies showed that the Ph-negative cells that reappeared in one such patient did arise from non-clonal, presumably normal, stem cells (30).

Acute Non-lymphocytic Leukemia

When patients with ANLL who have chromosomal abnormalities in marrow cells enter remission, there is often a return to normal karyotypes. However, this fact does not necessarily indicate that there is a repopulation of the marrow by normal stem cells. G6PD studies suggest that there are at least two patterns of remission in patients with ANLL, perhaps depending on the level of stem cell involvement.

Six patients whose ANLL showed unipotent stem cell differentiative expression were studied. In each case, during remission there was a return to a normal double-enzyme phenotype in granulocytes and the ratio of A:B colonies derived from CFU-C was more similar to that found in normal tissue (Table 2, upper panel). There was also a return to normal karyotypes in those patients who had marrow chromosome abnormalities.

Each of the long-term marrow cultures established from three of these patients with unipotent differentiative expression appeared morphologically normal and was still producing CFU-C-derived colonies at the time of sacrifice 4 to 23 weeks after initiation of the cultures. Supernatant cells and colonies cultured from them showed A and B G6PD activities

TABLE 2 - G6PD in normal tissues, blast cells, granulocytes, and blood cell colonies from eight patients with ANLL.

Patient		G6PD (Ratio of variant-type B enzyme)*			
		Prior to chemotherapy		Remission	
No.	Age (yrs)	Normal tissue**	Blast cells	Granulocytes	CFU-C-derived colonies+
Restricted Differentiative Expression					
1	2	60:40	100:0	60:40	7:6
2	10	50:50	100:0	50:50	6:7
3	11	50:50	0:100	50:50	NG
4	2	40:60	100:0	50:50	15:8
5	18	75:25	100:0	65:35	NG
6	34	60:40	100:0	50:50	10:5
Multipotent Stem Cell Expression					
7	69	40:60	0:100	25:75	6:15
8	67	50:50	0:100	5:95	0:15

NG - No growth.

* Patient 2 was heterozygous for B-type G6PD and a slowly migrating variant. The other patients were heterozygous for B- and A-type enzymes.

** Skin or pooled cultured T lymphocytes.

\+ Number of colonies showing variant enzyme:number showing B-type enzyme.

in ratios similar to those found in normal tissues (Table 3, upper panel). No evidence for a shift in ratio with time was noted, suggesting that if residual leukemic cells were present, they possessed minimal, if any, growth advantage in vitro. The data indicate that in these six patients with ANLL involving progenitors with restricted differentiative expression, during remission the marrow was largely repopulated by normal granulocyte progenitors.

The pattern of "remission" in the two patients with ANLL involving stem cells with multipotent differentiative expression was different. When Patient 7 entered remission, excess of B-type G6PD was present in granulocytes and platelets, as well as in granulocytic and erythroid colonies (Table 2, lower panel) (12). All of these preparations showed A:B G6PD

TABLE 3 - G6PD in hemopoietic cells and CFU-C-derived colonies grown from hemopoietic cells in long-term cultures of marrow from four patients with ANLL in remission.

	G6PD (Ratio of variant-type to type B enzyme)			
Patient No.	ANLL blast cells	Week of culture	Supernatant cells	CFU-C-derived colonies*
Restricted Stem Cell Expression				
1	100:0	0	-	16:9
		5	50:50	NT
		8	50:50	NT
		18	50:50	NT
		23	50:50	NT
4	100:0	0	-	15:8
		1	NT	7:4
		8	NT	10:10
6	100:0	0	-	9:5
		1	50:50	NT
		4	50:50	NT
		6	50:50	NT
Multipotent Stem Cell Expression				
8	0:100	0	-	0:15
		1	NT	0:15
		2	0:100	0:15
		3	5:95	1:14
		5	10:90	NT

NT - Not tested.
* Number of colonies showing variant enzyme:number showing B-type enzyme.

ratios of approximately 1:3, whereas pooled cultured T cells, cells not involved by the leukemic process, had a ratio of 1:1. One possible explanation for the imbalance of G6PD enzymes in the myeloid cells is that clonal stem cells capable of producing morphologically normal progeny coexisted with non-clonal normal stem cells. Thus, rather than regenerating entirely normal hemopoiesis, chemotherapy may have suppressed a sub-clone of blastic cells and restored a partially clonal preleukemic, partially non-clonal normal state.

The suggestion that chemotherapy in ANLL can induce a clinical "remission" without repopulation of the marrow by normal stem cells receives firm support from observations in Patient 8 (20). After induction therapy, the patient entered a clinical remission with normal blood and marrow morphology, and the distinctive chromosomal abnormalities found in 80% of marrow cells at diagnosis were no longer demonstrable. Nonetheless, the single-enzyme G6PD phenotype in granulocytes persisted during remission and only type B colonies from CFU-C were observed. Although the long-term marrow culture appeared morphologically normal and was still producing CFU-C at the time of sacrifice five weeks after initiation, predominantly type B G6PD was found in the supernatant cells and almost all CFU-C harvested from the long-term culture were G6PD type B (Table 3, lower panel). Although other possibilities exist, these data suggest that chemotherapy greatly reduced an overtly leukemic sub-clone but did not lead to repopulation of the marrow by normal stem cells. The situation is reminiscent of therapy-responsive blast crisis in CML: the acute leukemic subclone is greatly reduced and the patient is restored to what might be described as a preleukemic state. The findings also suggest that morphologic and cytogenetic observations alone are not sufficient to determine if normal hemopoiesis has been restored following antileukemic therapy. Furthermore, the data suggest that this patient's ANLL may have had a multi-step pathogenesis (see below).

EVIDENCE FOR A MULTI-STEP PATHOGENESIS OF MYELOID LEUKEMIAS

Multi-step pathogeneses have been suggested in the development of neoplasms, but there is little reported direct experimental evidence to support these postulates in human malignancies. The G6PD system provides an opportunity to approach this problem. One can ask, for example, what the temporal relationship is in the evolution of human myeloid neoplasms between development of a dominant clone of pluripotent stem cells and acquisition of some other attribute, such as a distinctive chromosome abnormality. Observations from three informative patients are described.

Chronic Myelocytic Leukemia

As discussed above, the observation that Ph was generally absent in mitoses from populations of non-E-rosetting lymphocytes from $\underline{Gd}^B/\underline{Gd}^A$ heterozygotes with CML, despite the fact that these cell populations showed only the single-enzyme types found in the leukemic clones, suggested that not all cells arising from the abnormal clones were necessarily Ph-positive. An alternate explanation, however, is that the single-enzyme

G6PD type reflected the phenotype of the dominant cell population, but not necessarily the only population. For example, a subset of cells with a double-enzyme phenotype might have been missed if it contributed less than 5% of the total activity. The mitogen-stimulated mitoses that lacked Ph reflected only the very small number of cells in metaphase, one that might have represented less than 5% of the whole cell population.

In order to examine this question further, we established from a single patient a large number of EBV-transformed B lymphoid cell lines that were homogeneous with respect to G6PD and cytoplasmic Ig. We then studied the chromosomes and G6PD of the lines to determine if there was an abnormal clone of Ph-negative cells in this patient (10). With conventional methods it is not possible to determine simultaneously the Ig class, G6PD type, and chromosomal composition of a single cell. With these homogenenous B cell lines, however, we were able to examine the progeny of one or a few cells for all three markers and thus infer the phenotypic expression of the progenitor(s) for each line.

In non-leukemic subjects, the proportions of type A and type B G6PD activities in mesenchymal tissues, including skin and blood lymphocytes, granulocytes, and erythrocytes, are highly correlated. Since the ratio of A:B enzyme in skin from this patient was 1:1, it was assumed that the frequency of normal B cell progenitors that expressed A-type G6PD should be equal to the frequency of progenitors that expressed B enzyme. However, 71% of the 63 Ph-negative lines manifested type B G6PD, the same single enzyme found in the patient's leukemic clone. This figure of 71% is significantly different from the expected 50% (X^2, $p < 0.001$). For reasons discussed elsewhere (10), it is unlikely that the discrepancy between the observed and expected frequencies of lymphoid cell lines showing only B-type G6PD resulted from a selective advantage in culture for progeny of abnormal precursors. It is more likely that the excess of lines that expressed type B enzyme is explained by the existence in this patient of B lymphoid cells that were derived from a clonal stem cell population that was abnormal, yet was also Ph-negative.

This conclusion was supported by results of detailed chromosomal studies on the lines. EBV-transformed B lymphoid lines established from the blood of normal donors generally are chromosomally normal during the first year of growth in vitro. In contrast, chromosomal abnormalities were detected in 8 of the 47 studied Ph-negative B lymphoid lines from our patient after only 15 to 45 days of growth in culture. Furthermore, the aberrations were not found at random, but were detected only in cells from lines that expressed the same G6PD (type B) as the CML clone ($p < 0.05$). We do not know if these chromosomal abnormalities arose in vivo or in vitro, but in either case the findings indicate that there existed in this patient an abnormal population of B lymphoid cells that was Ph-negative, had the same G6PD type as the leukemic clone, and was genetically unstable. Thus, formation of Ph may not be the sole event in the pathogenesis of CML. Compatible with this conclusion are the findings in patients in whom the marrow was reportedly entirely Ph-negative at diagnosis but was Ph-positive during subsequent follow-up (refs. in (10)).

One possibility is that Ph occurs secondarily in cells of an already leukemic clone as the disease progresses. However, the facts that Ph is generally detected in 90 to 100% of dividing marrow cells in patients with the leukemia, that it is very specific and characteristic of the disease, and that it has been found in several cases years before overt leukemia has developed make it unlikely that Ph is an entirely secondary occurrence. We favor the possibility that at least two steps were involved in the evolution of the leukemia in this patient - one causing proliferation of a clone of genetically unstable pluripotent hemopoietic stem cells and the other inducing Ph in one or more descendants of this progenitor clone. It is the preexisting genetic instability that predisposes both to formation of Ph and to the chromosomal abnormalities observed in the B lymphoid lines in vitro. The variety of karyotypic abnormalities detected in these cell lines suggests that formation of Ph was but one of many cytogenetic changes that could occur in cells of a genetically unstable clone. Once Ph occurs, however, it confers upon a subpopulation of cells a further selective growth advantage, since it is Ph-positive cells that generally greatly predominate in patients with Ph-positive CML. One possibility to explain this selective advantage is altered expression of an oncogene on the rearranged chromosome 22 or 9. A further step(s) in the evolution of CML presumably is responsible for the emergence of blastic crisis. In three of the cases of Ph-positive lymphoid blastic crisis of CML discussed above, a single class of Ig light chain was found in the leukemic blasts, suggesting that the cells originated from a single B lymphoid precursor, perhaps as the result of a mutation(s) in a single clonally derived cell already committed to B lymphoid differentiation. The frequent acquisition of additional cytogenetic abnormalities during progression towards blastic crisis may be another reflection of genetic instability in cells of the CML clone.

Although blastic crisis has been thought to occur by clonal evolution of already Ph-positive cells, the existence of clonally derived Ph-negative cells raises other possibilities. For example, blastic crisis could arise through de novo formation of Ph and further clonal evolution occurring in clonally derived cells that were originally Ph-negative. Such an occurrence could account for the occasional reports of "disappearance" of Ph and acquisition of other karyotypic abnormalities in CML blastic crisis (e.g., (18)), of a patient in whom both Ph-positive and Ph-negative blast cells were noted (1), and of a patient with constitutional mosaicism for 46,XY and 47,XYY cells in whose chronic phase and early blastic transformation CML cells, Ph was detected only in the 46,XY line, but who later manifested Ph only in 46,XYY,-C cells (26).

Myelodysplasia

The relationship of chromosomal abnormalities to clonality of pluripotent stem cells was also evaluated in the 61-year-old woman with myelodysplastic refractory anemia involving pluripotent stem cells discussed above. Cultured skin fibroblasts and PHA-stimulated lymphocytes from this patient were karyotypically normal. However, two chromosomal abnormalities were found in marrow - 46,XX,+8 and 46,XX,del(11)(q23) (29). These aberrations are nonrandom and are found in patients with preleukemia and ANLL. Non-E-rosetting blood lymphocytes obtained when 17 of 18 marrow metaphases revealed the $11q^-$ deletion were EBV-transformed. The blood cell clone in this patient showed B-type G6PD. As discussed above, twenty-four B lymphoid cell lines that expressed a single Ig were recovered, and twenty-one of them showed G6PD type B, suggesting that the pluripotent stem cells involved by the disease could differentiate to B lymphocytes. None of the 14 type B G6PD lines from which at least five metaphases could be analyzed in detail contained the karyotypic abnormalities observed in marrow. Thus, it is likely that not all cells that arose from the abnormal clone in this patient were chromosomally abnormal and that development of the nonrandom chromosomal aberrations was not the sole step in the development of the clonal myelodysplastic disorder. We hypothesize that at least two steps were involved in the pathogenesis of this patient's refractory anemia, one conferring genetic instability and a selective advantage on a clone of pluripotent stem cells and another inducing chromosomal abnormalities in its descendants. As opposed to the findings in the patient with CML discussed above, chromosomal aberrations were not detected in the B lymphoid cell lines from this patient in vitro. However, evidence for genetic instability was provided by the demonstration of two independent karyotypic abnormalities in marrow cells in vivo, 46,XX,+8 and 46,XX,del(11)(q23). Furthermore, since it is likely that this patient's disease is preleukemic, additional steps may occur and lead to development of ANLL.

Acute Non-lymphocytic Leukemia

In the patient described above whose ANLL involved a multipotent stem cell and in whom the single-enzyme G6PD type persisted in blood cells during clinical remission, over 80% of marrow metaphases had a distinctive complex chromosomal karyotype (20). It is generally assumed that when patients with ANLL enter complete clinical remission, marrow karyotype returns to normal. This indeed was the case in this patient. Two months after chemotherapy was instituted and at a time when the patient was felt to be in complete clinical remission, none of fifty-nine marrow metaphases had the chromosomal rearrangements found on initial presentation. However, despite this return to normal marrow karyotypes, the single-enzyme G6PD type persisted in blood and marrow cells and in cultured myeloid blood cell precursors. Thus, it can be concluded that the distinctive chromosomal abnormality in this patient was not a necessary requisite for the clonal proliferation of marrow stem cells, although it may have been necessary for clinical leukemia to become manifest.

In addition to its direct cytotoxic effects, the possibility cannot be excluded that the chemotherapy induced terminal differentiation in some of the myeloid blast cells. Nonetheless, the marked reduction in the prevalence of the chromosomally abnormal leukemic cells suggests that chemotherapy greatly decreased or eliminated a frankly leukemic subclone and restored the patient to a "preleukemic" state which persisted for eight months. Banding studies revealed no abnormalities in the chromosomes 22 nor any other evidence for the presence of a "masked" Ph. Nonetheless, this situation may be similar to what sometimes occurs in chemotherapy-responsive blastic crises of CML - the "remission" is associated with disappearance of the additional karyotypic abnormalities and a return to Ph-positive, clonal marrow stem cells which differentiate to mature blood cells. Thus, it seems very likely that at least two steps were also involved in the pathogenesis of this patient's overt leukemia - one leading to proliferation of a clone of genetically unstable pluripotent hemopoietic stem cells and the other inducing a chromosome abnormality in one or more descendants of that stem cell.

Acknowledgements. Supported in part by Grants CA 16448 and CA 18029 from the National Cancer Institute, Department of Health and Human Services, and by the Veterans Administration.

REFERENCES

(1) Appelbaum, F.R.; Najfeld, V.; and Singer, J.W. 1983. Prolonged survival with spontaneous decline in the frequency of Ph^1-positive cells and subsequent development of mixed Ph^1-positive and Ph^1-negative blast crisis. Cancer 51: 149-153.

(2) Bernheim, A.; Berger, R.; Preud'Homme, J.L.; LaBaume, S.; Bussell, A.; and Barot-Ciorbaru, R. 1981. Philadelphia chromosome positive blood B lymphocytes in chronic myelocytic leukemia. Leukemia Res. 5: 331-339.

(3) Blackstock, A.M., and Garson, O.M. 1974. Direct evidence for involvement of erythroid cells in acute myeloblastic leukaemia. Lancet 2: 1178-1179.

(4) Brouet, J.-C.; Vainchenker, W.; Blanchard, D.; Testa, U.; and Cartron, J.-P. 1983. The origin of human B and T cells from multipotent stem cells: a study of the Tn syndrome. Eur. J. Immunol. 13: 350-352.

(5) Dexter, T.M.; Allen, T.D.; and Lajtha, L.G. 1977. Conditions controlling the proliferation of hematopoietic stem cells in vitro. J. Cell Physiol. 91: 335-342.

(6) Fialkow, P.J. 1976. Clonal origin of human tumors. Biochim. Biophys. Acta 458: 283-321.

(7) Fialkow, P.J. 1980. Clonal and stem cell origin of blood cell neoplasms. In Contemporary Hematology/Oncology, eds. J. Lobue, A.S. Gordon, R. Silber, and F.M. Muggia, pp. 1-46. New York: Plenum Press.

(8) Fialkow, P.J.; Denman, A.M.; Jacobson, R.J.; and Lowenthal, M.N. 1979. Chronic myelocytic leukemia: origin of some lymphocytes from leukemic stem cells. J. Clin. Invest. 62: 815-823.

(9) Fialkow, P.J.; Jacobson, R.J.; and Papayannopoulou, T. 1977. Chronic myelocytic leukemia: clonal origin in a stem cell common to the granulocyte, erythrocyte, platelet and monocyte/macrophage. Am. J. Med. 63: 125-131.

(10) Fialkow, P.J.; Martin, P.J.; Najfeld, V.; Penfold, G.K.; Jacobson, R.J.; and Hansen, J.A. 1981. Evidence for a multistep pathogenesis of chronic myelogenous leukemia. Blood 58: 158-163.

(11) Fialkow, P.J.; Singer, J.W.; Adamson, J.W.; Berkow, R.L.; Friedman,

J.M.; Jacobson, R.J.; and Moohr, J.W. 1979. Acute nonlymphocytic leukemia: expression in cells restricted to granulocytic and monocytic differentiation. N. Engl. J. Med. 301: 1-5.

(12) Fialkow, P.J.; Singer, J.W.; Adamson, J.W.; Vaidya, K.; Dow, L.W.; Ochs, J.; and Moohr, J.W. 1981. Acute nonlymphocytic leukemia: heterogeneity of stem cell origin. Blood 57: 1068-1073.

(13) Gartner, S., and Kaplan, H.S. 1980. Long-term culture of human bone marrow cells. Proc. Natl. Acad. Sci. USA 77: 4756-4759.

(14) Goto, T.; Nishikori, M.; Arlin, Z.; Gee, T.; Kempin, S.; Burchenal, J.; Strife, A.; Wisniewski, D.; Lambek, C.; Little, C.; Jhanwar, S.; Chaganti, R.; and Clarkson, B. 1982. Growth characteristics of leukemic and normal hematopoietic cells in Ph+ chronic myelogenous leukemia and effects of intensive treatment. Blood 59: 793-808.

(15) Gown, A.M.; Gordon, D.; and Vogel, A.M. 1983. Analysis of smooth muscle cell-specific cytoskeletal antigens with monoclonal antibodies. Fed. Proc. 42: 502.

(16) Greaves, J.F. 1982. "Target" cells, differentiation and clonal evolution in chronic granulocytic leukaemia: a "model" for understanding the biology of malignancy. In Chronic Granulocytic Leukaemia, ed. M.T. Shaw, pp. 15-47. New York: Praeger.

(17) Griffin, J.D.; Tantravahi, R.; Canellos, G.P.; Wisch, J.S.; Reinherz, E.L.; Sherwood, G.; Beveridge, R.P.; Daley, J.F.; Lane, H.; and Schlossman, S.F. 1983. T-cell surface antigens in a patient with blast crisis of chronic myeloid leukemia. Blood 61: 640-644.

(18) Hagemeijer, A.; Smit, E.M.E.; Lowenberg, B.; and Abels, J. 1979. Chronic myeloid leukemia with permanent disappearance of the Ph^1 chromosome and development of new clonal subpopulations. Blood 53: 1-14.

(19) Jacobson, R.J.; Salo, A.; and Fialkow, P.J. 1978. Agnogenic myeloid metaplasia: a clonal proliferation of hematopoietic stem cells with secondary myelofibrosis. Blood 51: 189-194.

(20) Jacobson, R.J.; Temple, M.J.; Singer, J.W.; Raskind, W.; Powell, J.; and Fialkow, P.J. 1984. A clonal complete remission in a patient with acute nonlymphocytic leukemia originating in a multipotent stem cell. N. Engl. J. Med. 310: 1513-1517.

(21) Jensen, J.K., and Killmann, S.-A. 1971. Additional evidence for chromosome abnormalities in the erythroid precursors in acute

leukaemia. Act. Med. Scand. 189: 97-100.

(22) Kaye, F.J.; Najfeld, V.; Singer, J.; Cuttner, J.; and Fialkow, P.J. 1984. Confirming evidence for the clonal development and stem cell origin of Philadelphia chromosome-negative chronic myelogenous leukemia. Am. J. Hematol. 17: 93-96.

(23) Keating, A.; Singer, J.W.; Killen, P.D.; Striker, G.E.; Salo, A.C.; Sanders, J.; Thomas, E.D.; Thorning, D.; and Fialkow, P.J. 1982. Donor origin of the in vitro haematopoietic microenvironment after marrow transplantation in man. Nature 298: 280-283.

(24) Martin, P.J.; Najfeld, V.; Hansen, J.A.; Penfold, G.K.; Jacobson, R.J.; and Fialkow, P.J. 1980. Involvement of the B-lymphoid system in chronic myelogenous leukaemia. Nature 287: 49-50.

(25) Messner, H.A.; Lim, B.; Jamal, N.; and Takahashi, T. 1983. Lymphoid cells in multilineage colonies. In Haemopoietic Stem Cells, eds. SV.-AA. Killmann, E.P. Cronkite, and C.N. Muller-Berat, pp. 338-345. Copenhagen: Munksgaard.

(26) Moore, M.A.S. 1975. Agar culture studies in CML and blastic transformation. Ser. Haematol. 8: 11-27.

(27) Omary, M.B.; Trowbridge, I.S.; and Battifora, H.A. 1980. Human homologue of murine T200 glycoprotein. J. Exp. Med. 152: 1842-1852.

(28) Prchal, J.T.; Throckmortin, D.W.; Carroll, A.J. III; Fuson, E.W.; Gams, R.A.; and Prchal, J.F. 1978. A common progenitor for human myeloid and lymphoid cells. Nature 274: 590-591.

(29) Raskind, W.H.; Tirumali, N.; Jacobson, R.; Singer, J.; and Fialkow, P.J. 1984. Evidence for a multistep pathogenesis of a myelodysplastic syndrome. Blood 63: 1318-1323.

(30) Singer, J.W.; Arlin, Z.A.; Najfeld, V.; Adamson, J.W.; Kempin, S.J.; Clarkson, B.D.; and Fialkow, P.J. 1980. Restoration of nonclonal hematopoiesis in chronic myelogenous leukemia (CML) following a chemotherapy-induced loss of the Ph^1 chromosome. Blood 56: 356-360.

(31) Singer, J.W.; Keating, A.; Cuttner, J.; Gown, A.; Jacobson, R.; Killen, P.D.; Moohr, J.W.; Najfeld, V.; Powell, J.; Sanders, J.; Striker, G.W.; and Fialkow, P.J. 1984. Evidence for a stem cell common to hematopoiesis and its in vitro microenvironment: Studies of patients with clonal hematopoietic neoplasia. Leuk. Res. 8: 535-545.

Leukemia, ed. I.L. Weissman, pp. 223-234. Dahlem Konferenzen 1985. Berlin, Heidelberg, New York, Tokyo: Springer-Verlag.

The Preleukemic State in Virus-induced Leukemia

M. Essex
Dept. of Cancer Biology, Harvard University
School of Public Health, Boston, MA 02115, USA

INTRODUCTION

The evidence that retroviruses cause naturally occurring leukemia in species such as cats, wild mice, cattle, gibbon apes, and chickens is overwhelming. In most cases, but not all, the type of leukemia induced is lymphoid in origin. Recently, extensive evidence has accumulated which strongly suggests that another retrovirus, the human T cell leukemia virus (HTLV), may cause a particular type of lymphoid tumor in man, the adult T cell leukemia (ATL).

In all of these species the viruses infect the host by a horizontal route, although extrachromosomal vertical transmission can occur via egg albumin in the chicken. In all cases the leukemia that ultimately develops is monoclonal or oligoclonal. In all cases the induction period or period of preleukemia is prolonged, usually encompassing from 20% to 50% of the normal life span of the animal. During this time, DNA provirus remains integrated in numerous target cells and presumably continues to move to different sites within the DNA of the target cells. The biology and epidemiology of the leukemia virus infection is best understood in three species of higher mammals: the cat, the cow, and man. In all three species the final event of leukemia development is unusual, occurring in only 1% to 10% of the persistently infected animals that would live out their normal life span. The implication of this observation is that preleukemia as a distinct entity is difficult to define. Should all that become persistently infected be classified as preleukemic? If not, what distinguishes the few that become leukemic from the majority that do not? Obviously, the answer to the last question is largely unknown but is an important topic for discussion.

FELINE LEUKEMIA

The feline leukemia (FeLV) virus is spread primarily by saliva (11). When crowding occurs and cats have cause for extensive grooming, such as when infected mothers clean their kittens, transmission of FeLV occurs more readily. After exposure most young cats develop persistent viremia, as do a smaller proportion of adults. The rest resist persistent viremia, presumably due to an efficient virus-neutralizing antibody response. However, while it was formerly believed that the non-viremic exposed cats were uninfected, it now appears that most maintain the viral genome in a small proportion of bone marrow cells and/or lymph node cells (30). In either case, bone marrow cells appear to provide the primary focus for infection. Even in young cats that are inoculated with large doses of FeLV, infection is restricted to the bone marrow for a period of several weeks before viremia is seen. Following the viremia is a dramatic atrophy of the thymus and, at least in kittens inoculated with highly leukemogenic strains of virus, the replacement of the thymus with a developing thymic lymphoma (20).

Although all cats maintain a complete provirus of an inherited xenotrophic retroviral agent in their normal cell DNA, no evidence has emerged to suggest that this agent has anything to do with the development of disease. In addition, partial genomic sequences related to FeLV are also present in normal cat cell DNA. Since these sequences lack the long terminal repeat (LTR) regions characteristic of replicating FeLV, they cannot be activated. However, the possibility that newly infecting exogenous FeLV's could recombine with endogenous FeLV-related sequences remains open. Although most feline lymphomas appear to be monoclonal by Southern blot analysis, no evidence for preferred integration sites or frequent expression of known <u>onc</u>-related RNA's has been forthcoming.

In the feline system it appears that an active immune response by the host may play an important role in leukemia development. Aside from the role of the neutralizing antibody response in diminishing or eliminating the viremia, it has been noted that a humoral immune response directed to antigens at the surface of virus-producer leukemia cells can prevent the outgrowth of such cells, even in the presence of viremia (9). The absence of such an immune response, directed to the tumor antigen, feline oncornavirus-associated cell membrane antigen (FOCMA), signals a high risk for leukemia development. Although the identity of FOCMA antigen is not fully established, it appears to contain peptides related to the envelope (env) gene product of one particular subgroup of FeLV as well as cellular sequences that are distinct from all virus structural proteins (Snyder, personal communication). One logical hypothesis is that the FOCMA antigen is encoded by some combination of the endogenous FeLV-related cell sequences and non-FeLV related cell sequences after specific activation by FeLV.

About one third of the leukemias that occur in FeLV-exposed cats develop in non-viremic animals. Epidemiological evidence suggests that these tumors might also be caused by FeLV (17). Since immune responses to virion proteins that occur at the surface of virus-producer cells can serve as targets for lysis of both tumor and non-tumor cells, we hypothesized that an immunoselection phenomenon might be responsible for the development of the FeLV-nonproducer tumors (5). In this scenario, the presence of an effective antiviral response in the absence of an effective anti-FOCMA response might allow nonproducer tumor cells to "sneak through."

BOVINE LEUKEMIA

Leukemias or lymphomas of cattle caused by retroviruses feature several differences from feline leukemia caused by FeLV. Also, the bovine leukemia virus (BLV) is only distantly related to FeLV. The two viruses are not serologically cross-reactive. While feline leukemia is usually a disease of T cells, bovine leukemia is a disease of B cells. Bovine leukemia is often, though not always, preceded by a stage of polyclonal persistent lymphocytosis, a syndrome that has not been evident in feline leukemia. Whether the lymphocytosis should be considered as a more refined state of "preleukemia" is unclear.

The mechanism by which BLV infects the host is also unclear, but it is clear that provirus is not present in normal cell DNA, indicating that it must be horizontally acquired (2). Milk and biting flies have been suggested as vehicles and it is clear that high titers of free infectious virus, as is seen in infected plasma or saliva from cats, is not found in infected cattle. BLV appears to be highly cell-associated. Even though high titers of free virus are not found, the spread of the virus seems to be relatively efficient under conditions for housing dairy cattle, because entire herds frequently become infected in endemic regions.

The rate of replication of BLV in vivo appears to be severely limited, at least in cells that have good access to blood plasma. Nevertheless, periodic and/or limited replication must occur in some restricted focal areas of cells (e.g., bone marrow) to provide antigen to generate the levels of antibodies usually present in infected animals. Interestingly, when lymphoid cells of peripheral blood origin are removed from infected animals and cultured in vitro they generally produce readily measurable amounts of virus, at least when cultured in media that lacks serum from leukemic cattle (16). Conversely, the addition of serum from virus-infected cattle to such BLV-producer cultures shuts off virus production. Surprisingly, the factor involved in this suppression of replication does not appear to be an antibody, but rather a protein that acts to inhibit transcription of any BLV-related RNA.

Lymphoma cells taken from cattle with BLV-induced disease regularly have provirus integrated at the same site in each cell of the tumor, though in different sites with different tumors (21). This suggests that the viral genome plays an important role; however, attempts to identify transcription products related to known onc genes have been unsuccessful, as have attempts to find common integration "domains," using cloned probes from host-flanking DNA sequences in cross-hybridization studies (22). In still another enigma, while BLV is regularly associated with B cell tumors in cattle, it appears to induce primarily tumors of T cell lineage when inoculated into sheep. Although there is no evidence that the two phenomena are related, the tumors in cattle have a very prolonged induction period while the tumors in sheep occur at a much higher frequency and with a more restricted induction period.

HUMAN ADULT T CELL LEUKEMIA

The adult T cell leukemia (ATL) is a tumor of terminal transferase negative T cells that occurs at greatly elevated rates in southwestern Japan and in the Caribbean basin, where it is called lymphosarcoma cell leukemia (33). The disease is highly lethal and it occurs primarily in adulthood, though not in old age. The virus that appears to cause this tumor, the human T cell leukemia virus (HTLV), was recently isolated and characterized by Gallo and his colleagues (12, 26, 27). Several features of the virus and the virus-host relationship appear particularly important in reference to both of the other animal retroviruses mentioned above and in reference to the preleukemic stage.

HTLV is very difficult to transmit, but again, it is not genetically inherited. The relationship of HTLV proviral DNA to the normal cell DNA is somewhat analagous to that seen with BLV in cattle, although a small region of the env gene appears to resemble closely certain normal cell HLA genes, and expression of certain alien HLA haplotypes has been observed in HTLV-infected tumor cells (4, 23). The rates of infection with the virus vary from less than 1% in the United States and Western Europe to 5-20% in the Caribbean basin and southwestern Japan (1, 19, 29). The mechanism(s) by which the virus is transmitted are unknown. It appears that the agent can be transmitted by blood transfusion (25, 31), from males to females by sexual intercourse, and perhaps from mothers to children (32). Either way, the virus is not ordinarily present at meaningful levels as infectious virus in plasma, and transmission is probably associated with whole cells or cell debris. Whether or not an "inhibitory factor" that prevents virus replication at the transcriptional level is also present in plasma from infected people is unclear.

The tumor cells have a clear pattern of monoclonality in respect to the presence of the virus in a given tumor, although there is no evidence as yet for specific integration sites (13, 35). However, the presence of the provirus at the same site in all cells of a given tumor, but in different sites in different tumors, indicates that the agent was present in the cell before that particular cell grew out as a tumorous clone. This information, when taken in combination with the remarkably close geographical association between the prevalence rates of HTLV in a given population, and the rates for development of ATL in the same population, makes a strong case that HTLV may cause ATL. Within Japan, for example, high prevalence rates for antibodies only occur on the islands of Kyushu and Shikoku, where the rates of ATL are also greatly increased.

The leukemic cell found in ATL is classified as an OKT4 or Leu 3A T cell (6, 28). Despite this phenotype, which is supposed to be indicative of a helper or helper-inducer population, the tumor cells themselves demonstrate suppressor cell-type characteristics when assayed in vitro (18). While this may seem surprising, it seems conceivable that the relative tropism observed by HTLV for OKT4-positive cells may be limited to a subpopulation of those cells that already possess suppressor-type characteristics.

As in the case of cows and cats, HTLV appears to set up a permanent latent infection in a small proportion of the cells in some secluded population in the bone marrow or other lymphoid organs (34). Studies done on age-specific prevalence rates for the presence of antibodies are compatible with the evidence that most antibody-positive individuals appear to possess virus that can be activated under appropriate conditions (24). Whether the cell that harbors this virus is of the OKT4 phenotype or represents an earlier stage of a lymphoid cell that subsequently differentiates to the OKT4 phenotype after infection is unclear.

One property characteristic of HTLV is the ability to immortalize target lymphocytes (28). The mechanism involved in this activity is unclear. After successful immortalization the cells become independent of their need for T cell growth factor (TCGF) or interleukin 2 (IL 2), presumably because they become constitutive producers. The immortalized cells do express increased levels of the TCGF receptor. Whether immortalization is related to proviral insertion in the domain of the TCGF receptor gene or via another mechanism remains to be determined.

Since HTLV does not replicate very efficiently in vivo, exposure to the virus is best monitored at the seroepidemiologic level using tests for antibodies. Among the tests that have been used are fixed cell immunofluorescence, living cell membrane immunofluorescence, radioimmunoassays for the gag proteins p19 and p24, and immunoprecipitation for antibodies to gp61, the major protein that occurs at the surface of infected tumor cells that are positive for HTLV-related membrane antigens (HTLV-MA). Using membrane immunofluorescence tests for HTLV-MA as well as immunoprecipitation tests for gp61, we found that patients with the acquired immune deficiency syndrome (AIDS) had significantly higher rates of detectable antibodies than matched homosexual controls (7). Healthy hemophiliacs also had higher prevalence rates for HTLV exposure as compared to various control groups, and antibody-positive hemophiliacs had reduced levels of T4 cells as compared to antibody-negative hemophiliacs from the same area (8, 10). In other recently reported studies, HTLV-related proviral sequences were found in cells from two AIDS cases and virus was isolated from another case (14, 15). Furthermore, studies conducted with infectious disease patients in the endemic regions of Japan suggested that such individuals were infected with HTLV significantly more often than healthy adults from the same city (24). These results are compatible but certainly do not prove the hypothesis that a variant of HTLV could be involved in the etiology of AIDS. It has been firmly established that FeLV can cause immunosuppression in cats, an event that predisposes the animals to various lethal opportunistic infections (3).

SUMMARY AND CONCLUSIONS

In the three systems considered where retroviruses have been linked to naturally occurring leukemias, several common features emerge. All the viruses are horizontally acquired and most of the infected individuals do not develop leukemia. When leukemia (or lymphoma) does occur, it is only after a prolonged and variable induction period and the tumors that develop are monoclonal. Despite the fact that only a minority of the infected animals develop leukemia, most or all develop persistent latent infections in a limited population of hematopoietic cells. Some clear differences exist between the systems: in the FeLV-cat system, for example, high levels of free virus are present in the circulatory system, while this is not the case in BLV-infected cattle or HTLV-infected people. In cattle the BLV-associated tumors are of the B cell type, while in people and cats the retrovirus-associated tumors are primarily of T cell type. Also, in FeLV-infected cats and HTLV-infected people there are indications of immunosuppression, while this has not been reported for BLV-infected cattle.

Although much has been learned about the epidemiology and general biology of retrovirus infections, we know very little about many aspects of the disease process. Among the questions that seem important for future attention are the following:

1) How can we define the state of "preleukemia"? Should all individuals with persistent retroviral infections be considered potentially preleukemic?

2) Do differences in virus strains or genetics of the host determine which persistently infected individuals will develop leukemia, or is this only due to chance mutational events? Does immune surveillance directed to virus-infected cells play a role?

3) How do the changes of lymphoid cells associated with in vitro immortalization, such as those induced by the Epstein-Barr virus (EBV) in B cells or HTLV in T cells, relate to the leukemic process?

4) What is the importance of the integration site or domain for leukemogenic retroviruses? What is the significance of chromosomal translocations? How specific are these for a given type of leukemia? Does the 8 14 type of <u>myc</u> activation-translocation that occurs in most B cell lymphomas have the same effect as the same translocation as observed in a minority of HTLV-associated T cell lymphomas? Why are the types of chromosomal variations seen in HTLV, FeLV, and BLV-associated tumors so variable?

5) Do replication defective <u>onc</u>-carrying retroviral genomes ever play

a role in naturally occurring leukemias? If so, why are the resulting tumors monoclonal?

6) How common are the replication-inhibiting factors such as those that appear to play a role in the prevention of transcription of the BLV provirus in leukemic cattle?

7) Does retrovirus-induced immunosuppression play a role in leukemogenesis? Is the ability of a given strain of retrovirus to cause immunosuppression associated in any way with leukemogenic activity?

REFERENCES

(1) Blattner, W.A.; Kalyanaraman, V.S.; Robert-Guroff, M.; Lister, T.A.; Galton, D.A.G.; Sarin, P.S.; Crawford, M.A.; Catovsky, D.; Greaves, M.; and Gallo, R.C. 1982. The human type-C retrovirus, HTLV, in blacks from the Caribbean region, and relationship to adult T-cell leukemia/lymphoma. Int. J. Cancer 30: 257-264.

(2) Burny, A.; Bruck, C.; Chantrenne, H.; Cleuter, Y.; Dekegel, D.; Ghysdael, J.; Kettman, R.; Leclercq, M.; Leunen, J.; Mammerickx, M.; and Portetelle, D. 1980. Bovine leukemia virus: Molecular biology and epidemiology. In Viral Oncology, ed. G. Klein, pp. 231-290. New York: Raven Press.

(3) Cerny, J., and Essex, M. 1979. Mechanisms of immunosuppression by oncogenic RNA viruses. In Immunosuppressive Factors of Biological Significance, ed. R. Neubauer, pp. 233-256. Boca Raton: CRC Press.

(4) Clarke, M.F.; Gelmann, E.P.; and Reitz, M.S., Jr. 1983. Homology of human T-cell leukaemia virus envelope gene with class I HLA gene. Nature 305: 60-62.

(5) Essex, M. 1980. Feline leukemia and sarcoma viruses. In Viral Oncology, ed. G. Klein, pp. 205-229. New York: Raven Press.

(6) Essex, M. 1982. Adult T-cell leukemia/lymphoma: Role of a human retrovirus. J. Natl. Cancer Inst. 69: 981-985.

(7) Essex, M.; McLane, M.F.; Lee, T.-H.; Falk, L.; Howe, C.W.S.; Mullins, J.; Cabradilla, C.; and Francis, D.P. 1983. Antibodies to cell membrane antigens associated with human T-cell leukemia virus in patients with AIDS. Science 220: 859-862.

(8) Essex, M.; McLane, M.F.; Lee, T.-H.; Tachibana, N.; Mullins, J.I.; Kreiss, J.; Kasper, C.K.; Poon, M.-C.; Landay, A.; Stein, S.F.; Francis,

D.P.; Cabradilla, C.; Lawrence, D.N.; and Evatt, B.L. 1983. Antibodies to human T-cell leukemia virus membrane antigens (HTLV-MA) in hemophiliacs. Science 221: 1061-1064.

(9) Essex, M.; Sliski, A.; Cotter, A.M.; Jakowski, R.M.; and Hardy, W.D., Jr. 1975. Immunosurveillance of naturally occurring feline leukemia. Science 190: 790-792.

(10) Evatt, B.L.; Stein, S.F.; Lawrence, D.N.; McLane, M.F.; McDougal, J.S.; Lee, T.-H.; Spira, T.J.; Cabradilla, C.; Mullins, J.I.; Francis, D.P.; and Essex, M. 1983. Antibodies to human T-cell leukemia virus associated membrane antigens (HTLV-MA) in hemophiliacs: Evidence for infection prior to 1980. Lancet II: 698-701.

(11) Francis, D.P.; Essex, M.; and Hardy, W.D., Jr. 1977. Excretion of feline leukaemia virus by naturally infected pet cats. Nature 269: 252-254.

(12) Gallo, R.C.; Kalyanaraman, V.S.; Sarngadharan, M.G.; Sliski, A.; Vonderheid, E.C.; Maeda, M.; Nakao, Y.; Yamada, K.; Ito, Y.; Gutensohn, N.; Murphy, S.; Bunn, P.A.; Catovsky, D.; Greaves, M.F.; Blayney, D.W.; Blattner, W.; Jarrett, W.F.H.; Hausen, H. zur; Seligmann, M.; Brouet, J.C.; Haynes, B.F.; Jegasothy, B.V.; Jaffe, E.; Cossman, J.; Broder, S.; Fisher, R.I.; Golde, D.W.; and Robert-Guroff, M. 1983. Association of the human type C retrovirus with a subset of adult T-cell cancers. Cancer Res. 43: 3892-3899.

(13) Gallo, R.C.; Mann, D.; Broder, S.; Ruscetti, F.W.; Maeda, M.; Kalyanaraman, V.S.; Robert-Guroff, M.; and Reitz, M.S., Jr. 1982. Human T-cell leukemia-lymphoma virus (HTLV) is in T but not B lymphocytes from a patient with cutaneous T-cell lymphoma. Proc. Natl. Acad. Sci. USA 79: 5680-5683.

(14) Gallo, R.C.; Sarin, P.S.; Gelmann, E.P.; Robert-Guroff, M.; Richardson, E.; Kalyanaraman, V.S.; Mann, D.; Sidhu, G.D.; Stahl, R.E.; Zolla-Pazner, S.; Leibowitch, J.; and Popovic, M. 1983. Isolation of human T-cell leukemia virus in acquired immune deficiency syndrome (AIDS). Science 220: 865-867.

(15) Gelmann, E.P.; Popovic, M.; Blayney, D.; Masur, H.; Sidhu, G.; Stahl, R.E.; and Gallo, R.C. 1983. Proviral DNA of a retrovirus, human T-cell leukemia virus, in two patients with AIDS. Science 220: 862-865.

(16) Gupta, P., and Ferrer, J. 1982. Expression of BLV genome is blocked by a nonimmunoglobulin protein in plasma from infected cattle. Science 215: 405-407.

(17) Hardy, W.D., Jr.; McClelland, A.J.; Zuckerman, E.E.; Snyder, H.W., Jr.; MacEwen, E.G.; Francis, D.P.; and Essex, M. 1980. Development of virus nonproducer lymphosarcomas in pet cats exposed to FeLV. Nature 288: 90-92.

(18) Hattori, T.; Uchiyama, T.; Toibana, T.; Takatsuki, K.; and Uchino, H. 1981. Surface phenotype of Japanese adult T-cell leukemia cells characterized by monoclonal antibodies. Blood 58: 645-647.

(19) Hinuma, Y.; Komoda, H.; Chosa, T.; Kondo, T.; Kohakura, M.; Takenaka, T.; Kikuchi, M.; Ichimaru, M.; Yunoki, K.; Sato, I.; Matsuo, R.; Takiuchi, Y.; Uchino, H.; and Hanoaka, M. 1982. Antibodies to adult T-cell leukemia-virus-associated antigen (ATLA) in sera from patients with ATL and controls in Japan: a nation-wide sero-epidemiologic study. Int. J. Cancer 29: 631-635.

(20) Hoover, E.A.; Olsen, R.G.; Mathes, L.E.; and Schaller, J.P. 1977. Relationship between feline leukemia virus antigen expression and viral infectivity in blood, bone marrow, and saliva of cats. Cancer Res. 33: 145-152.

(21) Kettman, R.; Cleuter, Y.; Mammerickx, M.; Meunier-Rotival, M.; Bernardi, G.; Burny, A.; and Chantrenne, H. 1980. Genomic integration of bovine leukemia provirus: Comparison of persistent lymphocytosis with lymph node tumor form of enzootic bovine leukosis. Proc. Natl. Acad. Sci. USA 77: 2577-2581.

(22) Kettman, R.; Deschamps, J.; Cleuter, Y.; Couez, D.; Burny, A.; and Marbaix, G. 1982. Leukemogenesis by bovine leukemia virus: Proviral DNA integration and lack of RNA expression of viral long terminal repeat and 3' proximate cellular sequence. Proc. Natl. Acad. Sci. USA 79: 2465-2469.

(23) Mann, D.L.; Popovic, M.; Sarin, P.; Len, P.; Murray, C.; Reitz, M.S.; Strong, D.M.; Haynes, B.F.; Gallo, R.C.; and Blattner, W.A. 1983. Cell lines producing human T-cell lymphoma virus show altered HLA expression. Nature 305: 58-60.

(24) McLane, M.F.; Tachibana, N.; de-The, G.; Howe, C.; Lee, T.-H.; Azocar, J.; Kalyanaraman, V.; Gallo, R.C.; and Essex, M. 1983. Distribution of antibodies to human T-cell leukemia virus-associated cell membrane antigen (HTLV-MA). In Leukemia Reviews International, ed. M.A. Rich, pp. 103-104. New York: Marcel Dekker.

(25) Miyoshi, I.; Fujishita, M.; Taquchi, H.; Ohtsuki, Y.; Akagi, T.; Morimoto, Y.M.; and Nagasaki, A. 1982. Caution against blood transfusion from donors sero-positive to adult T-cell

leukaemia-associated antigens. Lancet I: 683.

(26) Poiesz, B.J.; Ruscetti, F.W.; Gazdar, A.F.; Bunn, P.A.; Minna, J.D.; and Gallo, R.C. 1980. Detection and isolation of type-C retrovirus particles from fresh and cultured lymphocytes of a patient with cutaneous T-cell lymphoma. Proc. Natl. Acad. Sci. USA 77: 7415-7419.

(27) Poiesz, B.J.; Ruscetti, F.W.; Reitz, M.S.; Kalyanaraman, V.S.; and Gallo, R.C. 1981. Isolation of a new type-C retrovirus (HTLV) in primary cultured cells of a patient with Sezary T-cell leukemia. Nature 294: 268-271.

(28) Popovic, M.; Sarin, P.S.; Robert-Guroff, M.; Kalyanaraman, V.S.; Mann, D.; Minowada, J.; and Gallo, R.C. 1983. Isolation and transmission of human retrovirus (Human T-Cell Leukemia Virus). Science 219: 856-869.

(29) Robert-Guroff, M.; Nakao, Y.; Notake, K.; Ito, Y.; Sliski, A.; and Gallo, R.C. 1982. Natural antibodies to the human retrovirus, HTLV, in a cluster of Japanese patients with adult T-cell leukemia. Science 215: 975-978.

(30) Rojko, J.L.; Hoover, E.A.; Quackenbursh, S.L.; and Olsen, R.G. 1982. Reactivation of latent feline leukaemia virus infection. Nature 298: 385-388.

(31) Saxinger, W.C., and Gallo, R.C. 1982. Possible risk to recipients of blood from donors carrying serum of human T-cell leukemia virus. Lancet I: 1074.

(32) Tajima, K.; Tominaga, S.; Suchi, T.; Kawagoe, T.; Komoda, H.; Hinuma, Y.; Oda, T.; and Fujita, K. 1982. Epidemiological analysis of the distribution of antibody to adult T-cell leukemia-virus-associated antigen: Possible horizontal transmission of adult T-cell leukemia virus. Gann 73: 893-901.

(33) Takatsuki, K.; Uchiyama, T.; Ueshima, Y.; and Hattori, T. 1979. Adult T-cell leukemia: further clinical observations and cytogenetic and functional studies of leukemic cells. Jap. J. Clin. Oncol. 9 (Suppl.): 317-324.

(34) Yamamoto, N.; Schneider, J.; Koyanagi, Y.; Hinuma, Y.; and Hunsmann, G. 1983. Adult T-cell leukemia (ATL) virus-specific antibodies in ATL patients and healthy virus carriers. Int. J. Cancer 32: 281-287.

(35) Yoshida, M.; Miyoshi, I.; and Hinuma, Y. 1982. Isolation and characterization of retrovirus from cell lines of human adult T-cell leukemia and its implication in the disease. Proc. Natl. Acad. Sci. USA 79: 2031-2035.

Leukemia, ed. I.L. Weissman, pp. 235-249. Dahlem Konferenzen 1985. Berlin, Heidelberg, New York, Tokyo: Springer-Verlag.

The Receptor-mediated Leukemogenesis Hypothesis: A Model of Retroviral Oncogenesis by Viral Stimulation of Cell-surface Receptors

I.L. Weissman, M.S. McGrath, and G. Tamura
Laboratory of Experimental Oncology
Dept. of Pathology, Stanford University School of Medicine
Standford, CA 94305, USA

INTRODUCTION

In our view the central lesion in oncogenesis is the sustained, apparently uncontrolled proliferation of malignant cells beyond the regulated number of their normal counterparts; these malignant cells would not differ in kind from normal cells, but mainly in the size of their proliferative compartments. Given this point of view, it is logical to assume that malignant cells utilize normal mitogenic pathways for their sustained proliferation, and that one must look to means by which a particular class of cells controls its proliferation if one wishes to understand how malignancy develops in that cell type.

For many if not all cells, the initial trigger for mitogenesis appears to be interaction of an extracellular growth factor with a cell surface growth factor receptor. Activation of the growth factor receptor leads in turn to yet undefined cytoplasmic signaling systems, but associated events may include the formation or degradation of particular cyclic nucleotides, as well as the activation of submembranous protein kinases which appear to phosphorylate amino acids at their tyrosine residues. The relationship of these cytoplasmic events to events leading to the activation of the nucleus and the initiation of DNA synthesis are still poorly understood but presumably involve the translocation of the signal to the nucleus, the interaction of signal-transmitting molecules with particular chromosomal regulatory genes, and the stimulation of a multi-enzyme DNA replication apparatus. It is obvious that oncogenesis could result from the sustained and inappropriate activation of either the surface receptor system or any of the internal events. It is possible that perturbation of the mitogenic apparatus at a single level is not sufficient, as regulation of events at a more central level might inhibit the oncogenic signal. In this view multiple genetic events must occur, perhaps providing an explanation for tumor progression.

The control of proliferation of antigen-specific lymphoid cells is an interesting case in point. These cells are usually small, G_0, long-lived cells and only enter proliferative cycles under the drive of antigenic stimulation. In general, interaction of antigens with a lymphocyte antigen-specific receptor is a necessary and, in some cases, sufficient condition for continued proliferation by these cells; in other cases, antigenic stimulation is necessary but not sufficient for continued proliferation. Some subsets of antigen-specific T lymphocytes are stimulated by cell-surface receptor-mediated recognition of antigens to express cell surface receptors specific for class-specific polypeptide growth factors (produced by other cells). An excellent example of this type of control of proliferation is shown by the subclass of T cells called T_c, or cytotoxic T cells. These cells possess as yet uncharacterized but exquisitely antigen-specific cell surface receptors, generally for foreign antigens placed somehow in the context of major histocompatibility complex (MHC) class I glycoproteins. Precursors of cytotoxic cells are small, G_0 circulating lymphocytes which, upon antigen recognition, express cell surface receptors for T cell growth factors such as interleukin 2 (TCGF or IL-2). IL-2 is sufficient to maintain proliferation by IL-2-sensitive T_c cells for extremely long periods, although maintenance of antigen recognition specificity and perhaps IL-2 receptor expression requires frequent restimulation of the cells by their inducing antigen. Several classes of helper T cells may act differently. These cells recognize and respond to antigen and continue to proliferate in the presence of antigen, but cease proliferation if antigen is removed. Conversely, after activation, it is likely that other classes of helper T cells may proliferate in response to IL-2 or other interleukins alone. It is not surprising then, that there is a heterogeneity in the control of T cell proliferation, as there is significant functional and receptor heterogeneity among subclasses of T cells, and even subclasses of helper T cells.

Similarly, antigen recognition in appropriate microenvironments by B lymphocytes occurs by antigen binding to receptor immunoglobulins, and these cells then express cell surface receptors for factors produced by some of the helper T cell classes. These factors, called B cell growth factors (BCGF's), drive the proliferation of antigen-activated B cells. The transition of proliferating B cells to terminally differentiated, antibody-secreting plasma cells is apparently controlled by the cell surface expression of receptors for B cell differentiation factors (BCDF's); these BCDF's are also produced by antigen-specific effector helper T lymphocytes. Whether the cessation of B cell proliferation is controlled by BCDF-induced B cell differentiation or whether other signals operate to regulate the BCGF-induced proliferative drive is unknown. From the above considerations, it is clearly possible that misregulation of the activation of antigen receptors, of growth factor receptors, or of differentiation factor receptors could each be involved in the malignant growth of lymphoid cells.

SLOWLY TRANSFORMING RETROVIRUSES AND MODELS FOR THEIR ONCOGENIC ACTION

If retroviruses cause malignant proliferation by utilizing the normal mitogenic apparatus, then the target of their action might be a) at the level of the cell surface antigen-specific receptor-mitogen complex, b) at the level of growth factor receptors on those cells which are sensitive to growth factors, c) at the level of regulation of the signal from cell-surface receptor-mitogen complexes to the activation of the gene program required for cell proliferation, d) reached by increasing one of the regulatory enzymes involved in cell proliferation, and e) reached by countermanding regulatory signals which suppress proliferation. Unlike rapidly transforming retroviruses, slowly transforming retroviruses apparently do not carry oncogenes whose direct expression leads to transformation of cells they infect. Elsewhere in this volume (Vogt et al., Hayman, Hayward et al., and Graf) the various rapidly transforming retroviruses and the oncogenes they contain are described in detail. In contrast, the slowly transforming retroviruses contain, in addition to their LTR's, the gag gene (encoding core proteins), the pol gene (encoding reverse transcriptase), and the env gene (encoding the cell surface envelope glycoprotein heterodimers). As a group, slowly transforming retroviruses can be distinguished from rapidly transforming retroviruses by their long latent period, their requisite in vivo action, and their absolute tissue specificity for transformation. Surprisingly, although several different histologically defined cell types may be infected by these viruses, only cells of one histologic type may be transformed by a particular retrovirus. For example, the lymphomagenic retroviruses may infect bone marrow cells, fibroblasts, and even several types of lymphocytes, but may only transform a particular subset of lymphocyte. Thus, there must be a particular match between a slowly transforming retrovirus and a target cell for oncogenesis to occur.

As outlined in other parts of this book, several events are correlated with lymphoid transformation by retroviruses. Included in the category of events in avian bursal lymphomagenesis is the almost constant retroviral insertion near and activation of c-myc genes (17), as well as the appearance in these cells of genetic elements - separate from retroviruses and c-myc genes - which reproducibly transfect and transform mouse 3T3 fibroblasts (3). Because the c-myc gene is expressed primarily as a nuclear protein, it might regulate events not in the cytoplasm or at the cell surface (19). The B-lym gene apparently encodes a genetic element structurally related to transferrin genes (5). Its level of action is unknown. (The bursal lymphoma genetic element is called B-lym.)

Where and how do these genes act? The direct evidence that expression of c-myc or any other cellular homologue of a viral oncogene in a particular cell is necessary for the transformed behavior of that cell is difficult to prove directly. At this point the nearly absolute correlation of these events in particular types of lymphomas must be taken as extremely strong support, but not proof, of their role in the induction and/or maintenance of the neoplastic state.

THE RECEPTOR-MEDIATED LEUKEMOGENESIS HYPOTHESIS (11, 13, 20)
Several years ago we proposed a hypothesis which postulated that proliferation of cells transformed by slowly transforming retroviruses was mediated through stimulation of antigen-specific receptors. Our specific model is: Each retrovirus should be considered to be a non-cytopathogenic virus with a potentially antigenic envelope. In hosts not tolerant of retroviral envelope antigens there should exist antigen-specific lymphocytes with receptors capable of binding these retroviral envelopes. If the interaction between receptor and antigen is strong, then the lymphocyte binding the virus should undergo cell division and/or express growth factor receptors. If these cells or associated antigen-presenting accessory cells are infected by that retrovirus, then their lymphoid progeny should both produce the antigen encoded by the viral env gene and the receptor specific for that antigen. These progeny cells should once again engage antigens via their antigen-specific receptor, and once again go through a round of antigen-driven or growth factor-driven proliferation (Fig. 1). If this process proceeded in the absence of any immune regulatory interaction or suppressive/cytotoxic functions, these cells could never escape the mitogenic drive provided by the antigen. In this view, each lymphoma

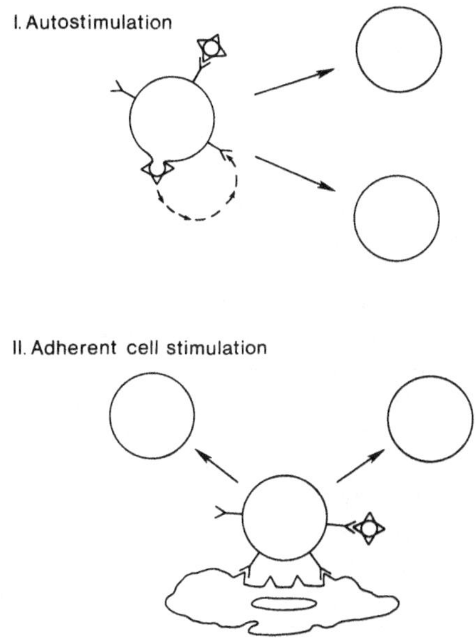

FIG. 1 - Receptor-mediated leukemogenesis.

should be a clone of cells bearing on their surface antigen-specific receptors directed toward the envelope of the retrovirus that induced them. Only those cells with high affinity receptors for virus should succeed to frank lymphomas, and surrounding cells with low affinity receptors (or no receptors) should not be in the target population for lymphomagenesis. Continued proliferation by these cells should remain dependent upon continued restimulation by virus and also, perhaps, by locally produced growth factors, unless a secondary malignant progression occurs. In this model, the oncogene should be the viral env gene, and not a host cellular gene.

It is also conceivable that the virus binds directly to the growth factor receptor (21). In that case one would expect that the receptor found on any tumor induced by a particular virus would be the same from tumor to tumor, given that the receptor might be for IL-2 or for another class of T or B cell growth factor. Ihle et al. (6) have proposed a variant of the receptor-mediated leukemogenesis hypothesis in which virus binding to antigen or mitogen receptors may initially cause prolonged proliferation of the cells, but that the oncogenesis requires a second event such as the inappropriate production of growth factors and their receptors by the same cell population. The distinction between these two similar hypotheses has been discussed previously (21).

The receptor-mediated leukemogenesis hypothesis has several predictions which are susceptible to experimental verification or exclusion. A brief summary of those experiments follows.

Each T Cell Lymphoma Expresses Surface Receptor Highly Specific for the Retrovirus Which Is Produced by It (9, 14, 15)
Using the fluorescence-activated cell sorter (FACS), we have demonstrated that each T lymphoma has surface receptors specific for murine retroviruses, and particularly for the virus which induces it. A typical experiment is shown in Fig. 2, wherein two retroviruses are simultaneously analyzed for their ability to bind to lymphomas induced by them, and to the lymphoma induced by the other. A high degree of specificity is shown. Similar results have now been shown for fifteen independent murine T cell lymphomas. Competitive binding assays with nonfluoresceinated virus of several types demonstrates that the fine specificity of binding is due to recognition of nonfluoresceinated envelope entities rather than the fluorescein (or rhodamine)-modified virions.

The Virus Receptor Is a Marker for Leukemia Cells and Distinguishes Them from Preleukemic Cells in the Same Thymus (14)
During the long latent period between first appearance of retroviruses and appearance of thymic lymphomas, AKR and C57BL mice first show infection of thymocytes by retroviruses and concomitant expression of cell surface gp70 and gag determinants (4). These cells do not bear detectable virus receptors (13, 14). However, at about the time that non-ecotropic recombinant or leukemogenic viruses are released from the thymus, there appears a population of lymphoblasts (starting in the thymic outer cortical regions) which are virus receptor-positive and which are extremely potent in giving rise to donor-derived leukemias upon transfer to Thy-1 congenic hosts (Fig. 3). Thus, these virus receptors are extremely accurate markers for newly arising leukemia cells, and there is no evidence for an increased frequency of thymocytes or peripheral lymphocytes with receptors for native, intact leukemogenic viruses during the preleukemic period.

Virus Receptor Binding May Regulate Lymphoma Proliferation (10, 12)
Several monoclonal antibodies to Thy-1 and T80 cell surface molecules

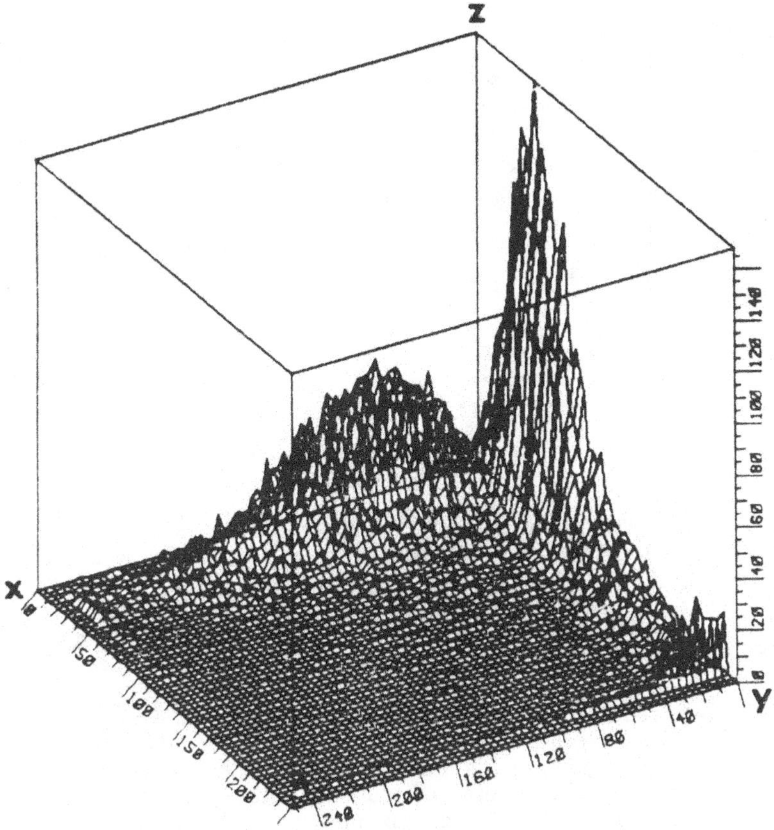

FIG. 2 - Two-color FACS Analysis: MCF-247 and RadLV/VL_3 Binding Specificities

This three-dimensional perspective plot shows rhodaminated MCF-247 and fluoresceinated RadLV/VL_3 binding to two different target cell populations. MCF-247-binding increases along the X axis, fluoresceinated RadLV/VL_3-binding increases along the Y axis, and the frequency of cells binding a particular level of fluorescence increases along the Z axis. In each case, 10^5 cells were analyzed, and the fluorescein and rhodamine backgrounds were equal to 30 units.

10^6 KKT-1 cells were added to 10^6 B1/VL_3 cells and were assayed for simultaneous binding of fluoresceinated RadLV/VL_3 and rhodaminated MCF-247. Cells with fluorescence greater than 250 units, representing $< 5\%$ of all cells analyzed, were collected and combined in the 250 unit computer channel, as represented by the ridges along the distal edges of the three-dimensional plots.

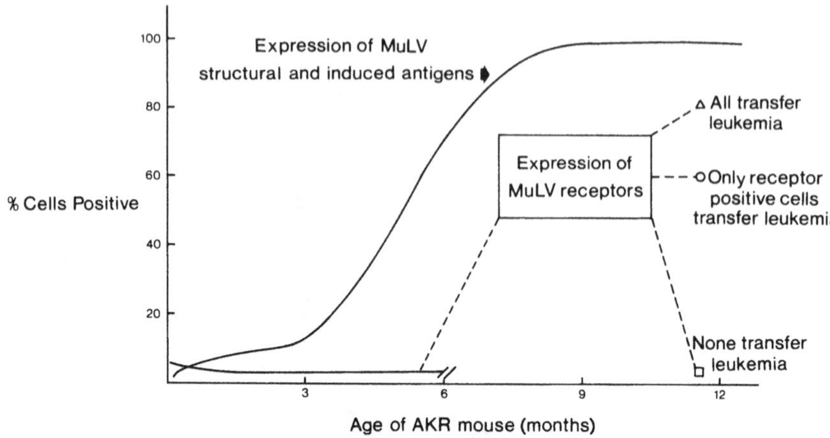

FIG. 3 - 10^5 AKR/Cum (Thy-1.2) virus antigen-positive MCF-binding negative thymocytes from five separate animals were injected intraperitoneally into groups of 4-10 one-month-old AKR/J (Thy-1.1) animals that had been given 400 Rads whole body X-ray just prior to transfer. In every case (n=26), the donor cells failed to cause leukemia or a lymphoma within a four month observation period. Similarly, 10^5 virus antigen-positive MCF-binding positive thymocytes from five separate animals were each injected intraperitoneally into independent groups of five irradiated one-month-old AKR/Cum mice; 18-40 days after transfer of 10^5 MCF-247-binding cells into irradiated one-month-old AKR/Cum hosts, all recipient animals died of leukemia. We used anti-Thy-1.1 antiserum to type the origin of the leukemia in these hosts; all were Thy-1.1-positive by absorption analysis (data not shown).

To determine whether animals possessing both MCF-binding positive and negative thymocytes also possessed intrathymic leukemic and non-leukemic cells, we sorted cells from animals bearing significant levels of both MCF-binding positive and negative fractions for adoptive transfer. Only MCF receptor-positive cells gave rise to donor-derived leukemias.

were found to block virus binding to KKT2 and S49 T lymphoma cells in vitro. These antibodies also inhibit lymphoma proliferation in vitro (Fig. 4). The Thy-1 molecule is not the virus receptor, because specific virus binding can be shown in Thy-1 negative variants of the S49 T lymphoma; that binding is inhibited in the presence of antibodies to the T80 but not to the Thy-1 molecule (8). That this growth inhibition was due to antibody blockade of virus binding was shown in several experiments

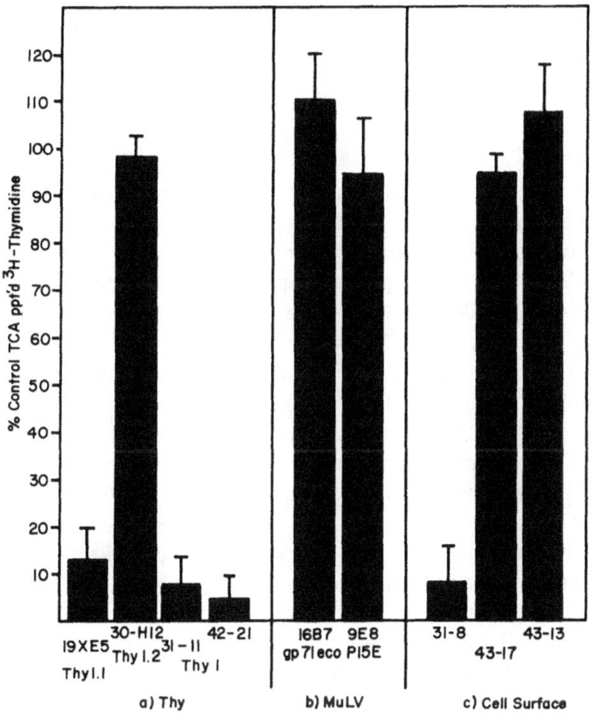

FIG. 4 - Lymphoma cell growth inhibition assay. KKT-2 lymphoma cells were pelleted from subconfluent cultures and were resuspended in serum-free growth medium (MEM, GIBCO) for 2h at 37°C at a density of 10^5 cells/ml. After repelleting, the cells were resuspended in cold tissue culture medium (MEM, 5% FCS) at a density of 2 x 10^4 cells/ml. Two and one half milliliters (5 x 10^4 cells) were placed in the bottom of 25 cm^2 Corning tissue culture flasks and monoclonal antibody was added for a 1:12 final dilution. After growing for 14h at 37°C, 0.1 ml of medium containing 10μ Ci [^{3}H] thymidine (NEN) was added to each culture for 2h. Labeled cells were washed, 5% TCA was precipitated, and percent growth inhibition was calculated using cells without antibody as equal to 100% growth, KKT-2 cells were tested for growth inhibition with a) anti-Thy-1 (19XE5, 30-H12, 31-11), b) anti-MuLV (16B7, 9E8), and c) anti-cell surface antibodies (31-8, 43-17, 43-13, 42-21). The above data represent five experiments ± standard deviations.

wherein virus presaturation of lymphoma cell surface receptors precluded the growth-inhibiting activity of the monoclonal antibody. Thus, in some way, virus receptor binding of envelope ligands appears to be obligatory for the proliferation of these lymphoma cells in vitro, and perhaps in vivo.

Virus Receptors on B Cell Lymphomas in Mice and Chickens

The biochemical nature of T cell antigen-specific receptors is still unknown. An opportunity to study a more well-defined virus receptor arose when we obtained BCL_1, a spontaneous BALB/c B cell lymphoma (from Strober and Slavin). This B cell lymphoma is largely spleen-dependent for its in vivo growth. Two lines of BCL_1 cells were available - an in vivo line which was incapable of in vitro growth, and an autonomously replicating variant in vitro line. The in vivo line could be maintained in culture for long intervals, so long as splenic surface adherent cells from the leukemic spleen were present. These splenic surface adherent cells produced retroviral particles at detectable levels. We postulated that the stromal cells were providing a virus which was the oncogenic stimulus for proliferation of the lymphoma cells (Fig. 1). If this were so, the autonomously replicating in vitro lymphoma line might also be producing that retrovirus. Indeed, the in vitro adapted lymphoma cells produced as much (or more) retrovirus as the splenic stromal adherent cells. We isolated both the stromal-produced virus and the in vitro lymphoma line-produced virus and found that these viruses bound to a high degree to BCL_1 lymphoma cells and to isolated BCL_1 immunoglobulin (21). Monoclonal antibodies recognizing idiotypic determinants on the isolated BCL_1 immunoglobulin blocked virus binding both to the isolated immunoglobulins and to BCL_1 cells. Thus, BCL_1 lymphoma cells express a surface immunoglobulin receptor with a high degree of specificity for a retrovirus associated with them.

In a similar study, we have obtained in vitro chicken bursal lymphoma lines, as well as ALV-injected chicken bursae at various stages in the pre-lymphomatous and lymphomatous progression. The (Rous associated virus) lymphomagenic viruses bind specifically to the in vivo and in vitro chicken lymphomas, but not to cells predominating in the pre-lymphomatous period. Monoclonal anti-chicken light chain antibodies block binding of these viruses to these chicken lymphoma cells, whereas antibodies to other cell surface structures of the chicken B cells do not. We are currently investigating in greater detail the nature of the binding site for viruses on these chicken immunoglobulins.

Thus, even the best model for retrovirus insertion and promotion of endogenous oncogenes, and the best model for transfecting DNA sequences also is one of the best models for the evidence of antigen-specific receptors which are retrovirus-specific. It is important at this point to consider the possibility that all three events correlate extremely well with the development of lymphomas in chickens, but that absolute proof of the necessary or sufficient nature of any one of these events in chicken lymphomagenesis is still lacking. Although it is possible to propose several models which would involve all three systems in an oncogenic progression, there is no clear evidence as to the importance and timing of each of these events during lymphomagenesis.

HUMAN MODELS

We have recently completed a preliminary set of experiments testing the possibility that human T cell leukemia virus (HTLV)-producing cells would have on their surface receptors specific for HTLV. HTLV binds to all HTLV-producing lines, and this binding shows saturation kinetics and blockade with unlabeled HTLV. Normal lymphocytes, in vitro human T cell lines, and several, but not all, non-HTLV-producing T and B cell lines lack the ability to bind the virus. Several experiments will be required to define the nature of the binding entity on these diverse cell lines, to test whether lymphomatous proliferation in vitro is dependent on virus rebinding, and whether HTLV receptors are markers for neoplastic transformation.

CONCEPTUAL PROBLEMS OF THE RECEPTOR-MEDIATED LEUKEMOGENESIS HYPOTHESIS

Although T cells have receptors of undefined biochemical nature, their antigen recognition appears to encompass the nominal antigen as well as host MHC (major histocompatibility complex) or immunoglobulin determinants. While it is conceivable that the diversity of retrovirus envelopes could match the diversity of structures recognized by T lymphocytes, until recently very little data were available to support that contention. Two bits of data may in fact be relevant: first, it has recently been demonstrated that the amino acid sequence of the HTLV env region shows some sequence homology to the human MHC class I genes, HLA-A, -B, and -C (2). Sequence comparison of murine retroviruses and murine MHC antigens has not yet been carried out. A second interesting correlation was found by Shinnick, Sutcliffe, and Lerner - the Moloney virus env region contains a short sequence which has a high degree of homology to the lambda immunoglobulin variable region (personal communication). Thus, it is conceivable that the retroviruses have produced envelopes which mimic the type of antigens usually recognized by antigen-specific T cells.

A second problem has to do with the incredible diversity of the viral env regions. Did the diversity preexist in the host, or was it generated by the rapid evolution of these retroviruses? In our view the generation of such diversity during ontogeny is required for the appearance of a retrovirus which is antigenic in the host of origin, and from that view we predict that the ecotropic viruses which are expressed early and throughout embryogenesis (e.g., in AKR mice) will not be oncogenic in the strain of origin, but could be oncogenic in other strains of mice. A strong argument that these particular envelope regions might themselves be restricting elements for cell-to-cell interactions comes from the work of Wecker (18) and Moroni (16): antigen-stimulated T and B lymphocytes apparently activate various endogenous env genes for cell surface expression, and, at least in some cases, antibodies to these env genes disrupt efficient cellular cooperation leading to antibody responses. Thus it is possible that the endogenous env genes preexist as a multigene family involved in important cell-cell interaction in the lymphoid system and perhaps in other systems as well (7). Thus, it shall be important in the future to try to understand the genetic diversity of these endogenous envelope regions and to develop experiments in which particular endogenous envelope genes are replaced by intentionally changed genes, either by standard genetic or molecular genetic techniques. The development of mice with such genes integrated in their germ line would be especially valuable for the study of lymphomagenesis, and also for the study of lymphoid cell interactions.

WHAT IS THE CRITICAL TEST FOR THE RECEPTOR-MEDIATED LEUKEMOGENESIS HYPOTHESIS?

The critical test is obvious - for T cell lymphomas the virus receptor must be either an antigen-specific receptor or a growth factor receptor. Recently, Allison et al. have defined a murine T cell lymphoma (C6VL) which expresses a T lymphoma clone-specific molecule which is one of the best candidates for a putative T cell receptor (1). The C6VL cells produce a virus related to Rad LV. The analysis of C6VL cells and of tumor models like C6VL should be carried out to determine whether the isolated virus receptor indeed turns out to be the antigen-specific T cell (or IL-2) receptor, and whether transfection of receptor structures to normal T cell clones will endow these cells with the property of leukemic transformation in the presence of the virus from the transfection donor cell.

Acknowledgements. Supported by grant IM 56 from the American Cancer Society and USPHS grant CA 32031.

REFERENCES

(1) Allison, J.P.; McIntyre, B.W.; and Bloch, D. 1982. Tumor specific antigen of murine T lymphoma cells defined with monoclonal antibody. J. Immunol. 129: 2293.

(2) Clarke, M.; Gelman, E.; and Reitz, M. 1983. Homology of human T-cell leukemia virus envelope gene with Class I HLA gene. Nature 350: 60.

(3) Cooper, G.M., and Neiman, P.E. 1981. Two distinct candidate transforming genes by lymphoid leukosis virus-induced neoplasms. Nature 292: 857.

(4) DeCleve, A.; Travis, M.; Weissman, I.L.; Lieberman, M.; and Kaplan, H.S. 1975. Focal infection and transformation in situ of thymic cell subclasses by a thymotropic murine leukemia virus (RadLV). Cancer Res. 35: 3585.

(5) Goubin, G.; Goldman, D.S.; Luce, J.; Neiman, P.E.; and Cooper, G.M. 1983. Molecular cloning and nucleotide sequence of a transforming gene detected by transfection of chicken B-cell lymphoma DNA. Nature 302: 114.

(6) Ihle, J.W., and Lee, J.C. 1982. Possible immunological mechanisms in C-type viral leukemogenesis in mice. Curr. Top. Microbiol. Immunol. 98: 85.

(7) Lerner, R.A.; Wilson, C.B.; and del Villano, B.C. 1976. Endogenous oncornaviral gene expression in adult and fetal mice. J. Exp. Med. 143: 151.

(8) McGrath, M.S.; Jerabek, L.; Pillemer, E.; Steinberg, R.A.; and Weissman, I.L. 1981. Receptor mediated murine leukemogenesis: Monoclonal antibody induced lymphoma cell growth arrest. Wilsede Meeting on Modern Trends in Human Leukemia IV, Haematology and Blood Transfusion, ed. R. Neth, vol. 26. Berlin, Heidelberg, New York: Springer-Verlag.

(9) McGrath, M.S.; Lieberman, M.; Decleve, A.; Kaplan, H.S.; and Weissman, I.L. 1978. The specificity of cell surface virus receptors on RadLV and radiation-induced thymic lymphomas. J. Virol. 28: 819.

(10) McGrath, M.S.; Pillemer, E.; Kooistra, D.; Jacobs, S.; Jerabek, L.; and Weissman, I.L. 1980. T lymphoma retroviral receptors and control of T-lymphoma cell proliferation. Cold Spring Harb. Symp. Quant. Biol. 44: 1297.

(11) McGrath, M.S.; Pillemer, E.; Kooistra, D.; and Weissman, I.L. 1980. The role of MuLV receptors on T lymphoma cells in lymphoma cell proliferation. Contemp. Top. Immunobiol. 11: 156.

(12) McGrath, M.S.; Pillemer, E.; and Weissman, I.L. 1980. Murine leukemogenesis: Monoclonal antibodies to T cell determinants which arrest T lymphoma cell proliferation. Nature 285: 259.

(13) McGrath, M.S., and Weissman, I.L. 1978. A receptor mediated model of viral leukemogenesis: hypothesis and experiments. In Cold Spring Harbor Symposium: Normal and Neoplastic Hematopoietic Cell Differentiation, Nr. 577. New York: Cold Spring Harbor Laboratory.

(14) McGrath, M.S., and Weissman, I.L. 1979. AKR leukemogenesis: Identification and biological significance of thymic lymphoma receptors for AKR retroviruses. Cell 17: 65.

(15) McGrath, M.; Weissman, I.L.; Baird, S.; Raschke, W.; Decleve, A.; Lieberman, M.; and Kaplan, H.S. 1978. Each T-cell lymphoma induced by a particular murine leukemia virus bears surface receptors specific for that virus. In The Molecular Basis of Cell-Cell Interaction. The National Foundation - March of Dimes Birth Defects: Original Article Series, eds. R. Lerner and D. Bergsma, vol. 14, p. 349. New York: Alan R. Liss.

(16) Moroni, C.; Stoye, J.P.; DeLamarter, J.F.; Erb, P.; Jay, F.; Jongstra, J.; Martin, D.; and Schuman, C. 1980. Normal B cell activation involves endogenous retroviral antigen expression: Implications for leukemogenesis. Cold Spring Harb. Symp. Quant. Biol. 44: 1205.

(17) Neel, B.G.; Hayward, W.S.; Robinson, H.L.; Fang, J.; and Astrin, S. 1981. Avian leukosis virus-induced tumors have common proviral integration sites and synthesize discrete new RNA's: oncogenesis by promoter insertion. Cell 23: 232.

(18) Wecker, E., and Horak, I. 1982. Expression of endogenous viral genes in mouse lym. Curr. Top. Microbiol. Immunol. 98: 27.

(19) Weiss, R. 1982. The myc oncogene in man and birds. Nature 299: 9.

(20) Weissman, I.L., and Baird, S. 1977. Oncornavirus leukemogenesis

as a model for selective neoplastic transformation. In Neoplastic Transformation: Mechanisms and Consequences, ed. H. Koprowski, vol. 7, p. 135. Berlin: Dahlem Konferenzen.

(21) Weissman, I.L., and McGrath, M.S. 1982. Retrovirus lymphomagenesis: Relationship of normal immune receptors to malignant cell proliferation. In Current Topics in Microbiology and Immunology, ed. W. Henle, pp. 103-112. Berlin, Heidelberg, New York: Springer-Verlag.

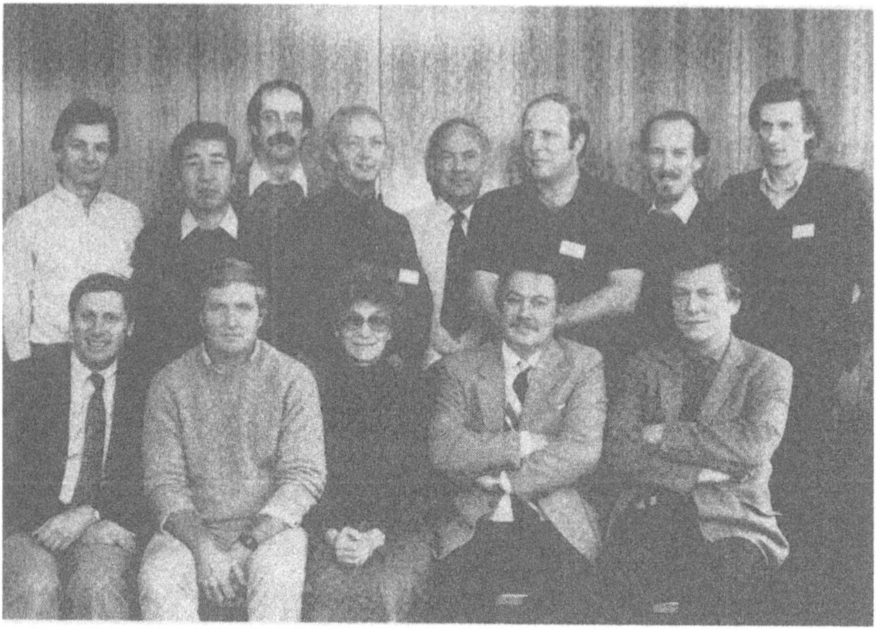

Standing, left to right:
Peter Meyer, Tadamitsu Kishimoto, Arnold Ganser, Frank Lilly, Don Metcalf, Peter Krammer, Norman Iscove, Marek Karpowicz.

Seated, left to right:
Bill Paul, Gary Fathman, Eva Klein, Malcolm Moore, Fritz Melchers.

Leukemia, ed. I.L. Weissman, pp. 251-260. Dahlem Konferenzen 1985. Berlin, Heidelberg, New York, Tokyo: Springer-Verlag.

Regulation of Hematopoietic Differentiation and Its Disruption
Group Report

C.G. Fathman, Rapporteur

A. Ganser	F. Lilly
N.N. Iscove	F. Melchers
M. Karpowicz	D. Metcalf
T. Kishimoto	P.A. Meyer
E. Klein	M.A.S. Moore
P.H. Krammer	W.E. Paul

INTRODUCTION

The purpose of this workshop was to examine the regulation of hematopoietic differentiation in an attempt to define possible sites of leukemogenesis. In particular, we were to examine the elements of normal differentiation and growth control within cells of the hematopoietic system. Emphasis was placed on those elements of growth regulation which might be particularly likely to play a role in the process by which these cells become leukemic. An additional item of discussion was possible therapeutic strategies based on these differentiation pathways. In order to address this theme, the group considered in detail several basic questions concerning normal pathways of hematopoietic growth and differentiation.

WHAT ARE THE NORMAL PATHWAYS OF HEMATOPOIETIC DIFFERENTIATION?

This question was examined in detail. The pathways were reviewed with special emphasis on regulatory factors involved in growth and differentiation. The possibility of aberrations in normal mechanisms controlling growth and differentiation, which might lead to leukemia, was discussed.

Cells of the hematopoietic series can be broadly categorized according to progressive states of differentiation. The earliest murine hematopoietic cell that can be studied experimentally is the "repopulating cell." This cell is characterized functionally as a cell derived from adult bone marrow that at the single cell (clonal) level can reconstitute a lethally irradiated recipient. There exists some controversy regarding the differentiation capabilities of this cell, but the evidence suggests that it can reconstitute both hematopoietic and lymphoid systems in the recipient mouse. This cell is thought to be responsible for the continuous maintenance of hemopoietic and lymphoid cell production. Unfortunately, there do not currently exist known markers for this cell type, it cannot be grown in culture in its nondifferentiated forms, and it can only be defined functionally.

The second cell in the hemopoietic lineage is the "pluripotential cell (CFU-S)." This cell is defined functionally as a cell capable of generating clones in spleen or in culture containing cells of all hemopoietic lineages. Pluripotential cell clones of mouse origin have not yet been shown to contain detectable cells of the lymphoid lineages. Pluripotential cell colonies of human origin grown in vitro have been suggested to contain lymphoid cells, but strong evidence of clonal derivation is lacking.

The third stage in this lineage is represented by "committed progenitor cells" which can be of one or more than one lineage specificity. One example would be the granulocyte/macrophage colony-forming cell in vitro. Finally, prior to end stage differentiation, there exist unipotential (committed progenitor) cells restricted to a single lineage.

Cells at particular stages have common characteristics. Most of the earliest (less mature) cells are noncycling under conditions of normal hemopoiesis. The signals for induction of proliferation and/or differentiation of the "repopulating" cells are not known. It has been shown that the multilineage growth factor (IL-3) is capable of induction of proliferation in the pluripotential cell. There is evidence that these early cells are the targets of events leading to chronic myelogenous leukemia (CML). A major problem in understanding normal function of the repopulating cells is their paucity in the bone marrow ($1/10^4$ cells), and the lack of known markers of differentiation and/or factors which allow their propagation with stable phenotypes. Responsiveness to known growth/ differentiation factors begins with the pluripotential cells and progresses through to end stage granulocytes and macrophages. These cells are dependent upon growth factors for proliferation. Removal of these factors leads to cell death in vitro. Known hemopoietic growth-promoting factors are discussed by Iscove (this volume).

One major obstacle to the characterization of these myeloid precursor cells is their limited growth potential. Although the "repopulating cell" may be immortal, there appear to be a finite number of divisions allowed the more differentiated progeny. Pluripotential cells can give rise to as many as 10^6 progeny in vitro, and the number of possible end stage cells that can arise from each successive stage along the differentiated myeloid stem cell lineage falls rapidly with unipotent precursor cells having only several thousand progeny in vitro.

What is known about the growth-promoting and differentiating factors of myeloid lineage cells? The factors which drive the growth of the early members of this lineage and which also seem to operate as differentiation factors on the more terminal members of the lineage, that is, the so-called colony stimulating factors (CSF) are factors which have been studied in very considerable detail. A substantial number of these factors have been purified to homogeneity.

CURRENT STATUS OF HEMOPOIETIC FACTOR CHARACTERIZATION

Sequencing Data

Partial sequencing data exist for human urine erythropoietin and murine GM-CSF, M-CSF, and Multi-CSF. For the small number of residues available (5-25), there is no significant homology between any of the above nor with T cell growth factor (TCGF; IL-2) (human) or any proteins on computer file. cDNAs for human IL-2 and erythropoietin, mouse IL-3 and GM-CSF have been cloned and no sequence homology has been noted between any, a situation of some interest in view of the many common functions shared by IL-3 and GM-CSF.

TABLE 1 - Factors purified to homogeneity.

Factor name	Apparent MW (glycosylated form)
Human Urine Erythropoietin	39,000
Human Urine CSF	45,000
Mouse M-CSF (CSF-1)	70,000
GM-CSF	23,000
G-CSF	25,000
Multi-CSF (IL-3) (1)	23,000
IL-2 (4)	15,000

Antibodies/Monoclonal Ab's

Both antibodies and monoclonal antibodies exist for human urine erythropoietin. Antibodies exist for murine M-CSF (CSF-1) that show limited cross-reactivities with certain human and murine M-CSF's and possibly some GM-CSF's, but no other known hormones or growth factors. Obviously, this now opens the possibility of detailed studies of the physiology of action of these agents, the identification of the membrane receptors for them, and, hopefully, the pathway of intercellular activation. It should be said that the understanding of the receptors for the colony-stimulating factors themselves is substantially less well advanced than is the status of the factors themselves, but the receptor for at least one of these factors, M-CSF, has been recently purified, and initial studies demonstrate that along with other growth factor receptors it shares the property of becoming rapidly phosphorylated after interaction with the ligand (J.R. Stanley, personal communication).

One interesting aspect of the hemopoietic cells and the factors required for their growth and differentiation concerns the multiple sites of action and multiple effects of purified growth factors. Not only do factors allow growth of hemopoietic cells in various states of differentiation, but the same factors can act on the end stage cells to drive effector function. Thus, although most of the factors have lineage specificity, they can act on cells at several levels of differentiation and result in different effects.

These factors are not only involved in normal growth and differentiation but are required for growth in vitro of primary myeloid leukemia cells. There is evidence that known hemopoietic growth factors act as assessed from their action in vivo. Not only can known hemopoeitic growth factors be detected in vivo, but they are in sufficient concentration to control growth of hematopoietic precursor cells in vitro. The majority of studies on known hemopoietic growth factors have been on those produced by activated lymphocytes or by non-hemopoietic tissues. The control of hematopoiesis in the bone marrow also could be under regulation of as yet unidentified factors. This is suggested by the scarcity of T cells in the bone marrow and the ability of Dexter cultures to support long-term growth of bone marrow cells with little growth-promoting activity detectable in the supernatants of such cultures.

The second major element of our consideration turned to the lymphoid cell population. In contrast to the hematopoietic system where there is a very great richness of understanding of the early precursors, our understanding of the earliest cells in the lymphoid system is substantially more primitive. It is very difficult to assay the noncommitted precursors in the lymphoid system. There is even some doubt that the so-called repopulating stem cell is, in fact, the precursor of the lymphoid system, although the majority of reports would favor that it is. Following this earliest cell, there is no well-defined maturational state prior to detection of early lymphoid cells defined as pre-B cells in the bone marrow or thymic cortical immature T cells. Although not studied, it is possible that early lymphocyte precursors may be under similar growth controls as are the early hematopoietic cells. By contrast, our understanding of the growth properties of the more mature members of the population are reasonably well advanced. This is particularly true for the cells of the T lymphocyte lineage in which it is now routinely possible to obtain members of at least several of the subsets of this lineage in long-term culture in a variety of functional forms. The best known growth-promoting factor in T lymphocyte lineage, interleukin II (IL-2 or TCGF), is perhaps the best characterized of any of the members of the hematopoietic family of growth factors. The protein has been purified to homogeneity by affinity chromatography, protein sequence has been obtained, the gene has been cloned (4), the entire sequence of the material is known, and it is being produced in substantial quantities in expression systems by several different commercial organizations. Furthermore, the receptor for interleukin II has been identified through the use of monoclonal antibodies in both human and mouse systems. In the human, the antibody is known as TAC (3); in the mouse, monoclonal antibodies identifying the receptor have been achieved both here, in Berlin, and at the NIH. This provides us with an elegant system for the analysis of at least one of the extracellular elements of the activation pathway.

Our understanding of the B lymphocyte system of cells is less well advanced than that of the T lymphocyte system. It is not yet possible routinely to grow large numbers of B cells, particularly antigen-specific B cells, in long-term culture. The factors which regulate growth of the B cell are the subject of great attention. There is one B cell growth factor which has been characterized to some extent chemically, and perhaps within the next year this material will also be brought to a stage of biochemical homogeneity. The B lymphocyte lineage is capable of very substantial alternative types of differentiation and provides us with a particularly elegant model for the study of the differentiated potential of such a cell.

An interesting feature of lymphocyte differentiation is the interposition of a resting stage (small B and T lymphocytes) prior to terminal growth and maturation to effector function. In contrast, growth in the hematopoietic lineages is continuous until terminal maturation. Only the resting end stage macrophage appears capable of reactivation to proliferation.

Small resting T cells do not display detectable growth factor receptors. The demonstration of the lack of TCGF receptors on resting T cells made use of antibodies to the IL-2 receptor and radiolabelled IL-2. Although we do not yet have the B cell growth factor (BCGF) gene cloned nor do we have anti-BCGF receptor antibodies to examine this question rigorously, experimental data obtained using activated B cells to absorb out BCGF activity suggest that resting B cells (like resting T cells) lack growth factor receptors. Resting precursor cells appear to be factor-sensitive, whereas the lymphoid cell growth factor receptors must be induced. This is accomplished by mitogen binding or by receptor cross-linking for the B cell and by mitogen presentation or antigen presentation to the T cell in the presence of class II major histocompatibility complex products (restricting elements).

We then considered the general question of growth regulation in hematopoietic and lymphoid cells and noted that there were certain "commonalities" that should not be overlooked, but also certain interesting differences. We reasoned that some of these differences stemmed from the logic of the systems. In particular, the lymphoid system has as its charge the ability to produce substantial numbers of cells and soluble products that are specific for foreign entities. It appears to do so by generating very large numbers of relatively mature cells which have already committed themselves to the particular specific product they will make, that is, T cell receptor or B cell receptor (antibody), and then apparently to store up and be able to utilize cells which are fundamentally resting. Upon contact with an appropriate activating agent, these cells then become sensitive to the growth-promoting activities of the system. In the immune system, the need for ability to store a repertoire in the form of resting cells and then selectively to activate these resting cells leads to this situation. At least two discrete sets of signals are thus required for the cell to proliferate: the first being an activation signal and the second a more traditional growth-promoting signal.

ARE GROWTH FACTORS INVOLVED IN AUTOCRINE FUNCTION IN LEUKEMIA?

The second major question addressed by our group concerned the potential autocrine function of the regulatory factors discussed above. One model of leukemogenesis would suggest that the leukemic cell makes its own growth-supporting factor and becomes independent of normal regulation. This is of particular importance in the examination of cells of the T lymphocyte lineage in which it appears that a physiologic example of potential autocrine function may exist. There is clear evidence in cloned, long-term T cell lines and very suggestive evidence from freshly explanted T cells that every T cell activated in vitro will express receptors for interleukin II. Although the precise incidence of the interleukin II-producing T cell is now known, it has been estimated to be as much as or perhaps in excess of 10% of the population. Therefore it seems inescapable that a percentage of T cells is capable of both producing a growth factor and possessing receptors through which it may respond to that factor. This is circumstantial evidence that suggests the possibility of autocrine function in leukemia. At least one example of T cell leukemia (adult HTLV) has been studied and found to be a candidate for such autocrine control (2). Most, if not all, HTLV cells express IL-2 receptors. Though not all HTLV cells can be shown to secrete IL-2, several have been shown to secrete detectable levels. If the potential for autocrine stimulation of the T cell population appears real, we may then ask, why does this cell not demonstrate unregulated growth? Indeed, why does this cell not express the properties of a transformed malignant leukemic population? First, if this analysis is correct, then the simple possession of autocrine function cannot be sufficient for expression of a malignant phenotype. Second, the physiology of the cells in the immune system provides an obvious example, an obvious reason why these cells may not be malignant, and that is that the expression of the growth factor receptor depends on prior activation of the cells. Presumably in each cell cycle an opportunity exists to break the cycle if the initial stimulus becomes exhausted. However, other regulatory mechanisms may exist, and we felt that the examination of the means by which the T cell escapes uncontrolled proliferation in view of its potential autocoid stimulation is one which should engage the efforts of many more colleagues in the future.

The second candidate cell with potential autocrine function is the mature macrophage. The macrophage has been demonstrated to secrete G-CSF under certain conditions. The possibility of autocrine control of more primitive myeloid leukemias is not simple to exclude. Some myelomonocytic leukemias (WEHI-3) are found to secrete certain CSF's which may be involved in their differentiation. Though most B cell tumors do not make BCGF, there was a suggestion that one B cell lymphoma (BCL_1) can, under certain circumstances, be shown to secrete a BCGF.

Thus, although not clearly demonstrated for any leukemia, autocrine function of growth factors remains one possible defect in a path leading to leukemia. Not only do these factors support proliferation of hematopoietic cells, they can additionally be shown to drive differentiation. The capacity of these factors to initiate differentiation commitment in the potential GM progenitor cells has been examined. Culturing such GM precursors with G-CSF or M-CSF for one-two divisions commits them irreversibly into that lineage, irrespective of the CSF used thereafter.

If growth and differentiation are controlled by extracellular signals (factors and receptors), how can we address the question of the internal pathway by which such factors/receptors deliver their signals? Clearly we do not yet understand the external pathways by which hematopoietic cells are activated. The internal signals received by the cell and the mechanism of differentiation or proliferation induction is not at all understood. If one can envision a final common pathway for induction of cellular divisions within the hematopoietic (and perhaps in other) cell lineages, is it possible to implicate oncogenes in this activation? Could c-myc encode a growth factor or a growth factor receptor? This question has added significance, when one considers the C-sis platelet-derived growth factor (PDGF) story. What do we know about c-myc that might have relevance to these questions?

Increased levels of c-myc mRNA are seen in most normal proliferating cells. Lymphocytes, following stimulation, greatly increase the expression of c-myc mRNA. Thus, it does not seem to define the "preleukemic" state. However, a rearranged and/or translocated c-myc gene is invariably associated with the majority of B cell lymphomas in man and plasmacytomas in mouse. c-myc is located on chromosome 8 in man and chromosome 15 in the mouse. It is possible that c-myc becomes an oncogene by translocations that join the coding sequences to positive control elements of other genes. Such a hypothesis seems to be borne out in the case of c-myc translocations in Burkitt's lymphoma.

The majority of Burkitt's lymphomas (~75%) have a c-myc translocation 8-14; ~18% have 8-22 translocations, and the remaining 7% 8-2 translocations. Each of these translocations is in the immunoglobulin variable region coding segments of either the heavy or the light chain. The suggestion is thus made that the hypervariable portions of the variable regions (?hyper-mutable) are in some way broken and translocated with c-myc following Epstein Barr virus (EBV) infection. Whereas the translocated c-myc gene is expressed (deregulated), the c-myc gene on the normal chromosome 8 is not.

Is c-myc a growth factor or receptor? The answer is not yet known. However, HL-60 cells, a promyelocytic leukemia line, are growth factor-dependent, despite having a rearranged c-myc. The factor dependence of HL-60 in vitro does not disprove the hypothesis, however. c-myc might function as a growth factor but require another signal or signals for proliferation.

The way in which c-myc acts to cause or be associated with leukemic transformation is not known. Simple experiments, such as using c-myc protein to attempt to induce proliferation or c-myc for transfection, are being attempted.

If we assume that leukemia is a multi-step process, is it possible to override the apparent maturational blockade? How are cells normally turned off? This question is addressed by Moore (this volume). If one assumes that no tumors have an absolute maturational arrest, is it possible to drive these tumors to terminal differentiation using any of the factors discussed above? Several experimental systems were described in which it seemed likely that terminal differentiation of myeloid leukemias might be possible. This includes several models of tumor suppression using CSF in vivo. WEHI-3 cells can be driven to terminal differentiation in vitro in the presence of G-CSF and lose their clonogenic potential. Other hematopoietic tumors, in particular certain plasmacytomas maintained in tissue culture, seemed incapable of terminal differentiation. That this may be due to a separate defect attributable to tissue culture adaptation was suggested by the inability of explants of fresh plasmacytomas to be transferred to recipients unless such recipients have been pretreated in a way that may well have activated growth factors (mineral oil ip).

In summary, leukemogenesis seems to be a multi-step process resulting in apparent maturational arrest and uninhibited proliferation of cells. It is not possible yet to understand either the number or sequence of "preleukemic" events. In order to understand more clearly the sequence of normal lymphoid and hematopoietic differentiation and to attempt to look for "preleukemic" events (such as c-myc rearrangement), we have devised the following wish list:

1. Monoclonals and/or markers that can select lineage-specific progenitor

cells and repopulating cells.

2. Cloned growth and maturation factors for production of quantities sufficient for in vivo application.

3. Isolation and characterization of factors involved in generation of primitive lymphoid cells and their markers.

4. Experiments which examine in situ replication and differentiation of thymic and bone marrow precursor cells.

5. Cloned cells of myeloid and lymphoid lineages.

6. An assay for c-myc translocations among non-transformed cells.

7. Does high c-myc mRNA indicate a preleukemic state? This can be tested in patient models.

8. Systems for transfection of normal human hematopoietic cells.

9. Knowledge of intracellular signals following growth factor receptor interactions.

REFERENCES

(1) Fung, M.C.; Hapel, A.J.; Ymer, S.; Cohen, D.R.; Johnson, R.M.; Campbell, H.D.; and Young, I.G. 1984. Molecular cloning of cDNA for murine interleukin-3. Nature 307: 233.

(2) Lando, Z.; Sarin, P.; Megson, M.; Greene, W.C.; Waldman, T.A.; Gallo, R.C.; and Broder, S. 1983. Association of human T-cell leukaemia/lymphoma virus with the Tac antigen marker for the human T-cell growth factor receptor. Nature 305: 733.

(3) Leonard, W.J.; Depper, J.M.; Uchiyama, T.; Smith, K.A.; Waldmann, T.A.; and Greene, W.C. 1982. A monoclonal antibody that appears to recognize the receptor for human T-cell growth factor: partial characterization of the receptor. Nature 300: 267.

(4) Taniguchi, T.; Matsui, H.; Fujita, T.; Takaoka, C.; Kashima, N.; Yoshimoto, R.; and Hamuro, J. 1983. Structure and expression of a cloned cDNA for human interleukin-2. Nature 302.

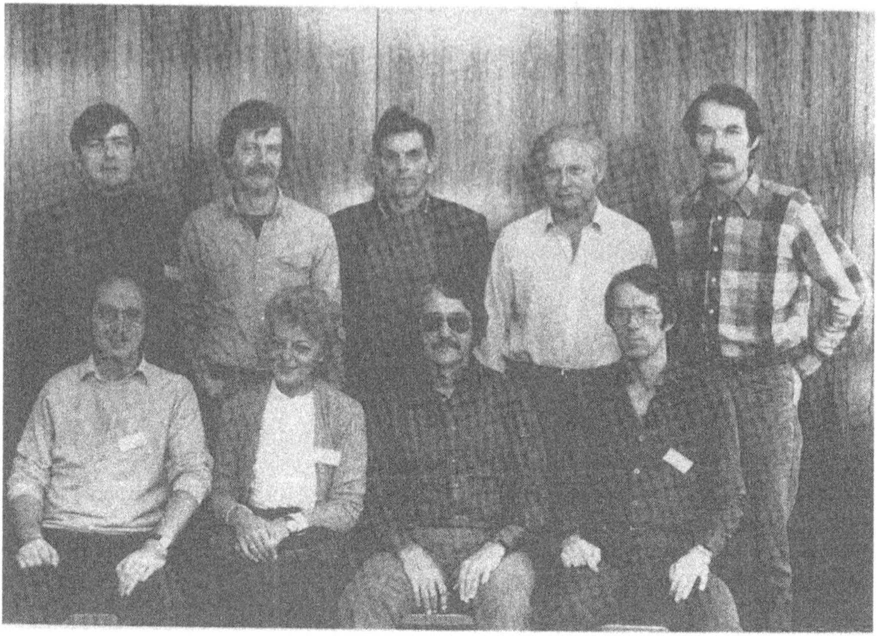

Standing, left to right:
Dick Lynch, Rudolf Jaenisch, Mike Potter, John Owen, Tom Graf.

Seated, left to right:
Mel Greaves, Antonia Harlozinska-Szmyrka, Max Cooper, David Boettiger.

Leukemia, ed. I.L. Weissman, pp. 263-272. Dahlem Konferenzen 1985. Berlin, Heidelberg, New York, Tokyo: Springer-Verlag.

Problems in Differentiation Pathways and Cellular Targets for Leukemogens
Group Report

D. Boettiger, Rapporteur
M.D. Cooper
T. Graf
M.F. Greaves
A.U. Harlozinska-Szmyrka
R. Jaenisch
R.G. Lynch
J.J.T. Owen
M. Potter

INTRODUCTION

The problem of the relationship between the normal processes of cell differentiation and leukemogenic transformation was examined by tracing the normal pathways for cell differentiation to identify potential targets for the leukemogenic transformation, as reflected in the characteristics of leukemic cells and by examination of the effects of introducing or activating specific oncogenes through infection with RNA tumor viruses.

Defining what is meant by the target cell population is complicated by the problem that the leukemogenic process is probably multi-step in most cases, and that practical usage tends to depend on the particular author's point of view. Essentially, the target cell population is the cell population at risk for a particular, potential transformating event. The final production of the leukemic phenotype may depend not only on the accumulation of potential transforming events, but also on the expression of particular normal cell programs. This is particularly apparent in the definition of the actual target cells for RNA tumor viruses carrying particular oncogenes. In a multi-step process, it is at the last step where the altered phenotype becomes recognizable. Where footprints of the successive processes such as oncogene activation or chromosomal rearrangements are left, it is possible to attempt a definition of the target cells for the potential preleukemic transformation. But in most cases, one is left making inferences as to the nature of the target cell population from the phenotype of the transformed or leukemic cell and relying on certain assumptions which may not always hold.

DIFFERENTIATION AND TRANSFORMATION IN THE T CELL LINEAGE

Pre-thymic Stem Cells

The differentiation pathway of the T cell lineage begins with an as yet undefined population of hemopoietic stem cells resident in the bone marrow. These stem cells produce progeny which are released from the bone marrow and seed the thymic cortex. Little is known about this bone marrow-derived cell population, though it is generally agreed that these cells lack T cell markers. It is not known whether commitment to the T cell lineage occurs in the bone marrow or only after arrival in the thymic cortex. Obviously, more information on the identification and characterization of this cell population is important for the understanding of the early events in T cell differentiation.

The seeding of the thymus with bone marrow-derived progenitors appears to be a slow and perhaps intermittent process. Most of the differentiation demand appears to be supplied by the multiplication of the pre-T stem cells resident in the thymic cortex. Clonal assays for cells at early levels in the T cell lineage would provide a more satisfactory analysis of T cell differentiation. The use of congenic mice which differ in specific T cell markers may provide such a system to analyze seeding and clonal expansion of the stem cells in the thymus: however, at present a demonstration of clonality for this assay is notably absent.

These pre-thymic stem cells do not appear to be targets which result in overt expansion and production of a recognizable T lineage leukemia. However, evidence from the chronic myelogenous leukemia (CML) model, discussed below, and from transplantation of bone marrow cells from irradiated mice suggests that some of the early or "preleukemic" events may occur in this cell population.

Pre-T Stem Cells Within the Thymus

Within a few hours of their arrival in the thymus these bone marrow-derived stem cells express Thy 1 antigen (for a more complete description of T cell markers in development, see Owen, this volume). This population localizes in the outer thymic cortex. These cells retain the stem cell qualities of extensive self-renewal capacity as demonstrated by serial transplantation in T cell-cleared thymuses in organ culture and by the ability to produce differentiated T cell progeny. No specific growth or differentiation factors which drive these processes in the stem cell population have been defined. It is generally thought that interactions with stromal epithelial cells may be important. In this regard the situation is similar to that for the hemopoietic stem cells in the bone marrow.

The dominant cell type in T cell acute lymphocytic leukemia (T-ALL) appears to have a pattern of cell surface markers essentially the same as these pre-T or T stem cells. This type of leukemia constitutes the major T lineage malignancy in children, suggesting that this is the major T cell compartment at risk, and hence provides the major target early in life (see Greaves, this volume).

T Cell Maturation in the Thymic Microenvironment

The presence of the thymic environment appears to be essential for the survival as well as the growth and differentiation of the pre-T cells, which may be serially passaged and proliferate in T cell-cleared thymuses but die rapidly when removed from this microenvironment. At least four cell types comprise the thymic stroma, and markers are available to distinguish them (see Owen, this volume). The functional nature and contribution of these cell populations to normal T cell maturation and their possible role in leukemogenic transformation remain to be determined. During differentiation, the T cells progress from the outer cortex to the cortical-medullary boundary, and in the process there is considerable cell loss. The differentiation process involves both the generation of T cell repertoire or diversity and the development of functional T subclasses. The generation of T cell repertoire or isotypes is associated with the diversity of the T cell receptor. While proof of actual identity is still lacking, the recent isolation of c-DNA clones which recognize genes which are rearranged in T cells and the production of antibodies which appear to identify an isotype determinant promise that progress in this area will be rapid. The overall strategy of the T cell diversification appears to parallel closely the generation of antibody diversity by B cells.

Since T cell neoplasms appear to require the presence of a functional thymus at least for some stages of their development, some of these thymus-dependent growth and differentiation processes may be critical in the development of these leukemias. Exposure of the thymus to either radiation, a leukemogenic virus, or a chemical carcinogen typically results in a degeneration-regeneration cycle of thymic cells. This provides circumstantial evidence that this stress and the transient alteration of the thymic microenvironment may play critical roles in the leukemogenic transformation.

Near the end phase of maturation in the thymus, the maturing T cells express a homing antigen which targets some of the mature T cells to Peyers patches. It is interesting to note that murine T cell lymphomas lacking this antigen remain at the site of innoculation, whereas those expressing it are dispersed.

The primary phenotype of the adult T cell malignancies appears to be of a mature T cell type, suggesting that the target population at risk in the adult is on average more mature than that available in children (see Greaves, this volume). The kind of postulated targets are the mature, immunocompetent T and B lymphoid compartments. Although these adult leukemias/lymphomas have mature cell phenotypes and may be normal with respect to B cell Ig expression, it cannot be excluded that the expansion of these lymphoid clones was preceded by early "predisposing events" in the lymphoid or pluripotent precursors. It would be very interesting to learn if the mature T cell lymphomas could be induced in mice deprived of T cell precursors or thymus (thymectomized), X-irradiated, and repopulated with syngeneic mature T cells.

THE IDENTIFICATION OF TARGET CELLS: ARGUMENT FROM PHENOTYPE

In the human system there is a wealth of data on the phenotypes of tumor cells, but most manipulative experiments to determine the origin of these tumor cells are ruled out. In this system the nature of the target cell population is inferred based on the observed phenotype of the leukemia and certain assumptions regarding the requirements for being a target cell. These assumptions generally include the following: a) The target cell is long-lived. In a multi-step process this is necessary to allow accumulation of the several steps involved in a single cell and to explain the long latent period. However, this is not necessary if the first step leads to an increased probability of the second step, or if the first step itself confers the longevity (as may be true for Burkitt's lymphoma). b) The target cell is capable of considerable proliferation (self-renewal). This is necessary to avoid entrapment in the terminal stages of differentiation which often are accompanied by a withdrawal from the cell cycle. c) Some fidelity in the continued expression of developmental markers is retained in the tumor cell. For this purpose it is usual to use the predominant cell phenotype and ignore much of the tumor cell heterogeneity (see Lynch, this volume). This assumption is necessary to allow a correspondence between the normal and tumor phenotypic markers. There seems to be general agreement that the tumor cells retain only markers of a single lineage and that the evidence for scrambling markers from different lineages in the same tumor cell is not convincing (see discussion of this point by Greaves, this volume). The fidelity of phenotype becomes more questionable when it is used to distinguish different stages of differentiation within a lineage.

Application of this comparison of phenotypic markers of normal and leukemic cell populations in the human system has led to the hypothesis that there are three distinct target cell populations for lymphoid malignancies: a) pluripotential stem cells for chronic granulocytic leukemia (CGL), b) committed progenitors restricted to the B or T cell lineage for (pre-B) or (pre-T) acute lymphocytic leukemias (ALL), and c) mature immunocompetent B or T lymphocytes for the chronic lymphocytic leukemias (Greaves, this volume).

MULTI-STEP LEUKEMOGENESIS: LESSONS FROM HUMAN CHRONIC MYELOGENOUS LEUKEMIA (CML)

Human CML provides one of the best examples of a multi-step leukemogenic process. The evidence for the various stages comes from studies using G6PD as a marker to identify clonal cell populations (see Fialkow and Singer, this volume), use of chromosomal markers (see Rowley, this volume), immunoglobulin gene rearrangement, and phenotypic markers. The steps which can be identified are as follows:

1. The appearance of a dominant hemopoietic cell clone which includes both the hemopoietic cell lineages and the bone marrow stromal cells. This implies an abnormal stem cell usage and produces a dominant clone. Although the stromal cells originate from the same clone, they do not appear to be part of the leukemia.

2. The appearance of the Philadelphia chromosome in a more restricted stem cell of the original clone which supplies only the hemopoietic lineages. Again, this sub-clone appears to be selectively utilized to supply the hemopoietic lineages. This alteration results in an over-expansion of the myeloid lineage producing CML. The lack of phenotypic abnormalities in both the erythroid and lymphoid lineages at this stage, in spite of the fact that they carry the Philadelphia chromosome and hence are derived from the same abnormal clone as the leukemic cells, suggests that the oncogenic event(s) are lineage-restricted in their expression. A similar lineage restriction in the action of known oncogenes is discussed below.

3. The third event alters the predominant phenotype of the leukemic clone and produces the blast crisis with the appearance of immature blasts. About 2/3 of the cases are myeloblasts, 1/3 are lymphoblasts, and about 10% are mixed. In the lymphoblastic cases the heavy chain immunoglobulin genes are rearranged and monoclonal, which implies that this population was derived from a single pre-B cell clone. In addition, a case of a single patient with two sequential blast crises has been reported in which the tumor cells of the first crisis contained a rearranged light chain gene, whereas tumor cells from the second crisis contained only germ-line light chain genes (2). Thus, it appears that the third event in this progressive disease occurred in the pre-B cells (or the myeloblasts for myeloid blast crisis) since only a subset of the potentially leukemogenic clone of pre-B cells was involved. It is also possible that two events are required at this level since the two blast crises represented subpopulations of the same pre-B cell clone. Presumably, different events are involved in the myeloid and the lymphoid blast crises.

The number of measurable events, timing of events, and their sequence can vary from patient to patient, but all occur within the same clone. In CML the early steps tend to confer a selective advantage either by increased proliferation or by a bias towards proliferation as opposed to differentiation within the stem cell population of the clone. This usually precedes the apparent arrest of differentiation. Finally, it is interesting to note the cellular specificity of the Philadelphia chromosome, which suggests that this rearrangement produces a selective advantage only at the stem cell level.

MODEL SYSTEMS EMPLOYING RNA TUMOR VIRUSES

Significance of Viral Replication: Murine T Cell Leukemia

Since all the leukemia virus and virus-mediated oncogene transformation models utilize viruses, at least as a vector for the oncogene, the limitations on the process of virus replication become important determinants of the oncogenic outcome. This is an area where information is limited, particularly in terms of which stages of developmental maturity within a lineage may be susceptible, and as to whether there are differences in the in vivo situation which are not adequately represented in the in vitro systems. In the situations which require promoter insertion to activate a resident cellular oncogene, it is not only the ability of the virus to replicate in the target cell population but also the efficiency of the process, since multiple rounds of replication increase the probability of integration in the appropriate site.

Based on the data from the rat system of specific integration sites in T cell leukemias (9), the biology of the system, and on the analogy with the avian B cell leukemias (10), it seems likely that the murine T cell leukemias also utilize the promoter insertion type of mechanism. An important event in the generation of the T cell leukemia in the AKR mouse is the generation of the recombinant virus. Recent results ((6), and Haseltine, personal communication) using molecular recombinants have demonstrated that the significant substitutions in the ecotropic virus lie in the enhancer regions of the LTR (long terminal repeat of the viral genome). These substitutions give the recombinant virus a replication advantage, particularly in the thymus. Additional insight may be derived from the BALB/Mo mouse model. This mouse strain has the highly oncogenic Moloney leukemia virus integrated into the germ line, and the mice develop a T cell leukemia. Virus replication occurs in all tissues as determined by the accumulation of additional provirus copies. However, unintegrated provirus can be recovered from the thymus but not from the spleen or bone marrow. This is consistent with continuous replication selectively in the thymus. It indicates that there may be a continuous generation of susceptible cells in the thymus, possibly as a result of T cell differentiation.

Model Systems for Oncogene-driven Leukemogenesis

The avian RNA tumor virus system offers a number of useful attributes for the analysis of target cells for specific oncogenes and for examination of the effects of these specific oncogenes on the processes of cell differentiation and on the expression of the differentiated phenotype. While some of these attributes also apply to some murine viruses, none of these carry oncogenes which are specific for the hemopoietic system, and the investigations of the effects of these genes on the differentiation of defined cell types is more restricted. The advantages of the avian model systems include: a) in vitro assay systems which utilize primary hemopoietic cell cultures, b) rapid transformation is achieved using defined oncogenes, c) temperature-sensitive transformation genes are available in several of the oncogenes, and d) the relative efficiency of the transformation system is high, though typically lower than that achieved with fibroblast systems. Much of the decreased efficiency may be due to the impure nature of the target cell populations used.

Using several avian viruses, it has been possible to demonstrate a lineage specificity for transformation by the oncogenes src, erbA+B, myb, and possibly myc. In the cases of Rous sarcoma virus (src) in macrophages (5, 7), and MC29 virus (myc) in erythroblasts (see Graf, this volume),

TABLE 1 - Cell-type specificity for transformation by specific oncogenes.

	Fibroblast	Erythroid	Macrophage
RSV (src)	+	+	+
AEV (erbA+B)	+	+	-
AMV (myb)	-	-	+
MC29 (myc)	(+)	-	+

( ) may require special circumstances

it has been possible to identify the oncogene product and determine that the cells were expressing the transforming protein but were failing to respond. The basis for this specificity is probably due to absence of normal cell products with which the oncogene product must interact.

The effect of oncogenes on the expression of cell differentiation depends on the oncogene involved and the particular cell system under investigation. We can tentatively suggest four different patterns of interaction between specific oncogenes and potential hemopoietic cell targets:

1. Apparent maturation block. This pattern is typified by the interaction of erbA+B in erythroid cells. This process has been investigated using temperature-sensitive mutants of erbB (see Graf, this volume). Erythroid cells infected with the AEV ts-mutant differentiate to mature erythrocytes in 4 to 5 days at non-permissive temperature. After 1 1/2 to 2 days at non-permissive temperature, cells shifted back to permissive temperature re-express the erbB gene product, but their continued differentiation is not affected. Hence the differentiation effects are not reversible.

2. Suppression of differentiation markers. This situation is typified by the action of myb in macrophage lineage cells. In this system infection of the committed progenitors or infection of the mature macrophages produces a similar transformed cell phenotype (3-5). Some, but not all, of the markers of the mature macrophage phenotype are suppressed (5). Isolation of temperature-sensitive mutants in E26 virus have demonstrated that the expression of the transformed phenotype is reversible to mature macrophage phenotype (see Graf, this volume). This situation parallels the effects of the src gene which has been studied in more detail in connective tissue cells (1, 8).

3. Increased proliferation with little effect on the expression of differentiated cell markers. This situation is typified by the interaction of myc with macrophages. These transformed cells still express most of the normal macrophage functions but display altered growth characteristics ((5), and Graf, this volume).

4. Failure to affect morphology, growth, or expression of differentiated cell functions. This has been most thoroughly investigated for macrophages expressing the src gene (5, 7).

PROBLEMS FOR FUTURE ANALYSIS

The major problems for future development involve devising systems for a more detailed analysis of the developmental processes in normal hemopoietic lineages, particularly at the stem cell and committed progenitor levels. Areas pinpointed for development include the development of markers specific for the stem cells and committed progenitors so that they may be recognized directly, and further development of in vitro culture conditions which would permit the growth and development of all the hemopoietic lineages. This would probably have to include the stromal cell types found in bone marrow and in the thymus.

REFERENCES

(1) Adams, S.L.; Boettiger, D.; Focht, R.; Holtzer, H.; and Pacifici, M. 1982. Regulation of the synthesis of extracellular matrix components in chondroblasts transformed by a temperature sensitive mutant of Rous sarcoma virus. Cell 30: 373-384.

(2) Bakhshi, A.; Minowada, J.; Arnold, A.; Cossman, J.; Jensen, J.; Whang-Peng, J.; Waldman, T.; and Korsmeyer, S. 1983. Lymphoid blast crises of chronic myelogenous leukemia represent stages in the development of B-cell precursors. New Engl. J. Med. 309: 826-831.

(3) Boettiger, D., and Durban, E.M. 1980. Progenitor cell populations can be infected by RNA tumor viruses, but transformation is dependent on the expression of specific differentiated cell functions. Cold S. H. Symp. Quant. Biol. 44: 1249-1254.

(4) Boettiger, D., and Durban, E.M. 1984. Target cells for avian myeloblastosis virus in embryonic yolk sac and the relationship of cell differentiation to cell transformation. J. Virol. 49: 841-847.

(5) Durban, E.M., and Boettiger, D. 1981. Differential effects of transforming avian RNA tumor viruses on avian macrophages. Proc. Natl. Acad. Sci. USA 78: 3600-3604.

(6) Lenz, J., and Haseltine, W.A. 1983. Localization of the leukemogenic determinants of SL3-3, an ecotropic, XC positive murine leukemia virus of AKR mouse origin. J. Virol. 47: 317-328.

(7) Lipsett, L.; Brugghe, J.S.; and Boettiger, D. 1984. Expression of the Rous sarcoma virus src gene in avian macrophages fails to elicit a transformed cell phenotype. Mol. Cell. Biol. 4: 1420-1424.

(8) Shanley, D.J.; Cossu, G.; Boettiger, D.; Holtzer, H.; and Pacifici, M. 1983. Transformation by Rous sarcoma virus induces similar patterns of glycosaminoglycan synthesis in chick embryo skin fibroblasts and vertebral chondroblasts. J. Biol. Chem. 258: 810-816.

(9) Tsichlis, P.; Strauss, G.; and Hu, L.F. 1983. A common region for proviral DNA intregration in Moloney murine leukemia virus induced rat thymic lymphoma. Nature 302: 445-449.

(10) Weiss, R.; Teich, N.; Varmus, H.; and Coffin, J. 1982. Molecular Biology of Tumor Viruses: RNA Tumor Viruses, 2nd ed. Cold Spring Harbor: Cold Spring Harbor Laboratory.

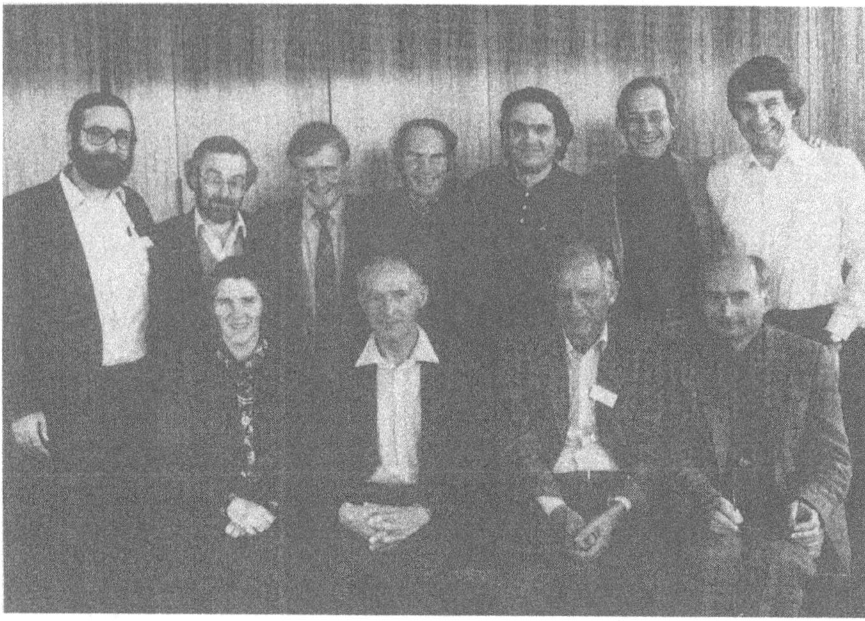

Standing, left to right:
Bill Hayward, Michael Hayman, Klaus Bister, Ian Pragnell, Carlo Croce, Bill Haseltine, Arsene Burny.

Seated, left to right:
Janet Rowley, George Klein, Rolf Neth, Peter Vogt.

(Not shown): Karin Moelling.

Leukemia, ed. I.L. Weissman, pp. 275-292. Dahlem Konferenzen 1985. Berlin, Heidelberg, New York, Tokyo: Springer-Verlag.

Genes and Viruses Able to Transform Hematopoietic Cells
Group Report

P.K. Vogt, Rapporteur
K. Bister
A.L. Burny
C.M. Croce
W.A. Haseltine
M.J. Hayman
W.S. Hayward
G. Klein
K. Moelling
R.D. Neth
I.B. Pragnell
J.D. Rowley

INTRODUCTION

Oncogenes are the common denominators of viral and of many (perhaps all) forms of nonviral leukemogenesis. Over the past few years oncogenes have been recognized as general and important determinants of carcinogenesis. An understanding of the leukemic state will have to include an understanding of oncogenes.

What are oncogenes? Oncogenes can be defined as eukaryotic genes that have been conserved in evolution and therefore presumably fulfill essential physiological functions in normal cells. All known oncogenes code for specific proteins. Oncogenes have the potential to act as dominant cancer-inducing determinants. This most outstanding characteristic of oncogenes requires quantitative or qualitative changes in gene function (Table 1).

Experimentally the carcinogenic potential of an oncogene is revealed by transfer of the gene into a susceptible normal cell where it induces oncogenic transformation. This genetic transfer can, for example, be accomplished in the course of transduction by a retrovirus or by transfection with oncogene DNA. Although oncogenes were originally defined

TABLE 1 - Definition of oncogenes.

An oncogene

(a) is a eukaryotic gene;

(b) is preserved in evolution and therefore presumably fulfills an important function in the normal cell;

(c) has the potential to become a dominant oncogenic determinant;

(d) codes for a protein.

---

as transforming genes in retroviruses, incorporation into a retrovirus vector is not an essential criterion of an oncogene. For instance, the B-lym gene has never been found in a retrovirus genome, yet it appears to qualify as an oncogene, being a eukaryotic gene that can be altered to become a dominant cell-transforming determinant. On the other hand, genes which are found to be affected by genetic rearrangement in cancer cells and may show elevated transcription are not ipso facto oncogenes. Sequences near the breakpoint in the chromosome t(11;14) translocation in human adult B cell lymphoma are actively transcribed as a result of the genetic rearrangement (C.M. Croce, personal communication). However, until it is shown that they have a dominant oncogenic effect in a normal cellular environment, they cannot be called oncogenes. A similar situation is found in mammary carcinomas induced by mouse mammary tumor virus: two loci near the integration site of the provirus show elevated transcription, but their effect in a normal cell has not yet been tested (36, 37, 39). The requirement for dominance in the action of an oncogene applies only to the appropriate cell type which permits expression of the gene. An active myc oncogene transfected from a leukemic cell into NIH3T3 fibroblasts is not expressed and therefore cannot act as an oncogenic determinant. The NIH3T3 cells would be the inappropriate environment to test for the dominant oncogenic potential of myc (C.M. Croce, personal communication).

Many oncogenes are maintenance genes. They are continuously expressed, and the transformed state of the cell can be sustained only as long as such expression persists. The src gene of Rous sarcoma virus is the classic example of such a maintenance oncogene. The erb B gene in erythroblastic leukemia also fits this pattern ((21, 50), and Hayward and Hayman, both this volume). However, continuous expression is not an absolute requirement for oncogenic action. For instance, tumors induced by Abelson murine leukemia virus can lose the abl gene without reverting to a normal phenotype (23). Presumably the initial transformation induced by Abelson virus has led to additional oncogenic changes that make the continued action of abl unnecessary and the viral genome dispensable.

LEUKEMOGENESIS INDUCED BY RETROVIRUSES CONTAINING ONCOGENES

Oncogenes become incorporated into retrovirus genomes almost always in exchange for viral replicative genes. The resulting rapidly tumorigenic agent can transform cells but has lost viral replicative information. For the production of infectious viral progeny, the same cell must be infected by helper virus with a complete set of replicative viral genes that can complement the defects in the transforming virus. Oncogenes in retroviruses are often fused with partial viral replicative sequences. A frequently encountered situation is the fusion with the 5' portion of the gag gene that then become the 5' end of the combined gag-onc gene and supplies initiator functions. Terminator functions are usually supplied by the residual viral sequences 3' to the onc insert. Signals for the packaging of viral RNA into particles are essential for the survival of the defective viral genome and are uniformly preserved in oncogene-containing retroviruses. onc genes may also be inserted into retrovirus genomes between viral genes. Their expression then requires appropriately positioned splice signals. Oncogenes in retrovirus genomes never form the terminus of the genome. They are always flanked on both sides by viral sequences. While cellular oncogenes usually consist of introns and exons, viral oncogenes have not yet been found to contain a complete intron. Therefore, the incorporation of a cellular oncogene into a retroviral genome probably includes an intermediate in which introns have been removed from cellular sequences. Varmus has proposed a mechanism by which cellular oncogenes can be acquired by a retrovirus genome (47). Although this mechanism as a whole has not been proven in experimental systems, its individual steps are well documented and have been shown to occur in retrovirus infections. As a first event, a retroviral genome without oncogene would integrate upstream from the cellular oncogene and in the same transcriptional orientation. This provirus would then suffer a deletion of its 3' end, creating a transcriptional unit which extends from the 5' promoter of the defective provirus to the terminator of the cellular oncogene. Enhanced transcription of the cellular oncogene will ensue, and the processed transcript, containing the packaging sequences of the virus, will be incorporated into viral particles. Full genome-length retroviral progeny RNA transcribed from a different provirus in the same cell could be packaged into the same particles, since retroviruses are diploid. Upon reverse transcription in the next cycle of infection, recombination between cellular oncogene sequences and the viral genome would take place, leading to the acquisition of the oncogene by the virus and probably resulting in the loss of viral-replicating sequences. Two recombinational events are required for this acquisition, one of these is illegitimate, involving nonhomologous sequences.

How many oncogenes are there? The widely held opinion that there are only a few (less than thirty) is based on two observations (49): first, the same oncogene has been isolated independently in different viruses. For instance, myc is found in MC29 virus (isolated in Bulgaria), in CMII (found in Germany), in OK10 (from Finland), and in MH2 (discovered in Great Britain). It is regarded as unlikely that a very large pool of different oncogenes would give rise to such multiple isolations. Second, many different oncogenes, for instance, all those with protein kinase activity and erb and mos show clear homologies, suggesting that they are derived from the same ancestral sequences (46, 52). It is, however, possible that these arguments lead to an underestimation of the total number of oncogenes. New oncogenes are still being described, and viruses may have a built-in bias for preferentially picking up certain oncogenes. Many more oncogenes may be revealed in tests that are independent of transduction by retroviruses.

As oncogenes are often fused into viral replicative genes, so are their products: they are proteins that contain viral and oncogene sequences on the same polypeptide chain ((4), and Hayman, this volume). The viral sequences provide a convenient antigenic marker that allows relatively easy detection of such oncogene products with appropriate antiviral antibody. Oncogene products without viral sequences are much more difficult to detect, because they are either unmodified or modified forms of cellular proteins and therefore are generally poorly antigenic. Besides providing an antigenic marker, the viral sequences may have an essential function in the leukemogenic effect of some fusion proteins, as has been recently shown with a gag-abl protein of Abelson murine leukemia virus (40). However, the fps oncogene, usually also expressed as a gag-linked protein, can induce transformation in vitro and tumors in vivo in the absence of the gag moiety (16).

A broad functional classification of oncogene products can be made by considering their localization in the cell: they are found at the cell surface, in the cytoplasm, and in the nucleus. An example of a cell surface onc protein is the product of erb B gene, important in avian erythroblastic leukemia. Homology of the erb B gene with onc genes coding for tyrosine-specific protein kinase raise the possibility that erb B may code for a molecule related to growth factor receptors and could provide a clue for a specific function (Hayman, this volume). Indeed, a striking homology between the erb B product and the EGF receptor has been found very recently (14). The abl and mil proteins show cytoplasmic localization in the transformed cell. The abl protein has tyrosine-specific protein kinase activity that, judged from mutant work, is important in leukemic transformation. The mil protein binds to DNA or RNA in vitro, a possible indicator of a regulatory function (5). Interestingly, it is also related by sequence to the kinase family although, like the erb B protein, it lacks kinase activity (Bister, private communication). The myc protein is localized in the nucleus and binds to double-stranded DNA in vitro. It is not known whether this binding is sequence-specific (12). Expression of this protein results in the transcriptional activation of the large block of cellular genes. More recent work suggests that the myc protein can at least partially substitute for the function of the E1A gene product of adenovirus and activate late gene expression of adenovirus as well as expression of a cellular heat shock protein (30, 42). There are, however, also some data which suggest the opposite: in vitro transcription can be turned off by myc protein. Whether this is a result of the binding to DNA is not known (K. Moelling, personal communication). In general, much less is known about the functions of onc gene products than about the structure of onc genes. And yet knowledge of these functions in the normal cell and of their possible modification in the leukemic cell is essential to an understanding of the transformed cellular phenotype. As the techniques for identifying and isolating onc gene products develop further, progress in the search for the essential transforming function of onc gene products will also be made.

Onc genes show a certain, albeit imperfect, tissue tropism. For instance, the erb B oncogene-containing viruses induce erythroblastic leukemia in the chicken. Myb-containing viruses cause myeloblastosis. The spectrum of tumors associated with the viral myc oncogene is much broader, including myelocytic elements as well as several different carcinomas. The abl oncogene transforms various types of lymphocytes. The basis for this tissue tropism is not understood. An interesting suggestion made by Graf and Beug is that onc gene products are stage-specific differentiation proteins that prevent further progression of the cell along a predetermined differentiation pathway ((20), and Graf, this volume).

LEUKEMOGENESIS INDUCED BY RETROVIRUSES WITHOUT ONCOGENES

Retroviruses without oncogenes can be leukemogenic, but instead of a latent period of days or weeks they require months to induce overt disease. The best studied example of this type of viral tumor is lymphoid leukosis in fowl. The tumors are B cell lymphomas, originating in the bursa of Fabricius, and are clonal with respect to viral integration site. In the vast majority of the tumors, a provirus is integrated upstream from the cellular myc oncogene in the same transcriptional orientation ((24, 35), and Hayward, this volume). This virus is usually defective and has lost the 5' portion of the genome. It appears that this defect activates the promoter in the 3' LTR of the provirus. The tumor cells show elevated levels of a cellular myc transcript that initiates in the defective provirus. Such promoter insertion is not the universal mechanism for activation of cellular onc genes. In a minority of the chicken lymphomas (and a majority of the mouse mammary carcinomas and of Moloney leukemia virus-induced lymphomas) the activation of the cellular onc sequences or of presumptive onc sequences appears to be effected through enhancer elements in the provirus. The provirus may then be integrated up- or downstream from the cellular onc locus. It does not need to be positioned in the immediate vicinity of the cellular onc gene, and it can be inserted in either transcriptional orientation (38). In feline leukemia, proviral elements have been found upstream of the cellular myc oncogene, although this observation is less common than that of transduction of myc by feline leukemia virus (J. Neil, personal communication). Although the activation of cellular myc in avian lymphoid leukosis appears to be a necessary step in leukemogenesis, it seems not to be sufficient. In transfection experiments with tumor DNA using NIH3T3 cells, the activated myc gene does not induce transformation, possibly because it is not expressed at an elevated level in NIH3T3 cells. There is a different gene, B-lym, that registers as dominant oncogenic marker in such experiments (9, 10). B-lym is not linked to the cellular myc gene. It appears that the activation of cellular myc leads directly or indirectly to a change of B-lym that makes it transforming. B-lym from normal cells does not transform.

Retroviruses without oncogenes are able to replicate in many tissues of the host, yet they may induce tumors only in certain target organs. Host factors play an important role in determining the kind of leukemia that is induced. For instance, the avian Rous-associated virus type 1 (RAV-1) induces B cell lymphomas in chickens of the SPAFAS genetic background, but in chickens of line 15I this virus causes an erythroblastic leukemia by activating the cellular erb B oncogene (17, 41). Evidence for viral factors determining tissue tropism also exists. The leukemogenicity of AKR murine leukemia virus and of Friend helper virus is strongly affected by the long terminal repeat (LTR) (7, 11). In the highly leukemogenic AKR viruses the LTR contains a thymotropic enhancer element that alone can convey leukemogenic potential to an otherwise congenic but non-leukemogenic viral variant. Recombination in the env region between non-leukemogenic murine retroviruses and endogenous viral sequences has been postulated to play an important role in leukemogenesis. However, it appears that such recombinants can replicate more efficiently, a property that may enhance leukemogenesis. The env recombinations are neither necessary nor sufficient for viral induction of murine leukemia (31).

Retroviruses without oncogenes may, however, not rely exclusively on the activation of cellular onc sequences in leukemogenesis. There is good evidence for viral gene products as active replicative signals. The Friend spleen focus-forming virus codes for a transmembrane glycoprotein that is generated from viral replicative genes by fusion of the 5' portion of the gp70 gene to the 3' end of the p15E sequences. Genetic evidence demonstrates that it is this aberrant viral glycoprotein that is essential for the factor leading to the proliferation of erythroblasts characteristic of Friend virus disease (43). A similar situation may exist with ring-necked pheasant virus which has recently been shown to cause an acute polyclonal proliferative disease and does not integrate in a specific region of the genome (W.S. Hayward, personal communication).

Two further leukemogenic retroviruses without oncogenes and without specific integration sites in the host genome are bovine leukemia virus and human T cell leukemia virus (18). They are related in their internal proteins and show many similarities in their biology. They spread mainly by horizontal transmission. They often induce a polyclonal lymphocytosis before the appearance of leukemia, which is almost always monoclonal. Leukemic cells contain the provirus but as a rule do not express viral sequences. Yet infected individuals have antibody against viral structural proteins, presumably a response to virus replication during the early phases of infection. The mechanism of leukemogenesis by bovine leukemia virus and human T cell leukemia virus is entirely unknown. One speculation centers on the open reading frames found 3' to the viral env gene (called px region in human T cell leukemia virus). These could code for nonstructural transforming proteins. The sequences in this region of the viral genome are not related to cellular sequences and thus, even if they proved to have a leukemogenic function, would not be considered as oncogenes in the sense of the (admittedly arbitrary) definition presented in the introduction of this report.

CELLULAR ONCOGENES ACTIVATED IN HEMATOPOIETIC NEOPLASMS BY CHROMOSOMAL REARRANGEMENT

Improved cytogenetic methods have revealed chromosomal rearrangements in many leukemias. The first example of such a chromosomal alteration was the Philadelphia chromosome found in the great majority of all chronic myelogenous leukemias. It derives from a reciprocal translocation between chromosomes 9 and 22. A consequence of this translocation is the movement of the cellular abl gene to chromosome 22, apparently resulting in altered transcriptional activity of this oncogene (Rowley, this volume).

Several translocations have been associated with acute non-lymphocytic leukemias. For instance, in a significant proportion (25%) of the myeloblastic leukemias, a t(8;21) translocation has been seen. In practically 100% of the promyelocytic leukemias, it is a t(15;17) translocation. Inversions and deletions in chromosome 16 are characteristic of myelomonocytic leukemia (M4), and in monocytic leukemia (M5) chromosome 11 is preferentially affected (Rowley, this volume). The frequencies and consistencies of these alterations argue for their importance in the leukemogenic process. Nevertheless, they may not represent the initial leukemogenic change in the cell. Observations reported in this workshop by Fialkow indicate that monoclonal expansion of bone marrow cells may precede a chromosomal rearrangement (Fialkow, this volume).

The best studied chromosomal translocations are those seen in Burkitt's lymphoma (2). All involve immunoglobulin genes and the cellular myc oncogene. The majority of the translocations are t(8;14). Translocations t(8;22) and t(2;8) occur less frequently. All three types of translocations bring the cellular myc gene from a transcriptionally silent area of the genome into the vicinity of immunoglobulin genes which are transcriptionally active in B cells. The result is transcriptional activation of the cellular myc gene. From the molecular analysis of these translocations, the following structual rules emerge: in the t(8;14) translocation the break in chromosome 8 is proximal to the cellular myc gene, and the cellular myc gene is translocated to the 5' end of the immunoglobulin region of chromosome 14. In the t(8;22) translocation the breakpoint of the chromosome 8 is distal to the cellular myc gene. The cellular myc gene remains on chromosome 8, but the C λ sequences are translocated to this breakpoint from chromosome 22. The 5' end of the C λ gene is then oriented toward the cellular myc gene. In the t(2;8) translocations the breakpoint in chromosome 8 is again distal to the cellular myc gene, leaving this gene behind. The translocation places the C kappa gene in the vicinity of myc. Thus, in all Burkitt's lymphomas the cellular myc gene is found oriented in either direction in the vicinity of the 5' end of an immunoglobulin gene. The breakpoints are imprecise. They occur within an area of forty to fifty kilobases. In the translocation the cellular myc gene may lose its first non-translated exon. Interestingly, the translocation usually involves the chromosome that is not active in immunoglobulin transcription. Only the rearranged cellular myc gene becomes transcriptionally active. Somatic hybridization experiments show that the transcription of c-myc on the normal chromosome 8 is not enhanced. The transcriptional activation of the rearranged cellular myc gene may be dependent on the cellular environment, as illustrated by the fact that the rearranged myc gene in NIH3T3 cells becomes transcriptionally silent. Transcriptional activation of cellular myc is also seen in lymphoblastoid cell lines transformed by Epstein Barr virus (EBV). However, the mechanism of this activation seems to be different from that in Burkitt's lymphomas. It does not involve chromosomal rearrangement. While rearranged myc remains active if fused into mouse plasmacytoma cells, the activated human cellular myc locus is shut down in this cellular environment. Chromosomal rearrangement of the cellular myc locus is seen in all Burkitt's lymphomas, whether they contain Epstein Barr virus or not. Therefore, it must have an important role in leukemogenesis.

The significance attributed to the translocations of cellular myc and immunoglobulin genes in Burkitt's lymphoma is strongly augmented by the occurrence of homologous translocations in mouse plasmacytomas and probably rat immunocytomas as well (27, 33). In mouse plasmacytomas the cellular myc gene is translocated from chromosome 15 to the IgH complex (usually the S μ region) on chromosome 12 in the typical, and to the kappa-carrying chromosome 6 in the variant translocations. In addition, mouse plasmacytomas have been found in which the cellular myc gene is rearranged and activated within chromosome 15 itself, due to an interstitial deletion. The activation of the cellular myc gene common to chromosomal rearrangements in Burkitt's lymphomas and mouse plasmacytomas is probably caused by transcriptional control elements of the immunoglobulin genes that have come in the vicinity of myc. These control elements have not yet been identified.

Trisomy of chromosome 15 is the most common and often the only chromosomal anomaly in murine T cell-derived leukemias, irrespective of etiology (26). In one 15-trisomic AKR lymphoma, a 33 kb rearranged Eco R1 segment containing cellular myc was found but no germ line segment. This segment is derived from chromosome 15; it contains a mink cell focus-forming (MCF) type provirus inserted 5' to the cellular myc gene. In two other T cell leukemias, defective retroviral sequences were found upstream from cellular myc. These observations raise the possibility that activation of cellular myc may have played a role in the genesis of these tumors. Chromosome amplification may lead to an abrogation of a transacting control emanating from the normal chromosome 15, a control that, judged from somatic hybridization studies, can counteract the phenotypic expression of oncogenicity.

ACTIVATION OF CELLULAR ONCOGENES BY POINT MUTATIONS AND AMPLIFICATION

Besides retroviral transduction, promoter or enhancer insertion, and chromosomal rearrangements, there are two other mechanisms by which cellular oncogenes can be activated: point mutations and amplification. The role of point mutations in changing a normal gene into an NIH3T3-transforming gene has been well documented with the human ras genes derived from colon, lung, and bladder carcinomas (45). The mutation appears to be site-specific and induces a functional alteration of the ras protein. A significance in the genesis of the primary tumor would require that it occurs in all, or a substantial fraction, of the tumors and is absent from the normal tissues of the patient. So far, point mutations have not been definitely implicated in the activation of a cellular onc gene involved in leukemogenesis. Amplification of the cellular myc gene has been reported in certain leukemias and some lung and colon carcinomas (1, 22, 28, 44). The amplified cellular onc gene is found in homogeneously staining regions of the chromosomes and in double minute chromosomes.

HOW DO CELLULAR ONCOGENES BECOME ONCOGENIC?

Cellular oncogenes do not normally induce cancer, rather they appear to have important, possibly regulatory functions in certain normal cell types. These functions are largely unknown. Their elucidation must be regarded as an important and urgent task of current cancer research. Expression of oncogenic potential reflects an alteration in the cellular onc gene. What is this alteration? Three possibilities can be considered.

They are not mutually exclusive, nor need one expect that activation of all oncogenes will follow the same mechanism. a) Increased transcription of the cellular oncogene leading to a qualitatively unchanged onc protein. Such increased transcription may be a result of qualitative change in the regulatory sequences of the gene or of gene amplification. b) Transcription of a cellular onc gene in an inappropriate cell, a cell whose replicative program would be altered by the presence of such an onc gene product. The same product may be innocuous in another cell type. c) A mutational change in the coding sequences of the onc gene leading to a change in protein function from physiological to carcinogenic.

Model a), the dosage hypothesis, seems applicable to the transcriptional activation of cellular onc sequences by promoter or enhancer insertion, or by chromosomal rearrangement. However, data on the sequence of the activated cellular myc gene in one case of avian lymphoid leukosis show point mutations in the coding sequences (51). Whether these point mutations are significant in the expression of oncogenic potential remains to be seen. The sequence studies on rearranged cellular myc in Burkitt's lymphomas do not have this proviso. Coding sequences of rearranged myc (three out of four) are identical to the non-rearranged cellular myc, and in some instances the transcripts contain the non-translated first exon of that gene as well ((3) and C.M. Croce, personal communication). The activation of cellular myc in Burkitt's lymphomas provides thus a good example for the dosage hypothesis. b) Little is known about the consequences of cellular oncogene expression in an inappropriate cell type. Verma has followed cellular onc gene expression in various tissues through embryonal development, and there are clear tissue-specific differences in transcriptional activity (34). Tissue-specific action of a normal oncogene product may also underlie the role of myc in lymphoid leukosis and Burkitt's lymphoma. c) Mutational changes in the coding sequences of cellular onc genes frequently accompany activation and are always found if the gene becomes part of a retroviral genome ((15) and Hayward, this volume). Not all of these mutations can be silent. Many must affect the function of the onc protein. In addition to numerous point mutations, major terminal deletions are frequent, especially in the cellular oncogenes inserted into retroviruses. Almost all viral oncogenes are truncated copies of their normal cellular counterparts. It is also a common observation that a retrovirus with an onc gene is less oncogenic at the time of its isolation and becomes more virulent and pathogenic with passage. These changes almost certainly result from mutation in the onc gene in conjunction with natural or experimental selective pressure.

LEUKEMOGENESIS AS A MULTISTAGE PROCESS, CONCERTED ACTION OF SEVERAL ONCOGENES

The clinical experience in humans and the experimental data in animals indicate that the development of leukemia proceeds through several distinct stages. It is of obvious importance to identify these stages and the factors which lead to the progression of tumor development. Avian B cell lymphomas and Burkitt's lymphomas have provided evidence that sequential activation of several oncogenes may be necessary for tumor development. In both tumors the cellular myc oncogene becomes transcriptionally activated either by integration of retroviral regulatory sequences in its vicinity or through chromosomal translocation to a transcriptionally active region of the genome. This activation of cellular myc appears a necessary and possibly early step in the development of these tumors, but at least one additional genetic change has been reported. In DNA transfection with avian or Burkitt's lymphoma DNA, the active NIH3T3-transforming gene is not myc but B-lym, a gene unrelated and unlinked to myc (19). The B-lym gene from lymphomas is mutated. B-lym from normal tissues lacks NIH3T3-transforming activity. Myc appears to be an enhancer of transcription, but the finding of a mutated B-lym gene would imply that myc can perhaps effect qualitative genetic changes as well. At present it is still unclear, however, whether B-lym actively contributes toward the transformed nature of the B cells in avian or Burkitt's lymphomas and whether the gene is indeed mutated only in the lymphomas. Evidence is needed on the expression of this gene in normal B cell development and in the tumors. Since the NIH3T3 transfection assay is sensitive to only certain transforming genes, other genetic elements may also be of importance in lymphoma development, but they would presently escape detection.

Evidence for the sequential activation of cellular genes in tumor progression is also found in mouse plasmacytomas. In addition to the common t(12;15) translocation resulting in myc activation, a t(10;6) translocation is seen sometimes and appears to lead to the transcriptional activation of genes in the region of chromosome 10 that is translocated to chromosome 6 (27, 33). Another secondary change in mouse plasmacytomas that may contribute to tumor progression is the insertion of an intracisternal A particle genome in the neighborhood of the cellular mos gene (6, 8). This insertion results in the activation of cellular mos as indicated by elevated transcription and acquisition of transforming ability for NIH3T3 cells.

Recent DNA transfection experiments suggest that some oncogenes may not be able to induce complete neoplastic transformation resulting in a tumorigenic cellular phenotype. However, such a frank oncogenicity can be achieved if two oncogenes are introduced in the same cell, presumably expressing complementary functions or acting in concert. The fact that two active oncogenes may confer a growth advantage on the transformed cell is reflected in the genetic structure of three avian acute leukemia viruses, each of which contains two oncogenes: avian erythroblastosis virus (AEV)-ES4 with erb A and erb B; E26 combining ets and myb; and MH2 recently found to contain mil and myc. While ets and erb A have so far not been isolated independently as transforming oncogenes, mil is homologous to the raf gene which is a transforming determinant in a murine sarcoma virus (25). The myb, myc, and erb B genes have been identified separately in other viral isolates as the only transforming genes. In each case, however, the virus with two oncogenes induces a more advanced state of transformation than a virus with only one oncogene. For instance, erythroblasts transformed by a virus containing only erb B are still dependent on erythropoietin, while erythroblasts transformed by a virus with erb A and erb B are erythropoietin-independent (21). Avian cells transformed by a virus containing only myc lack many of the characteristics of a fully transformed cell (increased hexose uptake, plasminogen activator), while cells transformed with mil and myc are more oncogenic in vivo (32). It is likely, but not proven, that the different onc genes combined in a single virus act on different cellular targets affecting cellular regulatory mechanisms in different places. These actions may be complementary rather than additive. In addition to an interaction between viral oncogenes, interactions between cells must occur in leukemogenesis. Retroviruses have been shown to induce the enhanced production of certain cellular growth factors (29). At least one retrovirus even carries the gene for a growth factor as an onc gene (13, 48). An autocrine stimulation of the originally infected cell could ensue, but the secretion of the growth factor may affect other cells as well, and these could proliferate without being necessarily infected or carrying an activated onc gene. This possibly indirect proliferation-inducing effect of onc genes and oncogenic viruses is often overlooked in experimental systems.

REFERENCES

(1) Alitalo, K.; Schwab, M.; Lin, C.C.; Varmus, H.E.; and Bishop, J.M. 1983. Homogeneously staining chromosomal regions contain amplified copies of an abundantly expressed cellular oncogene (c-myc) in

malignant neuroendocrine cells from a human colon carcinoma. Proc. Natl. Acad. Sci. USA 80: 1707-1711.

(2) ar-Rushdi, A.; Nishikura, K.; Erikson, J.; Watt, R.; Rovera, G.; and Croce, C.M. 1983. Differential expression of the translocated and the untranslocated c-myc oncogene in Burkitt lymphoma. Science 222: 390-393.

(3) Battey, J.; Moulding, C.; Taub, R.; Murphy, W.; Stewart, T.; Potter, H.; Lenoir, G.; and Leder, P. 1983. The human c-myc oncogene: Structural consequences of translocation into the IgH locus in Burkitt lymphoma. Cell 34: 779-787.

(4) Bishop, J.M. 1983. Cellular oncogenes and retroviruses. Ann. Rev. Biochem. 52: 301-354.

(5) Bunte, T.; Greiser-Wilke, I.; and Moelling, K. 1983. The transforming protein of the MC29-related virus CMII is a nuclear DNA-binding protein whereas MH2 codes for a cytoplasmic RNA-DNA binding polyprotein. EMBO J. 2: 1087-1092.

(6) Canaani, E.; Dreazen, O.; Klar, A.; Rechavi, G.; Ram, D.; Cohen, J.B.; and Givol, D. 1983. Activation of the c-mos oncogene in a mouse plasmacytoma by insertion of an endogenous intracisternal A-particle genome. Proc. Natl. Acad. Sci. USA 80: 7118-7122.

(7) Chatis, P.A.; Holland, C.A.; Hartley, J.W.; Rowe, W.P.; and Hopkins, N. 1983. Role for the 3' end of the genome in determining disease specificity of Friend and Moloney murine leukemia viruses. Proc. Natl. Acad. Sci. USA 80: 4408-4411.

(8) Cohen, J.B.; Unger, T.; Rechavi, G.; Canaani, E.; and Givol, D. 1983. Rearrangement of the oncogene c-mos in mouse myeloma NSI and hybridomas. Nature 306: 797-798.

(9) Cooper, G.M., and Neiman, P.E. 1980. Transforming genes of neoplasms induced by avian lymphoid leukosis viruses. Nature 287: 656-659.

(10) Cooper, G.M., and Neiman, P.E. 1981. Two distinct candidate transforming genes of lymphoid leukosis virus-induced neoplasms. Nature 292: 857-858.

(11) DesGroseillers, L.; Rassart, E.; and Jolicoeur, P. 1983. Thymotropism of murine leukemia virus is conferred by its long terminal repeat. Proc. Natl. Acad. Sci. USA 80: 4203-4207.

(12) Donner, P.; Greiser-Wilke, I.; and Moelling, K. 1982. Nuclear localization and DNA binding of the transforming gene product of avian myelocytomatosis virus. Nature 296: 262-269.

(13) Doolittle, R.F.; Hunkapiller, M.W.; Hood, L.E.; Devare, S.G.; Robbins, K.C.; Aaronson, S.A.; and Antoniades, H.N. 1983. Simian sarcoma virus onc gene, v-sis, is derived from the gene (or genes) encoding a platelet-derived growth factor. Science 221: 275-277.

(14) Downward, J.; Yarden, Y.; Mayes, E.; Scrace, G.; Totty, N.; Stockwell, P.; Ullrich, A.; Schlessinger, J.; and Waterfield, M.D. 1984. Close similarity of epidermal growth factor receptor and v-erb-B oncogene protein sequences. Nature 307: 521-527.

(15) Duesberg, P.H. 1983. Retroviral transforming genes in normal cells? Nature 304: 219-226.

(16) Foster, D.A., and Hanafusa, H. 1983. A fps gene without gag gene sequences transforms cells in culture and induces tumors in chickens. J. Virol. 48: 744-751.

(17) Fung, Y.-K.T.; Lewis, W.G.; Crittenden, L.B.; and Kung, H.-J. 1983. Activation of the cellular oncogene c-erbB by LTR insertion: Molecular basis for induction of erythroblastosis by avain leukosis virus. Cell 33: 357-368.

(18) Gallo, R.C.; Essex, M.E.; and Gross, L., eds. 1984. Human T-Cell Leukemia-Lymphoma Viruses. New York: Cold Spring Harbor Laboratory.

(19) Goubin, G.; Goldman, D.S.; Luce, J.; Neiman, P.E.; and Cooper, G.M. 1983. Molecular cloning and nucleotide sequence of a tranforming gene detected by transfection of chicken B-cell lymphoma DNA. Nature 302: 114-119.

(20) Graf, T., and Beug, H. 1978. Avian leukemia viruses. Interaction with their target cells in vivo and in vitro. Biochim. Biophys. Acta 516: 269-299.

(21) Graf, T., and Beug, H. 1983. Role of the v-erbA and v-erbB oncogenes of avian erythroblastosis virus in erythroid cell transformation. Cell 34: 7-9.

(22) Groudine, M. 1982. Amplification of endogenous myc-related DNA sequences in a human myeloid leukaemia cell line. Nature 298: 679-681.

(23) Grunwald, D.J.; Dale, B.; Dudley, J.; Lamph, W.; Sugden, B.; Ozanne, B.; and Risser, R. 1982. Loss of viral gene expression and retention of tumorigenicity by Abelson lymphoma cells. J. Virol. 43: 92-103.

(24) Hayward, W.S.; Neel, B.G.; and Astrin, S.M. 1981. Activation of a cellular onc gene by promoter insertion in ALV-induced lymphoid leukosis. Nature 290: 475-480.

(25) Jansen, H.W.; Lurz, R.; Bister, K.; Bonner, T.I.; Mark, G.E.; and Rapp, U.R. 1984. Homologous cell-derived oncogenes in avian carcinoma virus MH2 and murine sarcoma virus 3611. Nature 307: 281-284.

(26) Klein, G. 1981. The role of gene dosage and genetic transpositions in carcinogenesis. Nature 294: 313-318.

(27) Klein, G. 1983. Specific chromosomal translocations and the genesis of B-cell-derived tumors in mice and men. Cell 32: 311-315.

(28) Kohl, N.E.; Kanda, N.; Schreck, R.R.; Bruns, G.; Latt, S.A.; Gilbert, F.; and Alt, F.W. 1983. Transposition and amplification of oncogene-related sequences in human neuroblastomas. Cell 35: 359-367.

(29) Koury, M.J., and Pragnell, I.B. 1982. Retroviruses induce granulocyte-macrophage colony stimulating activity in fibroblasts. Nature 299: 638-640.

(30) Land, H.; Parada, L.F.; and Weinberg, R.A. 1983. Tumorigenic conversion of primary embryo fibroblasts requires at least two co-operating oncogenes. Nature 304: 596-602.

(31) Lenz, J., and Haseltine, W.A. 1983. Localization of the leukemogenic determinants of SL3-3, and ecotropic, XC-positive murine leukemia virus of AKR mouse origin. J. Virol. 47: 317-328.

(32) Linial, M. 1982. Two retroviruses with similar transforming genes exhibit differences in transforming potential. Virology 119: 382-391.

(33) Marcu, K.B.; Harris, L.J.; Stanton, L.W.; Erikson, J.; Watt, R.; and Croce, C.M. 1983. Transcriptionally active c-myc oncogene is contained within NIARD, a DNA sequence associated with chromosome translocations in B-cell neoplasia. Proc. Natl. Acad. Sci. USA 80: 519-523.

(34) Muller, R., and Verma, I.M. 1984. Expression of cellular oncogenes.

Curr. Top. Microbiol. Immunol. 113, in press.

(35) Neel, B.G.; Hayward, W.S.; Robinson, H.L.; Fang, J.; and Astrin, S.M. 1981. Avian leukosis virus-induced tumors have common proviral integration sites and synthesize discrete new RNAs: Oncogenesis by promoter insertion. Cell 23: 323-334.

(36) Nusse, R.; van Ooyen, A.; Cox, D.; Fung, Y.K.T.; and Varmus, H. 1984. Mode of proviral activation of a putative mammary oncogene (int-1) on mouse chromosome 15. Nature 307: 131-136.

(37) Nusse, R., and Varmus, H.E. 1982. Many tumors induced by the mouse mammary tumor virus contain a provirus integrated in the same region of the host genome. Cell 31: 99-109.

(38) Payne, G.S.; Bishop, J.M.; and Varmus, H.E. 1982. Multiple arrangements of viral DNA and an activated host oncogene in bursal lymphomas. Nature 295: 209-214.

(39) Peters, G.; Brookes, S.; Smith, R.; and Dickson, C. 1983. Tumorigenesis by mouse mammary tumor virus: Evidence for a common region for provirus integration in mammary tumors. Cell 33: 369-377.

(40) Prywes, R.; Foulkes, J.G.; Rosenberg, N.; and Baltimore, D. 1983. Sequences of the A-MuLV protein needed for fibroblast and lymphoid cell transformation. Cell 34: 569-579.

(41) Purchase, H.G.; Okazaki, W.; Vogt, P.K.; Hanafusa, H.; Burmaster, B.R.; and Crittenden, L.B. 1977. Oncogenicity of avian leukosis virus of different subgroups and mutants of sarcoma viruses. Infect. Immun. 15: 423-428.

(42) Ruley, H.E. 1983. Adenovirus early region 1A enables viral and cellular transforming genes to transform primary cells in culture. Nature 304: 602-606.

(43) Ruscetti, S., and Wolff, L. 1984. Spleen focus-forming virus: Relationship of an altered envelope gene to the development of a rapid erythroleukemia. Curr. Top. Microbiol. Immunol. 113, in press.

(44) Schwab, M.; Alitalo, K.; Klempnauer, K.-H.; Varmus, H.E.; Bishop, J.M.; Gilbert, F.; Brodeur, G.; Goldstein, M.; and Trent, J. 1983. Amplified DNA with limited homology to myc cellular oncogene is shared by human neuroblastoma cell lines and a neuroblastoma tumour. Nature 305: 245-248.

(45) Tabin, C.J.; Bradley, S.M.; Bargmann, C.I.; Weinberg, R.A.; Papageorge, A.G.; Scolnick, E.M.; Dhar, R.; Lowy, D.R.; and Chang, E.H. 1982. Mechanism of activation of a human oncogene. Nature 300: 143-149.

(46) Van Beveren, C.; Galleshaw, J.A.; Jonas, V.; Berns, A.J.M.; Doolittle, R.F.; Donoghue, D.J.; and Verma, I.M. 1981. Nucleotide sequence and formation of the transforming gene of a mouse sarcoma virus. Nature 289: 258-262.

(47) Varmus, H.E. 1982. Form and function of retroviral proviruses. Science 216: 812-820.

(48) Waterfield, M.D.; Scrace, G.T.; Whittle, N.; Stroobant, P.; Johnsson, A.; Wasteson, A.; Westermark, B.; Heldin, C.-H.; Huang, J.S.; and Deuel, T.F. 1983. Platelet-derived growth factor is structurally related to the putative transforming protein $p28^{sis}$ of simian sarcoma virus. Nature 304: 35-39.

(49) Weinberg, R.A. 1982. Fewer and fewer oncogenes. Cell 30: 3-4.

(50) Weiss, R.; Teich, N.; Varmus, H.; and Coffin, J., eds. 1982. RNA Tumor Viruses. New York: Cold Spring Harbor Laboratory.

(51) Westaway, D.; Payne, G.; and Varmus, H.E. 1984. Proviral deletions and oncogene base-substitutions in insertionally mutagenized c-myc alleles may contribute to the progression of avian bursal tumors. Proc. Natl. Acad. Sci. USA 81: 843-847.

(52) Yamamoto, T.; Nishida, T.; Miyajima, N.; Kawai, S.; Ooi, T.; and Toyoshima, K. 1983. The erbB gene of avian erythroblastosis virus is a member of the src gene family. Cell 35: 71-78.

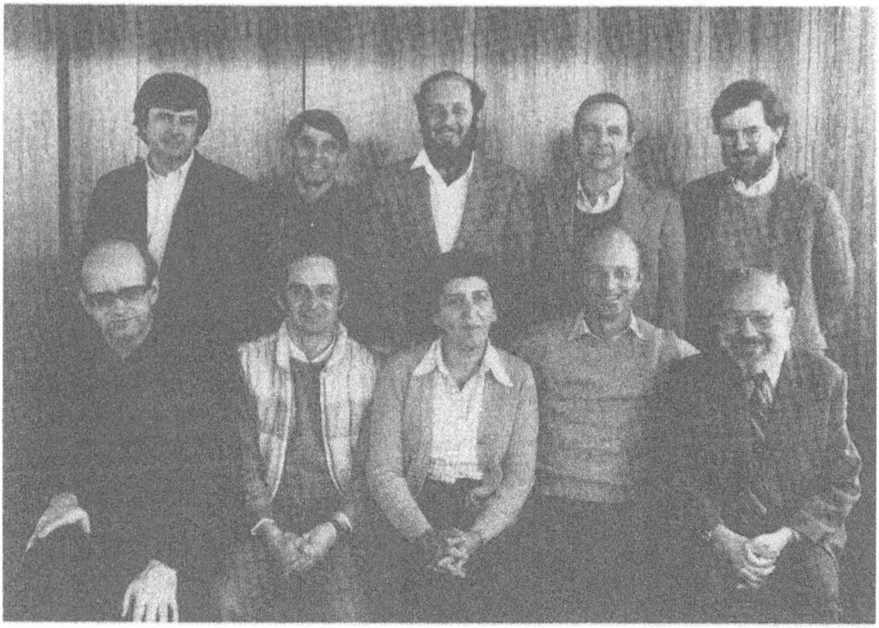

Standing, left to right:
Max Essex, Owen Witte, Irv Weissman, Hans Seidel, Jim Allison.

Seated, left to right:
Wolfram Ostertag, Jonathan Howard, Nechama Haran-Ghera, Volker Schirrmacher, Phil Fialkow.

Leukemia, ed. I.L. Weissman, pp. 295-300. Dahlem Konferenzen 1985. Berlin, Heidelberg, New York, Tokyo: Springer-Verlag.

Evolution of the Leukemic State
Group Report

O.N. Witte, Rapporteur
J.P. Allison
M. Essex
P.J. Fialkow
N. Haran-Ghera
J.C. Howard
W. Ostertag
V. Schirrmacher
H.J. Seidel
I.L. Weissman

INTRODUCTION

The study of any evolutionary process is experimentally limited by the time of the process and individual variation among members of populations, both at the whole organism and cellular levels. In leukemia, the survivors or tumors are the easiest cells to isolate and study, but the historical antecedents are the keys to understanding the mechanisms that developed or evolved this process.

In our attempt to define and measure some of the earlier steps in leukemic evolution we have utilized a wide range of natural and experimentally induced leukemia systems. Because of the variation in species of origin, inducing agents, and analytical methods there may be very common molecular mechanisms masked by simple experimental variables.

The general concept of stages in a leukemic progression finds support from many natural and experimentally induced systems. However, no precise definition of an intermediate or preleukemic cell has yet been accomplished. The correlation between an increased proliferation rate and the preleukemic state is a common but not global alteration in leukemic progression.

As most leukemia develops with the eventual outgrowth of a monoclonal cell population, secondary variations not essential for growth per se but important in pathogenesis frequently occur. A wide range of phenotypic alterations leading to altered cell distributions, invasiveness, and effects on normal hematopoietic and other cell lineages must be considered a part of the evolution. The overall concept of the preleukemic state must encompass the stochastic, sequential, and selective events we generally measure independently.

IS NORMAL HEMATOPOIESIS THE RIGHT FRAMEWORK FOR UNDERSTANDING LEUKEMOGENESIS?

The regulated balance of various hematopoietic differentiated elements arising from pluripotential stem cells in normal animals provides the framework for comparison to various leukemic systems. The native continuous proliferative property of pluripotential stem cells may set it apart from other hematopoietic elements as a preferred target for leukemic induction. The regulatory influences which control this cell balance (internal gene programs, microenvironments in close cell-cell interactions) can all be imagined as potential points of susceptibility. Such altered controls would be largely quantitative deviations exploiting resident pathways of hematopoietic cells' growth control. Qualitative changes, such as the expression of a new gene normally silent in stem cells, may be more difficult to relate to normal hematopoiesis but remain an important option for leukemia.

Although significant progress has been made in developing in vitro analogs of normal hematopoiesis (1), there are crucial milestones yet to be accomplished. Primary is the inability yet to culture cell populations significantly enriched for very early elements of any hematopoietic lineage in purity and numbers sufficient to biochemically characterize the stem cell phenotype. Clearly any reagent (monoclonal antibody, gene probe) specific for the pluripotent stem cell or other very early cells of any lineage would be extremely useful in the evaluation of these cell types following exposure to a leukemogen.

ARE PLURIPOTENT STEM CELLS THE INDUCTIVE TARGET FOR ALL LEUKEMIAS?

Although a number of experimental systems (for example, some acute transforming retroviruses) seem capable of using target cells progressed along one or another differentiated pathway, there are very few experiments that rule out the pluripotent stem cell as a preferred or alternative target for most experimental or natural leukemogens, with subsequent differentiation as part of the leukemic process. Interaction of a pure population of differentiated cells with an efficient leukemogen can provide counter-arguments to this idea.

In the spontaneous myeloid leukemias in man, X-chromosome inactivation glucose 6-phosphate dehydrogenase isozyme analysis has provided provocative data that stem cell alterations are a primary defect (Fialkow and Singer, this volume). Multiple lineages, including lymphoid, show the isozymic preference of the eventual frank leukemia clone. In chronic myelogenous leukemia (CML) and related diseases, the observation of macroscopic genetic alterations such as the Philadelphia chromosome translocation in the late clonal growth of leukemic cells (but not in all cells, probably derived from the same clone of pluripotential stem cells) suggests a multistage and active process. Data analysis for this system would be greatly aided by alternative biochemical markers for the X-chromosome, since currently only black female patients heterozygous for the two isozymic forms of G6PD are available for study.

What is striking is the extent and range of chromosomal abnormalities associated with human disease states in which clonal outgrowths of stem cells are observed. One possibility is a global alteration of the cells' genetic stability coupled with a higher proliferative rate that combines to generate first, overgrowth of cells derived from one clone, and later, secondary mutations (macroscopic or otherwise) generating malignant cells with overgrowth. This postulated genetic instability and proliferation change (perhaps one and the same) could take many mechanistic forms. The rare but independently reported occurrence of acute myeloblastic leukemia (AML) in the <u>donor</u> cells of bone marrow transplant AML recipients raises the possibility that a <u>transacting</u> mechanism could induce the instability in other cells. It is crucial to move such observations into either in vitro correlation for human disease or animal systems for further study. If a primary defect of genetic instability could be established, this would be a framework for comparing almost any model of leukemogenesis.

CAN WE IDENTIFY THE PRELEUKEMIA CELL IN THE PRELEUKEMIC STATE?

There is general agreement that most models of leukemogenesis are characterized by a latency period prior to frank disease which must be different from that of normal hematopoiesis and warrants definition. This preleukemic state, which can be subdivided into any number of experimental stages for different model systems, crucially depends on a statistical tendency for animals eventually to develop overt leukemia.

Changes in cell proliferation rates, new surface antigens, and suppression of normal cell populations including widespread immunodeficiency syndromes can all be correlated with the preleukemic state. However, the preleukemic state has not yet been defined sufficiently to pose specific experimental questions. Many of the events characteristic of a preleukemic state may not be causative for the ultimate leukemia. It is important for each defined type of leukemia to identify events which are necessary antecedents to the emergence of leukemic cells (2, 3). These events could even occur in cells which do not contain the targets for actual malignant progression. Obviously, the definition of a preleukemic cell should at least be that it is the lineal antecedent of the leukemic cell. Although it seems likely that preleukemic cells have been altered in a way which increases their leukemogenic potential, it is conceivable that they are merely the best targets for the leukemogenic event.

The common occurrence of an increased proliferation rate (for example, Epstein Barr virus (EBV) infection, bovine persistent lymphocytosis, and spleen focus-forming virus) and ability to culture in vitro cells from the preleukemic period in some systems may allow isolation of the preleukemic cell type. One major problem is how to allow such proliferation and yet experimentally "block" the subsequent changes selecting for a frank leukemic state. If possible, this would permit attempts to characterize biochemically such cell populations which could later be "unblocked" and tested for leukemia phenotype.

Unfortunately, some of the best characterized in vivo experimental systems for mapping leukemic progression (for example, avian leukosis viral bursal lymphomas) do not have in vitro culture systems for the early phases of the disease. If the wealth of molecular mechanisms (such as long terminal repeat (LTR) promoter insertion onc gene activation and secondarily activated onc genes) could be assessed in purified cell populations at these early stages and then related to subsequent leukemic phenotype in vivo, a better definition of the preleukemic cell might be forthcoming.

ARE THE NORMAL GROWTH RECEPTOR SYSTEMS OF HEMATOPOIETIC CELLS ESSENTIALLY INVOLVED IN LEUKEMIC EVOLUTIONS?

Many examples were provided to establish that alterations in growth control receptor systems are associated with leukemic cells. Every possible combination of too much, too little, altered, or inappropriate ligand or receptor molecules for both proliferative and differentiative systems was raised. In the special case of antigen-specific receptors for murine T and B cell lymphomas (Weissman et al., this volume), the added tenet of self-production of the putative ligand in an "autocrine" loop (MuLV in this case) complicates the analysis.

For this and other growth factor systems, the crucial development of molecular analysis of both the ligands and their receptors will provide the groundwork for testing their (essential) involvement in leukemogenesis. For example, experiments in which new or altered receptor molecules are transferred to test cells by DNA manipulations provide an approach for evaluating these interactions and relating them to subsequent leukemic progression. The technical barriers of DNA insertions into hematolymphoid cells are decreasing, and much progress should be possible in this area. It may be more difficult to obtain the appropriate test cells (enriched or purified subpopulations) for analysis, but improvements in in vitro culture systems (5) will complement these attempts.

ARE THE PROPERTIES OF ALTERED CELL DISTRIBUTION AND INVASIVENESS A PROGRAMMED PART OF LEUKEMIC EVOLUTION?

The normal mechanisms that require movements of hematolymphoid cells within the marrow, bloodstream, and peripheral sites were discussed as possible control points in leukemic evolution. Again, we first need to establish the nature of molecules that mediate specific cell-cell interactions (such as lymphocyte homing receptors) in order to test for their functions in leukemogenesis.

Since many of such normal, differentiated properties are lost during the growth and regrowth on passage of experimental tumors, it is difficult to assess their importance by correlation. Invasiveness and metastatic behavior may be a common property of many leukemic cell populations. This does not exclude normal homeostatic cell movements as important in the preleukemic state. For example, preleukemic cells from the bone marrow of some murine T cell lymphomas may need to migrate to the thymus to progress further in the leukemic phenotype.

There is a wide range of phenotypic changes associated with tumor systems of high metastatic capacity. Many of these changes have been mapped to surface alterations and secreted products (carbohydrate changes, neoantigens, proteases (4)). Any one of these could influence functional properties important for tissue invasion and metastasis, and multiple combinations may be the result of selection. What is not clear is if there is a single major dominant and obligate genetic change that occurs and facilitates the selection of these varied phenotypic traits that correlate with invasiveness. It will be important first to sort out these phenotypic traits and then to attempt to define a possible genetic trait that regulates the phenotype directly or through a chain of events. Gene transfer combined with in vivo selection using an organ-specific metastatic trait may be useful here.

SUMMARY

Future studies of the preleukemic state must focus on examining which molecular events are essential to the development of leukemia and whether one form of leukemia can progress through more than one preleukemic pathway.

REFERENCES

(1) Dexter, T.M.; Allen, T.D.; and Lajtha, L.G. 1979. Conditions controlling the in vitro proliferation of hemopoietic stem cells in vitro. J. Cell Physiol. 91: 335-340.

(2) Haran-Ghera, N. 1980. Pathogenesis of murine leukemia. In Viral Oncology, ed. G. Klein, pp. 161-185. New York: Raven Press.

(3) Haran-Ghera, N., and Peled, A. 1979. Induction of leukemia in mice by irradiation and radiation leukemia virus variants. Adv. Cancer Res. 30: 45-87.

(4) Schirrmacher, V. 1984. Cancer metastasis: clinical realities, experimental approaches and theoretical concepts. Adv. Cancer Res., in press.

(5) Whitlock, C.A., and Witte, O.N. 1982. Long term culture of B lymphocytes and their precursors from murine bone marrow. Proc. Natl. Acad. Sci. USA 79: 3608-3612.

List of Participants with Fields of Interest

ALLISON, J.P.
University of Texas
System Cancer Center
Science Park
Research Division
P.O. Box 389
Smithville, TX 78957
USA

Molecular immunology of the cell surface

BISTER, K.
Max-Planck-Institut für
Molekulare Genetik
Ihnestrasse 63-73
1000 Berlin (West) 33

Retroviral transforming genes and proteins and their cellular homologues

BOETTIGER, D.E.
Dept. of Microbiology
University of Pennsylvania
Philadelphia, PA 19104
USA

Tumor virus models to determine the relationship between normal hemopoietic cell differentiation and leukemogenesis

BURNY, A.L.
Dept. of Molecular Biology
University of Brussels
67, rue des Chevaux
1640 Rhoe-St.-Genèse
Belgium

Viral induction of leukemia in the bovine, ovine, and caprine species

COOPER, M.D.
224 Tumor Institute
University Station
University of Alabama
Birmingham, AL 35294
USA

Immunology - lymphocyte differentiation

CROCE, C.M.
The Wistar Institute
36th and Spruce Streets
Philadelphia, PA 19104
USA

Human and cancer genetics

ESSEX, M.
Dept. of Cancer Biology
Harvard School of Public Health
665 Huntington Avenue
Boston, MA 02115
USA

Lymphoma, leukemia, especially role of feline and human retroviruses and the immune response

FATHMAN, C.G.
Dept. of Medicine, S102A
Stanford University Medical School
Stanford, CA 94305
USA

T cell clones, immunoregulation, autoimmunity

FIALKOW, P.J.
Dept. of Medicine, RG 20
University of Washington
Seattle, WA 98195
USA

Use of cell markers to trace cell lineages and tumor development

GANSER, A.
Abt. Innere Medizin III
Universität Ulm
Steinhövelstrasse 9
7900 Ulm
Federal Republic of Germany

Hemopoietic stem cells, leukemia, clincis, differentiation

GRAF, T.
European Molecular Biology Laboratory
Meyerhofstrasse 1
6900 Heidelberg
Federal Republic of Germany

Mechanism of virus-induced leukemogenesis

GREAVES, M.F.
Leukemia Research Fund Center
Institute for Cancer Research
London SW3 6JB
England

Human leukemia cell biology and leukemia immunodiagnostics

HARAN-GHERA, N.
Dept. of Chemical Immunology
The Weizman Institute of Science
Rehovot 76100
Israel

Stages in the progression of murine T cell leukemias (using spontaneous RadLV, X-rays, or chemicals as leukemogens). Genetic control in leukemogenesis

HARLOZINSKA-SZMYRKA, A.U.
Dept. of Pathological Anatomy
Laboratory of Tumor Immunology
School of Medicine
ul. Marcinkowskiego 1
50 368 Wroclaw
Poland

Immunology of leukemias, especially differentiation markers of myeloid cells

HASELTINE, W.A.
44 Binney Street
Boston, MA 02115
USA

Molecular mechanisms of carcinogenesis

HAYMAN, M.J.
Imperial Cancer Research Fund Labs.
St. Bartholomew's Hospital
Dominion House, Bartholomew Close
London EC1A 7BE
England

Viral oncology

HAYWARD, W.S.
Sloan Kettering Institute for
Cancer Research, 406K
1275 York Avenue
New York, NY 10021
USA

Oncogenes and cancer

HOWARD, J.C.
A.R.C. Institute of Animal
Physiology
Babraham, Cambridge CB2 4AT
England

Immunogenetics

ISCOVE, N.N.
Basel Institute for Immunology
Grenzacherstr. 487
4005 Basel
Switzerland

Hematopoietic growth factors

JAENISCH, R.
Heinrich-Pette-Institut für
Experimentelle Virologie und
Immunologie an der
Universität Hamburg
Martinistrasse 52
2000 Hamburg 20
Federal Republic of Germany

Leukemia viruses

KARPOWICZ, M.
Dept. of Internal Medicine
Institute of Hematology
ul. Chocimska 5
00 957 Warsaw
Poland

Cell-mediated immunity in lymphomas and leukemias, cellular cooperation in immune response

KISHIMOTO, T.
The 3rd Dept. of Internal Medicine
Osaka University Medical School
Fukushima-ku
Osaka City 553
Japan

Immunology, especially B lymphocyte activation

KLEIN, E.
Dept. of Tumor Biology
Karolinska Institute
Box 60400
104 01 Stockholm 60
Sweden

Cell-mediated immunity, autoimmunity to tumors in man

KLEIN, G.
Dept. of Tumor Biology
Karolinska Institute
Box 60400
104 01 Stockholm 60
Sweden

Tumor immunology, virology, and cytogenetics. Special focus: the role of viral transformation vs. chromosomal translocations in the genesis of B lymphocyte tumors in mice and men

KRAMMER, P.H.
Institut für Immunologie und Genetik
Deutsches Krebsforschungszentrum
Im Neuenheimer Feld 280
6900 Heidelberg
Federal Republic of Germany

Immunobiology, activity and specificity of T lymphocytes, T cell clones, T cell-derived lymphokines, growth and differentiation of T cells, B cells and macrophages, antiviral immune responses

LILLY, F.
Dept. of Genetics
Albert Einstein College of Medicine
1300 Morris Park Avenue
Bronx, NY 10461
USA

Chemically induced lymphomagenesis in mice

LYNCH, R.G.
Dept. of Pathology (ML-144)
College of Medicine
University of Iowa
Iowa City, IA 52242
USA

The cellular and molecular mechanisms of immunoregulatory control of myeloma cell growth and differentiation

MELCHERS, F.
Basel Institute for Immunology
Grenzacherstrasse 487
4005 Basel
Switzerland

(Cellular cooperation in immune response. Differentiation of B lymphocytes from stem cells. Regulation of replication and maturation in normal and malignant B lymphocytes. T cell hybridoma with functions as helpers for B cells. Nature of mitogenic stimulation.) B lymphocyte development and growth control

METCALF, D.
The Walter and Eliza Hall Institute
Royal Melbourne Hospital P.O.
3050 Victoria
Australia

Control of myeloid leukemia cells by biological regulatory factors

MEYER, P.A.
Medizinische Poliklinik der
Universität Würzburg
Klinikstr. 8
8700 Würzburg
Federal Republic of Germany

Myelopoietic committed stem cells/ differentiation and regulation

MOELLING, K.
Max-Planck-Institut für
Molekulare Genetik
Ihnestrasse 63
1000 Berlin (West) 33

Transforming proteins of acute avian leukemia and sarcoma viruses

MOORE, M.A.S.
Memorial Sloan-Kettering
Cancer Center
1275 York Avenue
New York, NY 10021
USA

Experimental hematology/leukemia

NETH, R.D.
Abt. für Klinische Chemie der
Medizinischen Klinik
Universitäts-Krankenhaus Eppendorf
Martinistrasse 52
2000 Hamburg 20
Federal Republic of Germany

Clinical and experimental hematology

OSTERTAG, W.
Heinrich-Pette-Institut an der
Universität Hamburg
Martinistrasse 52
2000 Hamburg 20
Federal Republic of Germany

Influence of retroviruses on hematopoiesis (erythropoiesis); host range genes

OWEN, J.J.T.
Dept. of Anatomy
University of Birmingham
Vincent Drive
Birmingham B15 2TJ
England

Studies on the ontogeny of lymphocyte populations

PAUL, W.E.
Laboratory of Immunology
National Institute of Allergy
and Infectious Diseases
Building 10, Room 11N311
National Institutes of Health
Bethesda, MD 20205
USA

Immunology

POTTER, M.
National Cancer Institute
Building 8, Room B18
National Institutes of Health
Bethesda, MD 20205
USA

Plasma cell tumors in mice

PRAGNELL, I.B.
Beatson Institute for
Cancer Research
Garscube Estate
Switchback Road
Bearsden, Glasgow G61 1BD
Scotland

Hemopoietic growth factors and leukemia

ROWLEY, J.D.
Dept. of Medicine
University of Chicago
Chicago, Il 60637
USA

The identification of consistent chromosome abnormalities in the malignant cells of patients with leukemia and lymphoma and their correlation with particular biologic features of the diseases such as morphology, surface markers, and clinical course

SCHIRRMACHER, V.
Institut für Immunologie und Genetik
Deutsches Krebsforschungszentrum
Im Neuenheimer Feld 280
6900 Heidelberg
Federal Republic of Germany

Mechanism of cancer metastasis, in vitro investigation of cancer invasion; immunity and immunotherapy of cancer metastasis; aspects of cell differentiation in T and B cells and in respective leukemias

SEIDEL, H.J.
Abt. Klinische Physiologie der
Universität Ulm
Oberer Eselsberg
7900 Ulm
Federal Republic of Germany

T cell leukemogenesis in mice by chemicals, cellular aspects; the preleukemic state, T cell differentiation, NK cells. Hemopoietic stem cell regulation, friend leukemia

VOGT, P.K.
Dept. of Microbiology
University of Southern California
School of Medicine
2011 Zonal Avenue HMR 401
Los Angeles, CA 90023
USA

Virology

WEISSMAN, I.L.
Dept. of Pathology
Stanford University
School of Medicine
Stanford, CA 94305
USA

Normal and neoplastic lymphocyte maturation

WITTE, O.N.
Molecular Biology Institute
University of California
405 Hilgard Avenue
Los Angeles, CA 90024
USA

Mechanism of transformation by Abelson murine leukemia virus and in vitro differentiation of murine B cells

Subject Index

Abnormal clone, 91, 139, 182, 212, 215-219, 227, 267, 297
- karyotypes, 180, 185-190, 193, 195, 198, 199, 212, 217, 218
- marrow eosinophils, 179, 185, 189
Acid, Retinoic, 31, 42-47
Acquired Immunodeficiency Syndrome (AIDS), 2, 228
Activation, 14, 22, 23, 26, 43, 50, 69-80, 147-157, 224, 225, 229, 235-238, 246, 254-258, 263, 279, 280-286, 298
-, oncogene, 147-157, 280-286, 298
Acute leukemia viruses, avian, 131-143, 163-173, 287
- lymphoblastic leukemia, 41, 205
- - -, B cell, 179
- lymphocytic leukemia (ALL), 58, 59, 97-99, 102-104, 186, 191-198, 265, 267
- myeloblastic leukemia (AML-M2), 42, 97, 164, 167, 179, 181, 185-187, 196-198, 282, 297
- myeloid leukemia, 43, 203, 204
- non-lymphocytic leukemia (ANLL), 40-42, 58, 59, 179, 180, 185, 186, 189, 198, 206-209, 212-215, 218, 219, 282
- phase of CML, 183-185
Acute promyelocytic leukemia (APL-M3), 42, 43, 152, 154, 179, 181, 185-189, 196-198, 259, 282
Adipocytes, 55-58
Adult T cell leukemia, human, 223, 226-229, 257
AIDS, 2, 228
ALL, 58, 59, 97-99, 102-104, 186, 191-198, 265, 267
-, Ph^1 chromosome in, 194, 195
ALV, 148-151, 154, 155, 167, 244, 285, 298
AML-M2, 42, 97, 164, 167, 179, 181, 185-187, 196-198, 282, 297
AMMoL, 179, 181, 185
Anemia, aplastic, 35, 36
ANLL (see Acute non-lymphocytic leukemia)
Antibodies, 38, 47-57, 69-75, 85-90, 98, 104, 105, 118-121, 186, 210, 224, 227, 228, 240-244, 254-256, 259, 265, 278-283, 286, 287, 297
-, anti-Ig, 71-74
-, monoclonal (see Monoclonal antibodies)
Antibody, anti-idiotypic, 89, 90
Antigen recognition receptors, 114, 236, 237, 245
-/specific receptor, lymphocyte,

Antigen-specific receptor, lymphocyte (cont.), 236-239, 244-246, 299
Antigens, class I and class II MHC, 21-23, 117, 118, 122, 236
-, T cell surface, 22, 119
Anti-idiotypic antibody, 89, 90
-/Ig antibodies, 71-74
Aplastic anemia, 35, 36
APL-M3, 42, 43, 152, 154, 179, 181, 185-189, 196-198, 259, 282
Arrest, maturation, 96, 97, 100, 104, 142, 179, 259
Ataxia-telangiectasia, 186, 195
ATL, 223, 226-229, 257
Autocrine function, 166, 173, 256-260, 287, 299
Avian acute leukemia viruses, 131-143, 163-173, 287
- leukosis virus (ALV), 148-151, 154, 155, 167, 244, 285, 298

B cell acute lymphoblastic leukemia, 179
- - growth factor (BCGF), 69, 72-74, 78, 79, 237, 239, 255-257
- - neoplasms, 147-157
- cells, 21, 26, 69-80, 84, 87-90, 96, 98, 101-104, 133, 135, 139-142, 147-157, 171, 179, 184, 192-195, 199, 205, 216, 225, 226, 229, 237, 239, 244, 245, 255-258, 265-269, 276, 280-282, 286, 299
BCGF, 69, 72-74, 78, 79, 237, 239, 255-257
BFU-e, 33, 47, 48, 51, 58
Blockade, maturational, 259, 270, 298
BLV, 225, 226, 229, 230, 281
B-lym gene, 154-156, 171, 198, 238, 276, 280, 286
Bone marrow transplantation, 33-36, 48, 59, 113, 208, 264, 297
Bovine leukemia virus (BLV), 225, 226, 229, 230, 281
BPA, 6, 9
Burkitt's lymphoma, 100, 150-154, 179, 191-195, 198, 199, 258, 266, 282-286
Bursal lymphoma, 238, 244, 298
Burst Forming Units-erythroid (BFU-e), 33, 47, 48, 51, 58

Cell cycle, 33, 48, 70-73, 85-87, 120, 257, 266
- heterogeneity, tumor, 83, 84, 91, 266
-, pre-B, 88, 97-99, 101-104, 135, 184, 192, 205, 255, 267, 268
- specificity, target, 6, 135
-/surface receptors, 17, 235-246
Cells, dendritic, 22, 115-119, 122, 123
-, endothelial, 34, 52-55, 58, 171, 210, 211
-, Friend mouse erythroleukemic, 31
-, lymphoid tumor stem, 83-91
-, neoplasms of hematopoietic, 31, 163, 203, 219, 282-284
-, progenitor (see Progenitor cells)
-, stem (see Stem cells)
-, stimulatory, 21-26
-, target (see Target cells)
-, thymic epithelial, 117-123, 265
-, - nurse, 118
CFU, 33, 34, 39, 40, 45-54, 57, 58, 209, 212-215, 252
Chromosome changes, nonrandom, 151, 179-199, 218
- location of oncogenes, 196-199
- No. 12, extra, 195

Chromosomes, translocations of both No. 14, 195
Chronic lymphocytic leukemia (CLL), 87, 88, 97, 102, 105, 191 195, 198, 267
- myeloid leukemia (CML), 33, 40-42, 47, 54, 86, 87, 179, 180-186, 194-199, 203-219, 252, 257, 264, 267, 268, 282, 297
Class I and class II MHC antigens, 21-23, 117, 118, 122, 236
Classification of leukemia, 95-105
Clinical response, 59, 84, 103, 104, 215, 219
CLL, 87, 88, 97, 102, 105, 191, 195, 198, 267
Clonal deletion, 123, 124, 137, 169, 180, 181, 197, 199, 218, 277, 282, 285
Clone, abnormal, 91, 139, 182, 212, 215-219, 227, 267, 297
Clones, T cell, 25, 26, 122, 257
CML (see Chronic myeloid leukemia)
-, acute phase of, 183-185
c-myc gene, 100, 151, 152, 196, 199, 238, 258-260, 284, 285
Colony Forming Units (CFU), 33, 34, 39, 40, 45-54, 57, 58, 209, 212-215, 252
-/stimulating factors (CSF), 6-9, 12, 32, 37-40, 43-46, 134, 252, 254, 258, 259
CSF, 6-9, 12, 32, 37-40, 43-46, 134, 252, 254, 258, 259
Cycle, cell, 33, 48, 70-73, 85-87, 120, 257, 266

Deletion, clonal, 123, 124, 137, 169, 180, 181, 197, 199, 218, 277, 282, 285
Dendritic cells, 22, 115-119, 122, 123
Determinants, idiotypic, 244
Development of myeloma, 87
Diagnosis of leukemia, 103
Differentiation, 2, 3, 8, 13-15, 21-27, 31-59, 69-80, 83-85, 88-90, 95-103, 111-124, 131-143, 171, 203-209, 212, 213, 237, 251-260, 263-271, 280, 296-299
-/inducing factor, 27, 31, 32, 37-44, 59, 69-80, 88, 237, 252
- phenotypes, 120, 132-135, 138-143, 206, 269
-, regulation of hematopoietic, 31-59, 251-260
-, T cell, 111-124, 264, 269
Disorders, myeloproliferative, 54, 198, 211

Eclipse period, 91
Ecotropic viruses, 246, 269
11q23, 179, 185, 188-191
Endothelial cells, 34, 52-55, 58, 171, 210, 211
Endotoxin, 31, 32, 36-42
Enhancer, viral, 149-151, 269
Eosinophils, abnormal marrow, 179, 185, 189
Epidemiological studies, 1, 2, 105, 225
Epithelial cells, thymic, 117-123, 265
Epithelium, pharyngeal, 116
Evolution, 3, 91, 217, 218, 246, 275, 276, 295-300
Extra chromosome No. 12, 195
Extracellular growth factor, 235, 258

Factor, B cell growth, 69, 72-74, 78, 79, 237, 239, 255-257

Factor, differentiation-inducing, 27, 31, 32, 37-44, 59, 69-80, 88, 237, 252
-, extracellular growth, 235, 258
-, multilineage growth, 6, 7, 252
-, T cell growth, 228, 236, 239, 253-256
-, Tumor Necrosis, 31, 36-41
Factors, colony-stimulating, 6-9, 12, 32, 37-40, 43-46, 134, 252, 254, 258, 259
-, growth, (see Growth factors)
-, hemopoietic growth, 5-17, 254
Feline leukemia virus (FeLV), 224, 225, 228, 229, 280
Friend mouse erythroleukemic cells, 31
Function, autocrine, 166, 173, 256-260, 287, 299

Ganglioside, 119
Gene, B-lym, 154-156, 171, 198, 238, 276, 280, 286
-, c-myc, 100, 151, 152, 196, 199, 238, 258-260, 284, 285
-, myc, (see myc gene)
-, ras, 147-156, 171, 197, 198, 284
- rearrangements, immunoglobulin, 98-102, 137-139, 151, 152, 258, 267, 268, 282-284
Genetic instability, 217, 218, 297
GM-CSF, 32, 51, 252, 254, 257-259
GM-DF, 32, 36-41, 44
Growth factor, extracellular, 235, 258
- - receptor, 80, 165, 166, 172, 173, 235-240, 246, 256-260, 279, 298
- - , B cell, 69, 72-74, 78, 79, 237, 239, 255-257
- - , multilineage, 6, 7, 252
- - , T cell, 228, 236, 239, 252-256
Growth factors, 5-17, 21-26, 52, 69, 72-74, 78-80, 84, 100, 132-134, 140, 165, 166, 169, 172, 173, 228, 235-240, 246, 251-260, 279, 287, 298, 299
- - , hemopoietic, 5-17, 254

H-2 restriction, 121
Hematopoietic cells, neoplasms of, 31, 163, 203-219, 282-284
- differentiation, regulation of, 31-59, 251-260
- microenvironment, 33-36, 51-58, 203, 204, 208-211, 296
Hemopoietic growth factors, 5-17, 254
Heterogeneity, tumor cell, 83, 84, 91, 266
Histocompatibility-restricted T cells, 70, 71
Homing, 2
Hormones, thymic, 113, 114, 118, 119
HTLV, 1, 96, 97, 105, 119, 223, 226-228, 245, 257, 281, 282
Human adult T cell leukemia (ATL), 223, 226-229, 257
- T cell leukemia virus (HTLV), 1, 96, 97, 105, 119, 223, 226-228, 245, 257, 281, 282
- - - - - p 19, 119, 228
Hyperdiploidy, 181, 192-194

Ia-antigen, 33, 47-51, 55-57, 117, 118, 123
Idiotype, 86, 89
-/specific tumor immunity, 89
Idiotypic determinants, 244
Ig (see Immunoglobulin)
IL-1, 22, 23, 50, 72, 73

IL-2, 21-27, 51, 72, 73, 112, 113, 120, 228, 236, 239, 246, 252, 255-257
IL-3, 6, 7, 10, 24, 26, 252, 253
Immunity, idiotypic-specific tumor, 89
Immunoglobulin (Ig), 69, 70, 75, 77, 86-90, 96-102, 114, 121, 137-139, 151, 152, 179, 184, 195, 196, 199, 205, 207, 216-218, 236, 244, 245, 258, 266-268, 282-284
- gene rearrangements, 98-102, 137-139, 151, 152, 258, 267, 268, 282-284
- loci, 151, 152, 179, 195, 196
Immunoregulatory signals, 88, 89, 237
In vitro transformation, 268-271, 278
Insertion, promoter (proviral), 149-156, 228, 268, 269, 280, 284, 285, 298
Instability, genetic, 217, 218, 297
Interferon, 26, 31, 51, 78
Interleukin 1 (IL-1), 22, 23, 50, 72, 73
- 2 (IL-2), 21-27, 51, 72, 73, 112, 113, 120, 228, 236, 239, 246, 252, 255-257
- 2 (TCGF or IL-2), 228, 236, 239, 252, 255, 256
- 3 (IL-3), 6, 7, 10, 24, 26, 252, 253
Isoferritin, 33, 47-50
Inversion, 179, 181, 185, 189, 282

Karyotypes, abnormal, 180, 185-190, 193, 195, 198, 199, 212, 217, 218

Leukemic patient, occupation of, 190
Leukemogenesis, 2, 36, 76, 96, 100, 101, 131, 230, 235-246, 251, 257, 259, 263, 267-271, 275-287, 296-299
-, receptor-mediated, 76, 235-246
Leukemogens, 2, 31, 240, 245, 263-271, 296, 297
Leukosis virus, avian, 148-151, 154, 155, 167, 244, 285, 298
Lineage markers, T, 34, 111, 119, 121, 141, 264-267
Location of oncogenes, chromosome, 196-199
Loci, immunoglobulin, 151, 152, 179, 195, 196
Long terminal repeat (LTR), 149-152, 156, 224, 237, 269, 281, 298
Lymphoblastic leukemia, acute, 41, 205
- -, B cell acute, 179
Lymphocyte antigen-specific receptor, 236-239, 244-246, 299
Lymphocytes, 2, 9, 10, 26, 33, 48-51, 97, 101, 104, 111-124, 137, 191-195, 204-208, 215, 218, 228, 236-240, 244-246, 254, 255, 258, 279, 299
-, T (see T lymphocytes)
Lymphocytic leukemia, acute, 58, 59, 97-99, 102-104, 186, 191-198, 265, 267
- - , chronic, 87, 88, 97, 102, 105, 191, 195, 198, 267
- lymphoma, poorly differentiated, 193
Lymphoid neoplasms, 91
- tumor stem cells, 83-91
Lymphoma, 1-3, 23, 84-90, 95-101, 104, 149-155, 171, 179-199, 224, 226, 229, 238-246, 257, 258, 266, 267, 276, 280-286, 298, 299
-, Burkitt's, 100, 150-154, 179,

Lymphoma, Burkitt's (cont.), 191-195, 198, 199, 258, 266, 282-286
-, bursal, 238, 244, 298
-, poorly differentiated lymphocytic, 193
Lymphopoiesis, 113, 118

Macrophages, 6-17, 22, 31-38, 43-47, 55-58, 71, 72, 87, 133, 136-143, 169, 205, 210, 211, 252, 256, 257, 269, 270, 271
Major histocompatibility complex (MHC) restriction, 21-23, 74-77, 112, 117, 118, 121, 122, 236
Markers, T lineage, 34, 111, 119, 121, 141, 264-267
Marrow eosinophils, abnormal, 179, 185, 189
- transplantation, bone, 33-36, 48, 59, 113, 208, 264, 297
Maturation arrest, 96, 97, 100, 104, 142, 179, 259
-, T cell, 113-117, 121, 265, 266
Maturational blockade, 259, 270, 298
Metastasis, 2, 299, 300
MHC, 21-23, 74-77, 112, 117, 118, 121, 122, 236, 245, 256
- antigens, class I and class II, 21-23, 117, 118, 122, 236
- restriction, 21-23, 74-77, 112, 117, 118, 121, 122, 236
Mice, nude, 32, 112-118, 123
Microenvironment, hematopoietic, 33-36, 51-58, 203, 204, 208-211, 296
Mitogens, 235-239, 256
Monoblastic leukemia, 138, 179
Monoclonal antibodies, 48, 50, 54-57, 73, 85, 90, 98, 104, 105, 119, 121, 186, 210, 240, 243, 244, 254-256, 259, 296
MPD, 54, 198, 211
Multilineage growth factor (IL-3), 6, 7, 252
<u>myc</u> gene, 133, 136, 137, 142, 143, 147-156, 163, 164, 169-172, 179, 198, 229, 269, 270, 271, 276, 278-283, 286, 287
Myeloblastic leukemia, acute, 42, 97, 164, 167, 179, 181, 185-187, 196-198, 282, 297
Myeloid leukemia, 31, 36, 37, 41-44, 47, 59, 180, 186, 196, 199, 203-212, 215-219, 254, 257-260, 297
- -, acute, 43, 203, 204
- -, chronic (see Chronic myeloid leukemia)
Myeloma, 86-91, 97, 101, 102
-, development of, 87
Myeloproliferative disorders (MPD), 54, 198, 211

Neoplasms, B cell, 147-157
-, lymphoid, 91
- of hematopoietic cells, 31, 163, 203-219, 282-284
Neoplastic transformation, 3, 245, 287
No. 14 chromosomes, translocations of both, 195
Non-lymphocytic leukemia, acute (see Acute non-lymphocytic leukemia)
Nonrandom chromosome changes, 151, 179-199, 218
Nude mice, 32, 112-118, 123
Nurse cells, thymic, 118

Occupation of leukemic patient, 190

Oncogene activation, 147-157, 280-286, 298
Oncogenes, 2, 96, 100-102, 105, 131-133, 138, 139, 143, 147-157, 163-173, 196-199, 217, 226, 235-240, 244-246, 258, 263, 267-271, 275-287, 298
-, chromosome location of, 196-199
-, viral, 2, 138, 139, 147, 153-157, 165, 173, 268, 275-287

p19, human T cell leukemia virus, 119, 228
Period, eclipse, 91
Ph^1, 33, 47, 54, 97-103, 179-185, 194-196, 204-209, 212, 215-219, 267, 268, 282, 297
- chromosome in ALL, 194, 195
Pharyngeal epithelium, 116
Phase of CML, acute, 183-185
Phenotype of leukemia, 33, 51, 95-105, 263-268, 277, 298-300
Phenotypes, differentiation, 120, 132-135, 138-143, 206, 269
Philadelphia (Ph^1), 33, 47, 54, 97-103, 179-185, 194-196, 204-209, 212, 215-219, 267, 268, 282, 297
Plasmacytomas, 87-89, 151, 154, 258, 259, 283, 286
Poorly differentiated lymphocytic lymphoma, 193
Pre-B cell, 88, 97-99, 101-104, 135, 184, 192, 205, 255, 267, 268
Preleukemia, 35, 40-44, 119, 207, 214, 215, 218, 219, 223-230, 240, 258-260, 263, 264, 295-300
Progenitor cells, 2, 8, 33, 34, 36, 43, 47-51, 54, 57, 95, 98-102, 131-134, 184, 203, 206-208, 213, 216, 217, 252, 258-260, 264, 267, 270, 271
Prognostic significance, 103, 207
Progression of leukemia, 141, 229
-, tumor, 132, 142, 236, 239, 268, 280, 286, 299
Proliferation, 2, 3, 8, 10, 21-27, 31, 33, 47, 48, 51, 57, 59, 69-80, 83-89, 95-105, 114, 118, 131, 132, 137, 138, 143, 153, 179, 183, 203-206, 209-212, 217, 219, 235-245, 252, 256-259, 265-268, 271, 281, 287, 295-299
-, T cell, 21-27
Promoter (proviral) insertion, 149-156, 228, 268, 269, 280, 284, 285, 298
Promyelocytic leukemia, acute, 42, 43, 152, 154, 179, 181, 185-189, 196-198, 259, 282
Prostaglandin E, 31, 33, 44, 47, 48-51
Proto-oncogene, 147, 148, 151-157

<u>ras</u> gene, 147-156, 171, 197, 198, 284
Rearrangements, immunoglobulin gene, 98-102, 137-139, 151, 152, 258, 267, 268, 282-284
Receptor, growth factor (see Growth factor receptor)
-, lymphocyte antigen-specific, 236-239, 244-246, 299
-/mediated leukemogenesis, 76, 235-246
-, T cell, 124, 265
Receptors, 2, 14-17, 22, 24, 43, 44, 50, 69-80, 104, 114, 121, 124, 165, 166, 172, 173, 228, 235-246, 254-260, 265, 279, 298, 299
-, antigen recognition, 114, 236, 237, 245
-, cell-surface, 17, 235-246

Regulation of hematopoietic differentiation, 31-59, 251-260
Response, clinical, 59, 84, 103, 104, 215, 219
Restriction, H-2, 121
-, major histocompatability complex, 21-23, 74-77, 112, 117, 118, 121, 122, 236
Retinoic acid, 31, 42-47
Retroviruses, 148-151, 223-230, 235-246, 275-282, 285, 287, 296
-, slowly transforming, 148-151, 237, 238
Richter's Syndrome, 87

S^+, 21-26
Signals, immunoregulatory, 88, 89, 237
Significance, prognostic, 103, 207
16 (p13q22), 179, 189
Slowly transforming retroviruses, 148-151, 237, 238
Specificity, target cell, 6, 135
Stem cells, 2, 33, 36, 43, 54, 83-91, 97-104, 111-116, 119, 123, 132-135, 203-219, 252-255, 264-268, 271, 296, 297
- -, lymphoid tumor, 83-91
Stimulatory cells (S^+), 21-26
Strategies, therapeutic, 104, 251
Stroma, thymic, 111, 115-119, 124, 265
Studies, epidemiological, 1, 2, 105, 225
Surface antigens, T cell, 22, 119

t(8;21) (q22;q22), 179, 181, 185-191, 196-199, 282
t(9;22) (q34;q11), 179-182, 187, 196, 198
t(14;18) (q32;q21), 192-195
t(15;17) (q22;q21), 179, 181, 185-191, 196-199, 282
T cell, 2, 9, 13, 14, 17, 21-27, 32, 33, 36, 47-51, 69-71, 74-78, 88-90, 96-98, 101-105, 111-124, 141, 150, 152, 186, 203-206, 209, 214, 223-229, 236, 239, 240, 244-246, 252-257, 264-269, 281-284, 299
- - clones, 25, 26, 122, 257
- - differentiation, 111-124, 264, 269
- - growth factor (TCGF), 228, 236, 239, 252-256
- - leukemia, human adult, 223, 226-229, 257
- - - virus, human, 1, 96, 97, 105, 119, 223, 226-228, 245, 257, 281, 282
- - - - p 19, human, 119, 228
- - maturation, 113-117, 121, 265, 266
- - proliferation, 21-27
- - receptor, 124, 265
- - surface antigens, 22, 119
T cells, histocompatibility-restricted, 70, 71
- lineage markers, 34, 111, 119, 121, 141, 264-267
- lymphocytes, 2, 10, 26, 33, 48-51, 97, 101, 111-124, 205-208, 213, 236, 237, 245, 246, 255-257, 267
Target cell specificity, 6, 135
- cells, 6, 10, 12, 15, 16, 37, 43, 95-97, 101-103, 112, 115, 131-137, 142, 143, 148, 155, 164, 173, 223, 228, 238, 241, 252, 263-271, 287, 296-298
TCGF, 228, 236, 239, 252-256
Terminal deoxynucleotidyl transferase (TdT), 98, 99, 120
Therapeutic strategies, 104, 251
Thymectomy, 89, 111, 113, 266

Thymic epithelial cells, 117-123, 265
- hormones, 113, 114, 118, 119
- nurse cells, 118
- stroma, 111, 115-119, 124, 265
TNF, 31, 36-39, 41
Tolerance, 32, 38, 41, 114, 115, 119, 123, 124
Transformation, 3, 33, 69, 98, 102, 131-143, 148, 154, 163-173, 181-184, 191, 195, 237, 238, 245, 246, 257, 259, 263-271, 275-287, 296
-, in vitro, 268-271, 278
-, neoplastic, 3, 245, 287
Translocations, 24, 41, 147, 148, 151, 152, 156, 179-199, 229, 258, 260, 282, 283, 286, 297
- of both No. 14 chromosomes, 195
Translocations, variant, 182, 187, 192-197, 258, 283
Transplantation, bone marrow, 33-36, 48, 59, 113, 208, 264, 297
Tumor cell heterogeneity, 83, 84, 91, 266
- immunity, idiotype-specific, 89
- Necrosis Factor (TNF), 31, 36-41
- progression, 132, 142, 236, 239, 268, 280, 286, 299
- stem cells, lymphoid, 83-91

Units, Colony Forming, 33, 34, 39, 40, 45-54, 57, 58, 209, 212-215, 252
-/erythroid, Burst Forming, 33, 47, 48, 51, 58

Variant translocations, 182, 187, 192-197, 258, 283
Viral enhancer, 149-151, 269
- oncogenes, 2, 138, 139, 147, 153-157, 165, 173, 268, 275-287
Virus, avian leukosis, 148-151, 154, 155, 167, 244, 285, 298
-, bovine leukemia, 225, 226, 229, 230, 281
-, feline leukemia, 224, 225, 228, 229, 280
-, human T cell leukemia, 1, 96, 97, 105, 119, 223, 226-228, 245, 257, 281, 282
- p^{19}, human T cell leukemia, 119, 228
Viruses, avian acute leukemia, 131-143, 163-173, 287
-, ecotropic, 246, 269
Vitamin A, 42-47
- D, 42-47
- D_3, 44, 45, 47

Author Index

Allison, J.P.; 295-300
Bister, K.; 275-292
Boettiger, D.E.; 263-272
Burny, A.L.; 275-292
Cooper, M.D.; 263-272
Croce, C.M.; 275-292
Essex, M.; 223-234, 295-300
Fathman, C.G.; 251-260
Fialkow, P.J.; 203-222, 295-300
Ganser, A.; 251-260
Graf, T.; 131-145, 263-272
Greaves, M.F.; 95-110, 263-272
Haas, W.; 21-30
Haran-Ghera, N.; 295-300
Harlozinska-Szmyrka, A.U.; 263-272
Haseltine, W.A.; 275-292
Hayman, M.J.; 163-178, 275-292
Hayward, W.S.; 147-162, 275-292
Howard, J.C.; 295-300
Iscove, N.N.; 5-20, 251-260
Jaenisch, R.; 263-272
Karpowicz, M.; 251-260
Kishimoto, T.; 251-260
Klein, E.; 251-260
Klein, G.; 275-292
Krammer, P.H.; 251-260
Lilly, F.; 251-260
Lynch, R.G.; 83-94, 263-272
McGrath, M.S.; 235-249
Melchers, F.; 251-260
Metcalf, D.; 251-260
Meyer, P.A.; 251-260
Moelling, K.; 275-292
Moore, M.A.S.; 31-67, 251-260
Neth, R.D.; 275-292
Ostertag, W.; 295-300
Owen, J.J.T.; 111-130, 263-272
Paul, W.E.; 69-82, 251-260
Potter, M.; 263-272
Pragnell, I.B.; 275-292
Rowley, J.D.; 179-202, 275-292
Schirrmacher, V.; 295-300
Seidel, H.J.; 295-300
Singer, J.W.; 203-222
Tamura, G.; 235-249
Vogt, P.K.; 275-292
von Boehmer, H.; 21-30
Weissman, I.L.; 1-3, 235-249, 295-300
Witte, O.N.; 295-300

Dahlem Workshop Reports

Life Sciences Research Reports (LS)

LS 1 The Molecular Basis of Circadian Rhythms.
Editors: J. W. Hastings, H.-G. Schweiger

LS 2 Appetite and Food Intake.
Editor: T. Silverstone

LS 3 Hormone and Antihormone Action at the Target Cell.
Editors: J. H. Clark et al.

LS 4 Organization and Expression of Chromosomes.
Editors: V. G. Allfrey et al.

LS 5 Recognition of Complex Acoustic Signals.
Editor: T. H. Bullock

LS 6 Function and Formation of Neural Systems.
Editor: G. S. Stent

LS 7 Neoplastic Transformation: Mechanisms and Consequences.
Editor: H. Koprowski

LS 8 The Bases of Addiction.
Editor: J. Fishman

LS 9 Morality as a Biological Phenomenon.
Editor: G. S. Stent

LS 10 Abnormal Fetal Growth: Biological Bases and Consequences.
Editor: F. Naftolin

LS 11 Transport of Macromolecules in Cellular Systems.
Editor: S. C. Silverstein

LS 12 Light-Induced Charge Separation in Biology and Chemistry.
Editors: H. Gerischer, J. J. Katz

LS 13 Strategies of Microbial Life in Extreme Environments.
Editor: M. Shilo

LS 14 The Role of Intercellular Signals: Navigation, Encounter, Outcome.
Editor: J. G. Nicholls

LS 15 Biomedical Pattern Recognition and Image Processing.
Editors: K. S. Fu, T. Pavlidis

LS 16 The Molecular Basis of Microbial Pathogenicity.
Editors: H. Smith et al.

LS 17 Pain and Society.
Editors: H. W. Kosterlitz, L. Y. Terenius

LS 18 Evolution of Social Behavior: Hypotheses and Empirical Tests.
Editor: H. Markl

LS 19 Signed and Spoken Language: Biological Constraints on Linguistic Form.
Editors: U. Bellugi, M. Studdert-Kennedy

Physical and Chemical Sciences Research Reports (PC)

PC 1 The Nature of Seawater (out of print)

PC 2 Global Chemical Cycles and Their Alteration by Man.
Editor: W. Stumm

Distributor for LS 1–19 and PC 1 + 2:
Verlag Chemie, Pappelallee 3, 6940 Weinheim,
Federal Republic of Germany

GPSR Compliance
The European Union's (EU) General Product Safety Regulation (GPSR) is a set of rules that requires consumer products to be safe and our obligations to ensure this.

If you have any concerns about our products, you can contact us on

ProductSafety@springernature.com

In case Publisher is established outside the EU, the EU authorized representative is:

Springer Nature Customer Service Center GmbH
Europaplatz 3
69115 Heidelberg, Germany

www.ingramcontent.com/pod-product-compliance
Lightning Source LLC
Chambersburg PA
CBHW072312240926
51846CB00011B/131
* 9 7 8 3 6 4 2 6 9 7 2 4 1 *